Degenerative Disease of the Cervical Spine

AANS Publications Committee
Paul R. Cooper, MD, Editor

Neurosurgical Topics

American Association of
Neurological Surgeons

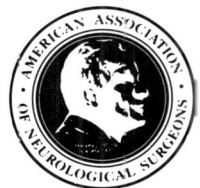

ISBN: 1-879284-04-9

Neurosurgical Topics ISBN: 0-9624246-6-8

Copyright © 1992 by American Association of Neurological Surgeons

Printed in U.S.A.

All rights reserved. None of the contents of this publication may be reproduced in a retrieval system or transmitted in any form or by any means (electronic, mechanical, photocopying, recording, or otherwise) without prior written permission of the publisher.

This publication is published under the auspices of the Publications Committee of the American Association of Neurological Surgeons (AANS). However, this should not be construed as indicating endorsement or approval of the views presented, by the AANS, or by its committees, commissions, affiliates, or staff.

Robert H. Wilkins, MD, Chairman
AANS Publications Committee

Linda S. Miller, AANS Staff Editor

AANS1.3M1292

Forthcoming Books in the *Neurosurgical Topics* Series

1993

Surgery of the Cranial Nerves of the Posterior Fossa
   Edited by Daniel L. Barrow, MD

Spinal Trauma: Current Evaluation and Management
   Edited by Gary L. Rea, MD

Current Management of Cerebral Aneurysms
   Edited by Issam A. Awad, MD

Spinal Instrumentation
   Edited by Edward C. Benzel, MD

Interactive Image-Guided Neurosurgery
   Edited by Robert J. Maciunas, MD

Neurosurgical Emergencies
   Edited by Christopher Loftus, MD

Contents

CONTRIBUTORS		vii
PREFACE		ix
PART I	**CLINICAL MANIFESTATIONS AND PATHOPHYSIOLOGY OF CERVICAL SPONDYLOSIS**	
Chapter 1	Clinical Manifestations of Myelopathy and Radiculopathy *Paul C. McCormick, MD*	1
Chapter 2	Pathophysiology of Bony and Ligamentous Changes in Cervical Spondylosis *Richard B. Raynor, MD*	9
PART II	**DIAGNOSTIC EVALUATION**	
Chapter 3	Imaging and the Diagnosis of Degenerative Disease of the Cervical Spine *Andrew W. Litt, MD*	17
Chapter 4	Diseases that Mimic Degenerative Diseases of the Cervical Spine *E. Wayne Massey, MD*	37
Chapter 5	Somatosensory Evoked Potential Monitoring in Cervical Spine Surgery *Nancy E. Epstein, MD*	49
PART III	**OPERATIVE MANAGEMENT OF CERVICAL SPONDYLOSIS AND DEGENERATIVE DISK DISEASE**	
Chapter 6	Cervical Spondylotic Myelopathy: Management with Anterior Operation *Paul R. Cooper, MD*	73
Chapter 7	Cervical Spondylotic Myelopathy: Posterior Surgical Approaches *Edward C. Benzel, MD*	91
Chapter 8	Cervical Spondylotic Radiculopathy: Management with Posterior Operation *Ulrich Batzdorf, MD*	105

| Chapter 9 | The Soft Cervical Disk: Natural History and Management
Regis W. Haid, Jr., MD | 113 |

PART IV   **OTHER DEGENERATIVE DISEASES**

Chapter 10	Rheumatoid Arthritis of the Cervical Spine *Michael G. Fehlings, MD, PhD, FRCS(C), Paul R. Cooper, MD, and Thomas J. Errico, MD*	125
Chapter 11	Ankylosing Spondylitis *Deborah A. Blades, MD, and Russell W. Hardy, MD*	141
Chapter 12	Ossification of the Posterior Longitudinal Ligament *Noel Perin, MD, FRCS*	151

PART V   **NONOPERATIVE MANAGEMENT OF CERVICAL SPONDYLOSIS**

| Chapter 13 | Natural History and Nonoperative Management
Harold J. Weinberg, MD, PhD | 159 |

INDEX   167

List of Contributors

Ulrich Batzdorf, MD
Professor of Neurosurgery
University of California
Los Angeles, California

Edward C. Benzel, MD
Chief, Department of Neurosurgery
University of New Mexico
Albuquerque, New Mexico

Deborah A. Blades, MD
Fellow in Spinal Surgery
New York University Medical Center
New York, New York

Paul R. Cooper, MD
Professor of Neurosurgery
and Orthopedic Surgery
New York University Medical Center
New York, New York

Nancy E. Epstein, MD
Associate Clinical Professor of Neurosurgery
North Shore University Hospital
Cornell Medical Center
New York, New York

Thomas Errico, MD
Assistant Professor of Neurosurgery
and Orthopedic Surgery
New York University Medical Center
New York, New York

Michael G. Fehlings, MD, PhD, FRCS(C)
Assistant Professor of Neurosurgery
Department of Neurosurgery
University of Toronto
Toronto, Ontario, Canada

Regis W. Haid, Jr, MD
Staff Neurosurgeon
Wilford Hall Medical Center
San Antonio, Texas
Assistant Professor of Neurosurgery
Emory University School of Medicine
Atlanta, Georgia

Russell W. Hardy, MD
Professor of Neurosurgery
Case Western Reserve University
Cleveland, Ohio

Andrew W. Litt, MD
Assistant Professor of Radiology
New York University Medical Center
New York, New York

E. Wayne Massey, MD
Professor of Neurosurgery
Duke University Medical Center
Durham, North Carolina

Paul C. McCormick, MD
Assistant Professor of Neurological Surgery
Columbia-Presbyterian Medical Center
New York, New York

Noel Perin, MD, FRCS
Assistant Professor of Neurosurgery
University of Cincinnati
Cincinnati, Ohio

Richard B. Raynor, MD
Clinical Professor of Neurosurgery
New York University Medical Center
New York, New York

Harold J. Weinberg, MD, PhD
Clinical Associate Professor of Neurology
New York University Medical Center
New York, New York

AANS Publications Committee

Robert H. Wilkins, MD, Chairman
Michael L.J. Apuzzo, MD
Issam A. Awad, MD
Daniel L. Barrow, MD
Edward C. Benzel, MD
Paul R. Cooper, MD

Howard H. Kaufman, MD
Oliver D. Grin, Jr., MD
Christopher M. Loftus, MD
Robert J. Maciunas, MD
J. Gordon McComb, MD
Setti S. Rengachary, MD

Preface:

Degenerative disease of the cervical spine is as old as the human race. Bony evidence of a variety of degenerative processes has been found in Egyptian mummies and skeletal remains of humans from even earlier eras. However, it has only been in the last 75-100 years that we have begun to understand the significance of cervical degenerative disease in producing neurologic symptoms. It is barely 20 years since the advent of computerized tomography has provided us with new insights regarding the diagnosis and most appropriate treatment for these conditions. Indeed, magnetic resonance imaging has been available for less than 10 years.

This volume, with contributions by a variety of experts in the field, reviews and places in perspective many of the major advances which have been made in the management of degenerative cervical disease. These include the revolutionary progress in our ability to image the spine, which has been noted above, as well as new insights into familiar rheumatoid conditions of the cervical spine, and less common entities such as ossification of the posterior longitudinal ligament (OPLL), which has only recently come to be recognized. The uses of evoked potential monitoring in the diagnosis and perioperative management of patients with cervical disease are extensively reviewed. New concepts of the pathophysiology, natural history, and differential diagnosis of spondylotic disease are discussed along with the implications for the correct choice of patient management. The basic operative approaches for the management of cervical degenerative disease discussed in this volume are not new. However, their correct application, refinements in technique which have the potential for markedly improving outcome, and the results of treatment are critically reviewed and thoughtfully discussed.

The state-of-the-art reviews contained in this volume have been contributed by an eclectic group of physicians — all of whom have a deep interest in degenerative cervical disease. The opinions expressed by the authors are not always in agreement but are all well thought out and will enable readers to reach their own conclusions. The material contained in this volume should prove useful to residents and practicing neurosurgeons, neurologists, rhematologists, physiatrists, and all others who care for patients with degenerative disease of the cervical spine.

Paul R. Cooper, MD
New York, N.Y.

CHAPTER 1

Clinical Manifestations of Myelopathy and Radiculopathy

Paul C. McCormick, MD

Disk degeneration and spondylosis of the cervical spine are a frequent cause of disability. The prevalence of neck pain has been estimated at about 10%; up to one-third of the adult population has experienced at least one episode of severe neck pain with or without arm radiation.[11] While the differential diagnosis of cervical pain, radiculopathy, and myelopathy is extensive, a dysfunctional cervical motion segment is by far the most common etiology.

Symptoms and signs of benign disk disease and spondylosis can be regarded as axial, radicular, or myelopathic in nature. Rarely, the presenting feature is represented, respectively, as vertebrobasilar vascular insufficiency or dysphagia from osteophyte compression from the vertebral artery or esophagus. This chapter reviews the common clinical features as well as some unusual clinical syndromes associated with cervical disk herniation and spondylosis.

Axial Symptoms

Axial complaints, usually pain, are the most common symptoms of benign cervical disk disease and spondylosis. They characteristically precede or coexist with radicular pain from nerve root compression caused by either a soft or hard disk. In many cases, pain or stiffness may constitute the only feature of a symptomatic event.

Chronic disabling neck pain, which may require surgical intervention, can be produced by a central or subligamentous disk herniation, as well as by single-level advanced disk degeneration as seen on magnetic resonance imaging (MRI), without evidence of nerve root or spinal cord compression (Figure 1).

The origin of axial pain has been the basis of much speculation and some study. Small radicles from ventral or dorsal rami of the spinal nerves innervate surrounding structures such as the annulus fibrosis, periosteum, ligaments, and facet joints and capsules. Primary muscle afferents also travel with motor nerves to the axial paraspinal, shoulder girdle, and scapular muscles. It seems reasonable to assume that axial pain may be produced either by direct compression of the spinal nerve or dorsal root, or by focal activation of a smaller peripheral sensory branch. Numerous investigators have reported a reproduction of axial pain during provocative procedures such as diskography or direct needle stimulation of the annulus fibrosis or facet joints.[4]

Axial pain associated with nerve root dysfunction probably reflects the myotomal and sclerotomal distribution of the affected nerve root. While axial complaints associated with nerve root dysfunction generally correspond to the side of involvement, they are somewhat less specific for the individual nerve root. There are, however, certain patterns which are commonly noted in clinical prac-

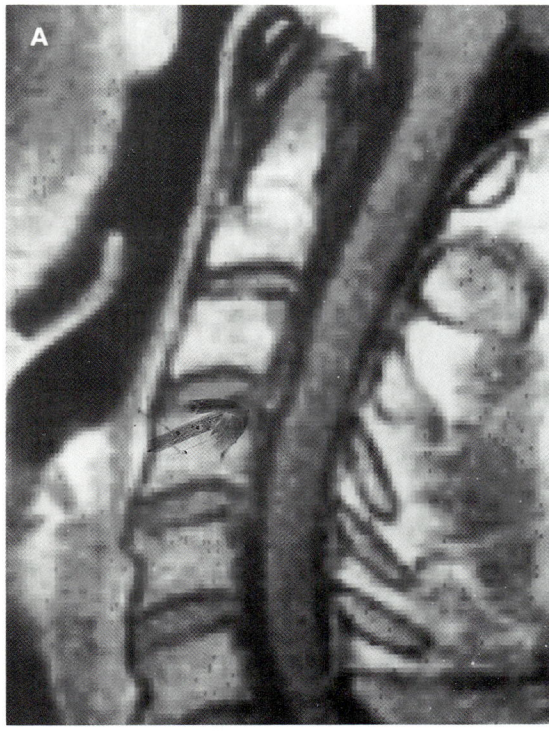

tice. Headache, other than from C2 entrapment, rarely accompanies lower root involvement. It is occasionally seen with chronic disabling neck pain of long duration, and in such cases is probably secondary to either a sympathetically mediated response or muscle tension. Pain radiation to the jaw and periauricular region, is typical of C3 or C4 compression.

Differentiation of C5-T1 root involvement on the basis of axial complaints is difficult because of overlap. Pain in the trapezius muscle is typical in most cases of C5, C6, or C7 root involvement. Radiation along the medial scapular border is seen primarily, although not exclusively, with C5 or C7 root compression. Pain radiation into the latissimus dorsi, pectoral muscles, and axilla are relatively specific for C7 root involvement although the latter two regions may be affected with C8 and T1 root dysfunction, respectively.

Figure 1. Sagittal (A) and axial (B) MRI show central subligamentous C3-4 disk herniation without spinal cord or nerve root compression in a 39-year-old man with disabling neck pain of 14-month duration. Symptoms resolved following anterior diskectomy and allograft fusion.

Radiculopathy

Radicular signs and symptoms are the hallmark of lateral cervical disk herniation and the foraminal spur (hard disk). Pain is pres-

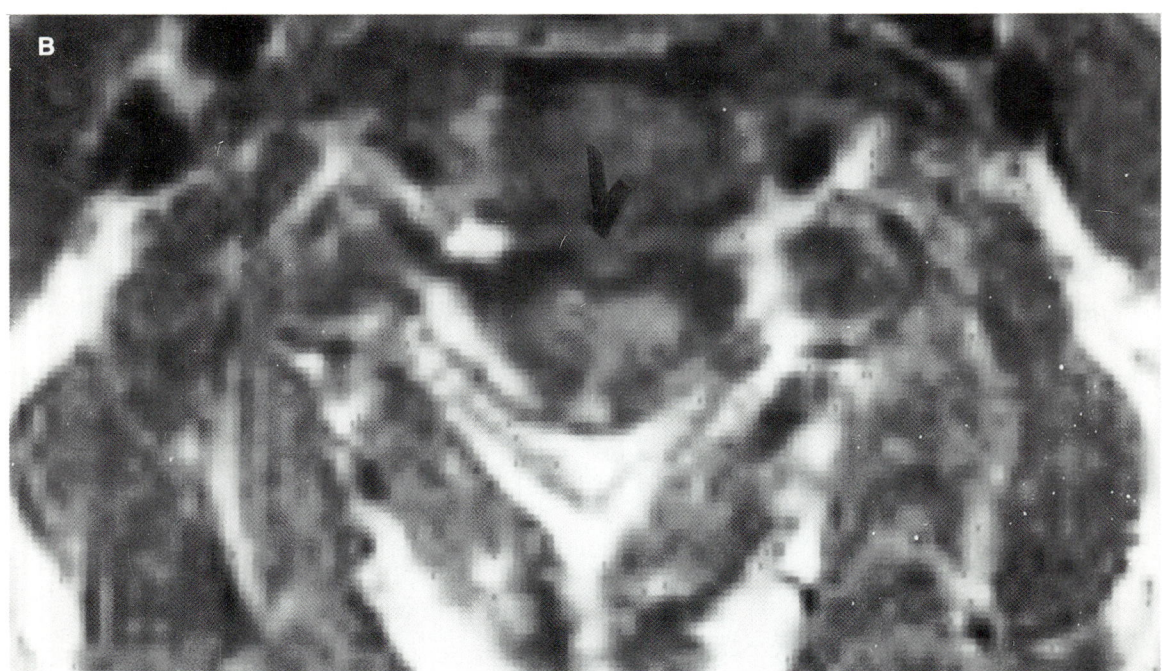

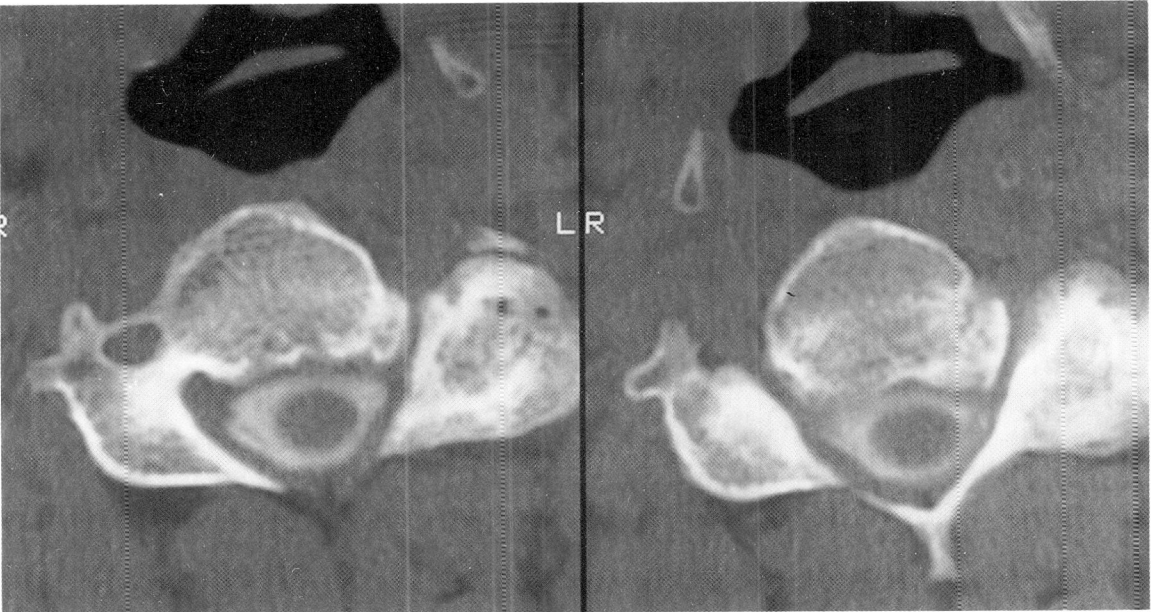

Figure 2. Postmyelographic computed tomography (CT) scan shows foraminal narrowing caused by facet overgrowth at C3-4 on the left. Symptoms of the left C4 radiculopathy in a 57-year-old man completely resolved following posterior "keyhole" foraminotomy.

ent and is the most prominent complaint in virtually all patients. Sensory complaints—numbness or paresthesias in the distal target distribution of the involved root—and motor weakness are somewhat less common.

The typical presentation is similar in most patients, irrespective of the root involved. The onset is heralded by a dull ache or discomfort in the neck or axial muscles which is often first noted upon awakening. Although the causal relationship of trauma to cervical disk herniation is a matter of much debate, there is frequently a recent history of strenuous or unaccustomed activity. After a variable period, classic radicular arm pain will appear. The distal sensory territory provides the clinical signature of the specific root involved.

History and examination usually disclose a number of features common to foraminal narrowing irrespective of both cause and level. Pain is often worsened by the recumbent position, presumably from increased epidural venous plexus pressure, which forces the patient to sleep in a seated position. Neck extension, rotation away from the affected side, and Valsalva maneuver characteristically exacerbate pain. A forward translation of the head with slight neck flexion is the preferred position in these patients. Forward translation of the head may be so marked as to create a slight anterolisthesis of one or more vertebral motion segments on lateral cervical spine x-rays. Raising the arm and placing the hand behind the head will usually temporarily relieve the pain caused by foraminal compression.

Symptomatic spondylotic or disk involvement of upper cervical roots (C3-4) is extremely rare and probably accounts for about 1% of cases of cervical radiculopathy.[10] Unlike the lower cervical levels, foraminal narrowing is more commonly secondary to facet arthropathy and overgrowth (Figure 2). Symptoms typically consist of pain, which radiates into the jaw, periauricular region, or anterior neck. The erroneous diagnosis of atypical facial pain and temporomandibular joint dysfunction is common. Objective sensory loss in these dermatomal regions may help to differentiate radicular involvement from the other disorders.

C5 root dysfunction usually produces pain

radiating over the shoulder to the lateral upper arm. The pain does not radiate beyond the elbow. Medial scapular or rhomboid muscle pain is the typical axial component of a C5 root syndrome. The motor distribution of C5 includes the shoulder girdle musculature and rhomboid muscle. Weakness of shoulder abduction and external rotation are characteristic of a C5 radiculopathy. There is no specific reflex change indicative of C5 root dysfunction, although the biceps reflex may occasionally be diminished.

Because most symptoms center around the shoulder, it may be difficult to differentiate a C5 radiculopathy from primary shoulder pathology such as osteoarthritis, acromial spur, bursitis, or rotator cuff tears. Point tenderness over the involved joint, pain with abduction or rotation of the shoulder, and weakness or limitation of shoulder rotation out of proportion to abduction abnormalities usually indicates shoulder pathology. A diagnostic periarticular or intra-articular block with local anesthesia may help to establish the diagnosis.

Entrapment neuropathy of the suprascapular nerve may mimic a C5 radiculopathy. Postosterolateral shoulder pain with weakness and wasting of the infra- and supraspinatus muscles are the clinical features produced by suprascapular nerve entrapment. The diagnosis is usually confirmed by electrical studies.[2]

Pain in the C6 root travels across the biceps muscles onto the radial half of the forearm and hand. The thumb, first dorsal web space, and index finger constitute the specific terminal territory of the C6 nerve root. Motor weakness typically involves the biceps, brachioradialis, pronator, and supinator muscles. Diminution of the biceps and brachioradialis reflexes are also clues to a C6 radiculopathy.

C7 root dysfunction results in pain radiating over the triceps muscle onto the dorsum of the forearm and hand. The middle finger is the specific terminal territory for C7, although the patient may note more pain on the ulnar side of the index finger. Axial pain radiates into the trapezius muscle and medial scapula but, unlike the other roots coming from the cervical enlargement, may also extend into the latissimus and, less commonly, pectoral muscles. The triceps muscle and reflex are the target of C7. Finger flexion and extension, and to a lesser extent wrist flexion and extension, may also be weakened with C7 root involvement.

The C8 nerve root is only rarely affected by degenerative disease of the cervical spine. Sensory symptoms are usually limited to the ulnar aspect of the forearm and hand. In the absence of axial symptoms, it may be difficult to differentiate C8 radiculopathy from ulnar nerve entrapment in the cubital tunnel. Electrical studies are usually helpful in differentiating root from peripheral nerve involvement. A C8 motor deficit includes weakness of long flexors and extensors of the fingers and thumb. It is the author's experience that the intrinsic muscles of the hand are more affected with C8 than with T1 root dysfunction.

A T1 radiculopathy produces pain radiating around the axilla and onto the inner aspect of the upper arm. Like C5, it does not radiate beyond the elbow. The terminal motor territory of T1 is inconsistent. It occasionally provides some contribution to the intrinsic muscles and the hand, particularly on the *ulnar* aspect. The T1 nerve root is sacrificed routinely during resection of superior sulcus (Pancoast) tumor with little functional consequence in upper limb or hand function in most patients.

Myelopathy

Cervical spondylosis is the most common cause of myelopathy in middle-aged and elderly patients. Nevertheless, despite the radiologic prevalence of spondylosis in this age group, even with significant spinal canal compromise and spinal cord deformation, surprisingly few people develop myelopathy.[16] Myelopathy develops in only 5% to 10% of patients with clinically symptomatic spondylosis.[17]

The symptoms of myelopathy may pro-

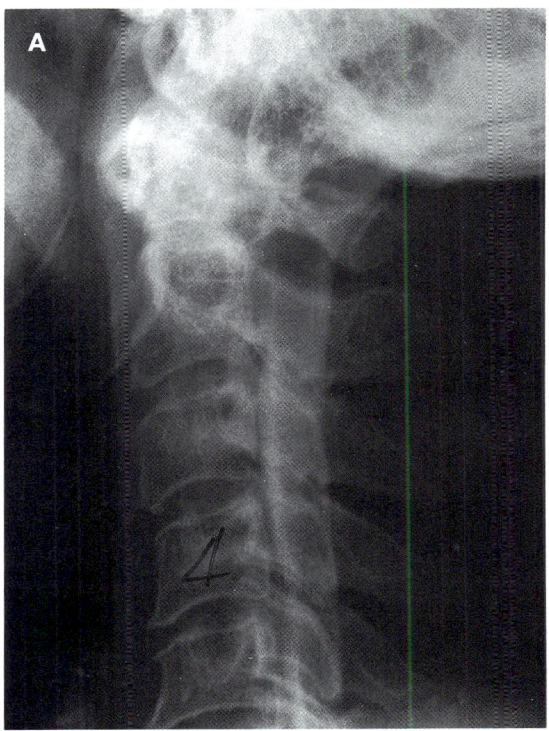 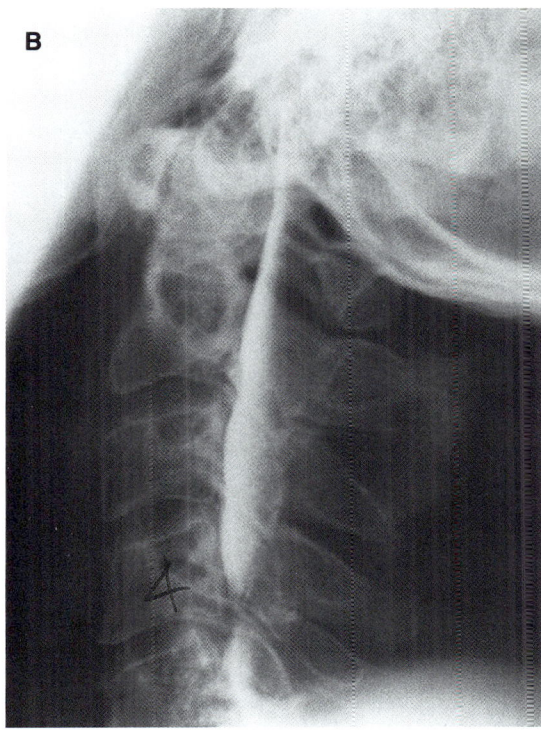

Figure 3. Lateral cervical myelogram in a 43-year-old man who acutely developed a central spinal cord syndrome following a fall down one flight of stairs. Note the marked degree of canal narrowing seen with neck extension (B) as compared with the routine view (A).

gress insidiously or in a step-wise episodic fashion, separated often by prolonged periods of stable or improving neurologic function. The natural history of spondylotic myelopathy in these patients has not been well studied, but perhaps one-third to one-half of them will experience long-term stabilization or even regression of their myelopathy.[9,12] Rarely, an acute onset or worsening of myelopathy may occur following trauma in patients with pre-existing congenital or spondylotic spinal canal narrowing (Figure 3). Frequently, no radiographic evidence of vertebral fracture is present, suggesting the absorbed force was relatively minor. The injury is probably the result of shear, as infolding of the ligamentum flavum during hyperextension produces a pincer-type compression of the spinal cord against the vertebral body or spondylotic ridge. Shear force is concentrated centrally within the cylindrical spinal cord, which may account for the frequent presentation of these patients with a syndrome of central spinal cord dysfunction.

The clinical features, time course, and natural history of spondylotic myelopathy vary considerably, probably because of their relation to mechanical (size and location of osteophyte), dynamic (neck movement), and perhaps vascular factors. Consequently, different patterns of myelopathy have been described to include transverse, central, hemicord, and motor syndromes.[5]

The classic presentation of cervical spondylotic myelopathy is segmental cervical cord deficit and long-tract symptoms and signs (see Figure 4). Although there may be a history of prior episodes of neck pain, it is unusual for the patient with spondylotic myelopathy to complain of anything more than mild neck stiffness. Coexistent radicular pain is also unusual.[3,9]

In fact, there does not appear to be any correlation with an episode or history of spondylotic radiculopathy and the subsequent development of myelopathy.[12] Thus, the classic clinical syndrome triad of cervicobrachalgia, radiculopathy, and myelopathy are only occasionally encountered.

Segmental deficits are manifested by lower motor neuron weakness with atrophy, discriminitive and epicritic sensory loss and/or paresthesias, and absent or diminished myotatic reflex arc. The segmental deficit is frequently unilateral or asymmetric in distribution. Fasiculations only infrequently involve segmentally weakened muscles in spondylotic

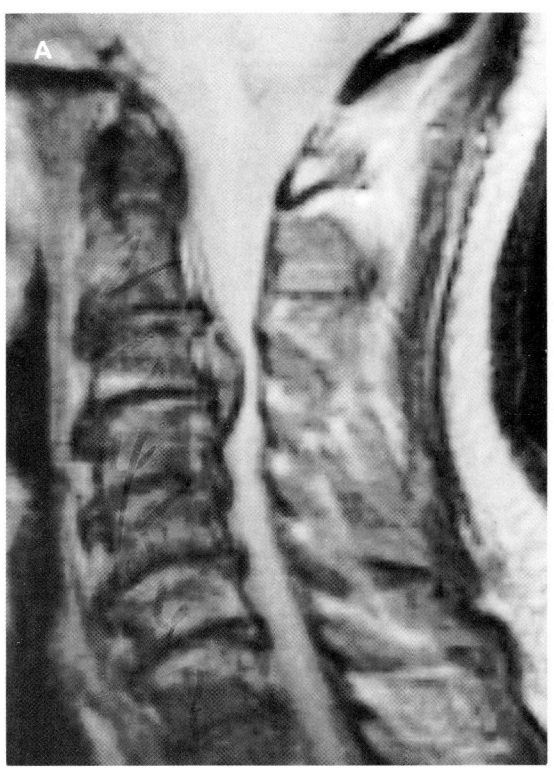

Figure 4. Sagittal *(A)* and axial *(B)* MRI demonstrate a large calcified osteophyte with predominately left-sided spinal cord compression at C3-4. Although this 59-year-old man had mild long-tract signs, his main presenting complaint was distal weakness with some wasting of the left arm and hand.

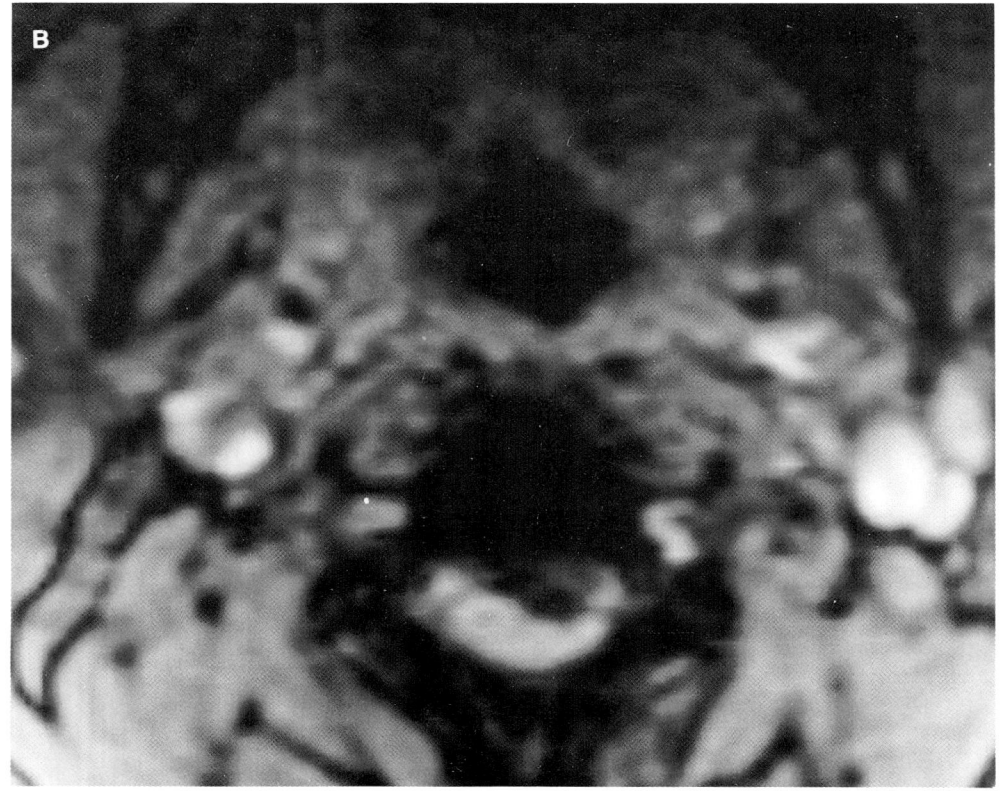

myelopathy. When fasiculations are prominent or diffuse, motor neuron disease should be suspected.

In the presence of segmental findings, there are commonly upper motor neuron signs in the cervical segments below the compression. Thus, spondylotic compression of the C6 cord segment may produce weakness and loss of the biceps and brachioradialis reflex in conjunction with a hyperactive triceps reflex and a Hoffman sign.

The presence of long-tract symptoms and signs represents the *sina qua non* for the diagnosis of myelopathy. While long-tract dysfunction frequently exists without significant segmental deficit, the reverse is rarely encountered. Motor complaints such as weakness, spasticity, or gait difficulties tend to predominate because of their functional consequence to the patient as well as the probable unique vulnerability of the corticospinal tracts which are located subjacent to the dentate ligament attachment. Lower extremity complaints such as increasing fatiguability, stiffness, or exertional weakness are prominent symptoms of motor myelopathy. Hyperreflexia with pathologic reflexes and spasticity which may be asymmetric are common findings on examination. Significant coexistent lumbar stenosis which occurs in about 15% of patients with cervical spondylotic myelopathy may mask the lower extremity signs of myelopathy.

Sensory complaints are usually minor, or absent; if present, they often consist of paresthesias or dysesthesias which can be segmental or confined to the hands or feet. In some patients, distal sensory and motor complaints may suggest carpal tunnel or cubital tunnel entrapment neuropathy.[7] It is hypothesized that proximal nerve root or spinal cord compression renders the peripheral nerve more susceptible to distal compartment entrapment, the so-called "double crush syndrome." Such a presentation is also seen in patients with intradural tumors, and should be suspected in patients with suboptimal results following peripheral nerve release with concomitant proximal symptoms.[13]

Rarely, a patient may present with progressive marked gait abnormality with remarkably little objective corticospinal or even posterior column deficit. The gait tends to be wide-based, and unsteady with frequent falls. This probably represents a sensory ataxia which is occasionally also seen with dorsal or dorsolateral intradural tumors.

In some patients, spondylotic myelopathy may present as a pure spastic paraparesis. There may be no definitive clinical, radiologic or electrophysiologic method (other than surgery) to differentiate this clinical syndrome from nonsurgical causes of paraparesis. This particularly applies to conditions such as multiple sclerosis or motor neuron diseases such as amyotrophic lateral sclerosis (ALS) and its rare primary lateral sclerosis (5%) variant. Symptomatic spondylosis may coexist with other myelopathic disorders.[1] About 5% of patients with ALS have undergone prior cervical decompression (L. Rowland, personal communication, 1991). Conversely, even optimistic reports of the results of operative decompression note between a 15% to 30% surgical failure rate.[6] While negative prognostic factors such as spinal cord atrophy, long-standing deficit, and intramedullary signal abnormalities on MRI have been defined, an incorrect diagnosis probably accounts for a significant number of poor outcomes.

A number of other unusual presentations of spondylosis render it difficult to establish a definitive preoperative diagnosis. This seems particularly true when spondylotic spinal cord compression occurs above the cervical enlargement. These patients often note numb, clumsy hands (with atrophy) as a predominant complaint.[8] This is similar to the clinical syndrome associated with ventrally located meningiomas of the foramen magnum.[15]

References

1. Burgerman RS, Rigamonti D, Fishman P, et al. The association of cervical spondylosis and multiple sclerosis. *Ann Neurol.* 1990;28:278. Abstract.
2. Callahan JD, Scully TB, Shapiro SA, et al. Suprascapular nerve entrapment: a series of 27 cases. *J Neurosurg.* 1991;74:893-896.

3. Clarke E, Robinson PK. Cervical myelopathy: a complication of cervical spondylosis. *Brain.* 1956; 79:483-510.
4. Cloward RB. Cervical diskography: a contribution to the etiology and mechanism of neck, shoulder and arm pain. *Ann Surg.* 1959;150:1052-1064.
5. Crandall PH, Batzdorf U. Cervical spondylotic myelopathy. *J Neurosurg.* 1966;25:57-66.
6. Epstein JA, Epstein NE. The surgical management of cervical spinal stenosis, spondylosis, and myeloradiculopathy by means of the posterior approach. In: Cervical Spine Research Society, ed. *The Cervical Spine.* 2nd ed. Philadelphia, Pa: Lippincott; 1989:625-669.
7. Epstein NE, Epstein JA, Carras R. Coexisting spondylotic myelopathy and bilateral carpal tunnel syndromes. *J Spinal Disorders.* 1989;2:36-42.
8. Goodridge AE, Feasby TE, Ebers GC, et al. Hand wasting due to mid-cervical spinal cord compression. *Can J Neurol Sci.* 1987;14:309-311.
9. Gregorius FK, Estrin T, Crandall PH. Cervical spondylotic radiculopathy and myelopathy: a long-term follow up study. *Arch Neurol.* 1976;33: 618-625.
10. Kessler LA, Abla A. Syndrome of the cervical plexus caused by high cervical nerve root compression. *Neurosurgery.* 1991;28:506-509.
11. Lawrence JS. Disc degeneration: its frequency and relationship to symptoms. *Ann Rheum Dis.* 1969; 28:121-138.
12. Lees F, Turner JWA. Natural history and prognosis of cervical spondylosis. *Br Med J.* 1963;2:1607-1610.
13. McCormick PC, Torres R, Post KD, et al. Intramedullary ependymoma of the spinal cord. *J Neurosurg.* 1990;72:523-532.
14. Metzger CS, Schlitt M, Quindlen EA. Small central disc syndrome: evaluation and treatment of chronic disabling neck pain. *J Spinal Disorders.* 1989;2: 234-237.
15. Stein BM, Leeds NE, Taveras JM, et al. Meningiomas of the foramen magnum. *J Neurosurg.* 1963; 20:740-751.
16. Teres LM, Lufkin RB, Reicher MA, et al. Asymptomatic degenerative disk disease and spondylosis of the cervical spine: MR imaging. *Radiology.* 1987; 164:83-88.
17. Young PH. Degenerative cervical disc disorders: pathophysiology and clinical syndromes. In: Young PH, ed. *Microsurgery of the Cervical Spine.* New York, NY: Raven Press; 1991;49-63.

CHAPTER 2

Pathophysiology of Bony and Ligamentous Changes in Cervical Spondylosis

Richard B. Raynor, MD

"Spondylosis, a term often applied more specifically to any lesion of the spine of a degenerative nature." Although this dictionary definition[36] appears quite clear upon first reading, more is left unsaid than said. It is not specified where in the spine the "lesion" occurs or how degenerative is defined. The dilemma of spondylosis, its causes and effects, is inherent in its definition.

A specific etiology of spondylosis has not been identified and there appear to be multiple factors that determine its presence and severity. There may be a genetic predisposition. In a study involving 23 pairs of twins, a close similarity was noted in the shape of cervical vertebrae, especially if the twins were monozygotic. When degenerative changes were present, these were similar in the pairs.[28] There is also good evidence that repeated stress or low-grade trauma causes degenerative disease in the cervical spine. When a group of rugby players was studied and matched against controls,[33] the degenerative changes noted radiographically showed premature and advanced changes in the players when compared to the control group.

Unless there is a definite history of trauma, normal "senescent" changes in the older age groups are difficult to distinguish morphologically from pathologic changes since spondylosis is common in the older age group.[19] The question arises if any of these changes should be considered pathologic in the absence of defined trauma. In many instances, x-rays of the cervical region reveal degenerative changes that are asymptomatic. In some circumstances, where more sophisticated techniques such as magnetic resonance imaging (MRI) have been done, cord and root involvement have been observed, again without patient complaints.[40]

To further confound the issue of normal versus pathologic changes and the interpretation of the radiographic changes, Gore et al followed 210 patients for a minimum of 10 years after the onset of neck pain. Forty-three percent were pain free while 79% had a decrease in pain. This group did include patients with a history of injury and these were the most likely to have symptoms. Of interest was the fact that the presence or severity of pain was not related to the presence of degenerative changes, the canal saggital diameter, the degree of lordosis, or any changes in these parameters during the observation period.[12]

In a general sense, cervical spondylosis involves a sequence of degenerative changes involving the intervertebral disks and vertebral bodies. The vertebral bodies may exhibit osteophytosis, facet hypertrophy, and laminal hypertrophy. Ligamentous changes occur in the facet and uncovertebral joints that alter strength and elasticity and result in segmental instability. The cartilaginous elements in the joints and disk are altered chemically and morphologically.

Cartilage

In the newborn, two layers of cartilage form the end plate separating the bone of the vertebra from the nucleus pulposus. An inner growth zone next to bone consists of parallel columns of proliferating and hypertrophic cells, while the outer or articular zone borders the disk and consists of spindle-shaped chrondrocytes scattered in a matrix. By age 15, there is a reduction in the width of the growth zone along with a decrease in the number of proliferating cells. Sometime between 17 and 20 years of age, the growth zone disappears and fissures appear in the cartilage.

A gradual mineralization of the articular cartilage begins at about age 20.[1] Since cartilage and its adjacent disk do not have an independent blood supply, but rely on diffusion through the central part of the cartilaginous end plate for nutritional support,[4] mineralization decreases the permeability of the cartilage and results in decreased diffusion through the end plates.[5] This in turn may be a mechanism that induces the chemical changes to be described. As the articular cartilage undergoes calcification, it also undergoes resorption and replacement by bone from the vertebral body.

By age 60, there may be only a thin layer of articular cartilage, which may be calcified, separating disk from vertebral body. If calcium is present, it will interfere with nutrient transfer. At the same time, the capillary walls in the adjacent vertebrae are thickening and developing degenerative changes that further decrease optimal nutritional support of the adjacent cartilage and disk.[1] These changes result in further degeneration as part of a cycle that may be difficult to break.

The earliest visible degenerative changes in spondylosis occur in the cartilaginous end plates attached to the vertebral bodies,[7] although even earlier changes are taking place at the molecular level. Proteoglycans, high molecular weight glycoproteins found in connective tissue, and essential for the transfer of water, decrease and predispose the disk and apophyseal joint cartilage to degeneration. Because neither the disk nor the end plates have an independent blood supply, but must rely on osmosis for their nutritional needs, a decrease in water transfer decreases their nutrition.[4]

Animal model data suggest the earliest measurable changes are an increase in chondroitin sulfate, decrease in keratin sulfate, and an increase in type II collagen syntheses in proportion to other collagen types.[6] Specific collagenase enzyme systems, some of which originate in the synovial membrane and fluid, are involved in controlling these chemical changes.[16] Inflammation of the joints also influences the metabolic activity of the articular cartilage and may enhance the chemical changes,[20] with synovial proliferation occurring as a late secondary event in osteoarthritis.[22]

Under the influence of chemical changes, fissures appear in the cartilaginous end plates. Although these fissures occur as part of the normal aging process, increasing with age,[39] an exact fissure/age correlation has not been determined. The distinction between normal and pathologic fissuring remains blurred.[19]

Extensive destruction of cartilage can be found without osteophyte formation, and may precede osteophyte formation by as much as two decades. Based upon their studies, ten Have and Eulderink[39] believe that irregularity of the vertebral end plates is not a necessary condition for osteophyte formation, nor is a reduction in disk height. However, they did note that paradiskal osteophytes almost always occurred if irregularity of the end plates was present. These authors also observed that the degree of cartilage loss in the apophyseal joints corresponded on both the right and left sides but, interestingly, there was no side-to-side correlation of osteophyte location in the joints.[38]

Disk

The intervertebral disk consists of two parts, the central nucleus pulposis and its peripherally encircling annulus fibrosis that retains the nucleus pulposis. A key function of these structures is to act as a shock absorber for applied forces created by normal and abnormal body motions. Their viscoelastic nature suits them well for this role.

The nucleus, which is a notochordal remnant, consists of a randomly distributed loose network of collagen fibers in a gelatinous fluid that is 85% to 90% water in the very young individual. The remainder of this matrix is about 25% to 35% collagen and 60% to 65% proteoglycans. With aging, the water content of the nucleus decreases, resulting in a relative increase of the proteoglycan and collagen content. The annulus is 60% to 70% water, with collagen constituting 60% of the remainder. The collagen fibers are arranged in a criss-cross pattern and are attached to the vertebral body. Unlike the nucleus, annulus water content does not change with age.[34] The cells are fibroblast-like, occurring singly or in groups, and are sparse. In the mature annulus there are a large number of degenerated cells and necrotic debris. The matrix is fine-textured with protein polysaccharide particles, and fine short and thicker longer collagen fibrils.[11]

Collagen types I and II predominate in the disk. Type I is suited to withstand tensile-type loading and is located in the annulus, along with type II which is suited to sustain tensile loads. The nucleus contains mostly type II. Collagen type remains constant, but other constituents of the disk change with age.[34] The proteoglycan content decreases while there is an increase in keratin 6 sulfate.

These changes indicate that there are active enzyme systems in the disk. Recent work has shown that there is a change in these enzymes when disk prolapse occurs. The normal disk contains enzymes active against type II collagen, while in the prolapsed disk the enzyme systems are active against type I collagen.[25] The prolapsed disk also contains agents active against elastin, whereas no such activity was observed in the normal disk. Whether these changes were the cause of, or the result of, the disk pathology, was not determined; the authors felt, from ancillary data, that the enzyme changes were probably the primary event.[14]

Elastic fibers are located in the annulus at the interface disk and vertebral body. The increased presence of enzyme in the annulus acting against elastin and type I collagen, both located in the annulus, suggests at least one mechanism for disk herniation.

The histological changes noted in disk degeneration are in the adjacent cartilaginous end plate where neovascularization, capillary wall thickening, and calcification are found.[26,41] By altering the local environment, they could initiate the enzyme changes. However, other factors such as mechanical and chemical changes discussed in other sections could initiate the events or, at least, contribute to them.

Bone

Bone is a living tissue that changes form in response to stimuli from its local environment. These stimuli may be either mechanical, such as local pressure and stresses, or chemical due to the peptides produced by adjacent hematopoietic cells, fibroblasts, and bone cells.[51] Both osteoblasts and osteoclasts occur in the calcified matrix of normal bone. The majority of these cells are in an inactive state, but localized discreet metabolic units are scattered throughout the normal structure. These are active bone structural units or bone metabolic units.

In the normal ongoing process of change, resorption takes about 7 to 10 days and is controlled by osteoclasts. In an intermediate period, called the reversal phase, the lacunae are occupied by mononuclear cells. These geographically localized pockets appear to be under control of local factors produced in the bone marrow microenvironment. Osteoblast precursors then appear in the lacunae and mature into active osteoblasts that lay down new bone. The regenerative phase lasts about three months under normal conditions.[23]

Under abnormal conditions the time frame and localization of the remodeling process can be altered, as can the process itself. An imbalance may develop between the various phases, resulting in pathologic remodeling due to excess absorption or proliferation

During resorption, bone mineral and degradation products are released simultaneously under the control of multinucleated osteoclasts. The osteoclasts are, in turn, under the influence of factors such as vitamin D, thyroid hormone, parathyroid hormone, cytokines, and prostaglandin, especially those of the E series.[23] PGE_2, an endogenously produced prostaglandin that causes bone resorption, can be blocked by drugs such as indomethacin.[35] Factors that inhibit resorptive activity are calcitonin, colchicine, phosphate, gamma interferon, and glucocorticoids. Chronic use of glucocorticoids causes osteoporosis. The resorptive process involves the release of collagenase and lysosomal enzymes, which in turn affect neighboring tissues. There is also a local production of acid that causes bone demineralization.[23]

The origin of the osteoclast has not been fully defined. It appears to be extraskeletal, and circulates, and probably originates, from a cell line similar to the line that produces the macrophage. Under certain conditions, monocytes are capable of direct bone resorption, a further indication of the origin of osteoclasts.[18]

Mechanical factors play a significant role in bone remodeling. Whether they are the originators of the process or responders to initial chemical alterations has not been determined, but most likely there is a critical interplay between factors. Since each functional segment is designed to move as a unit, an alteration in this segmental movement due to bone or soft-tissue change affects movement elsewhere.[6]

Mechanical stimulation causes normal bone growth and remodeling, and abnormal pressure or distortion stimulates abnormal osteoclast activity either directly or indirectly.[27,35] As a result of this remodeling the instantaneous center of motion for the segment may change during motion,[30] causing further distortion and pressure, which then results in further bone remodeling. In a study of patients who had undergone anterior cervical fusions, significant changes were found in the architecture of joints above and below the fused area although most of these changes were not clinically significant.[8] Elimination of the local traumatic factors by fusion may not result in resorption of the abnormal osteophytes.[24] Why these osteophytes sometimes disappear in fused segments and sometimes do not is unclear. If they are due to mechanical stimulation, immobilization should result in their resorption. However, remodeling is a dynamic process and the local surgical stress may have reduced the factors necessary to initiate and sustain it.

Factors in addition to trauma implicated in causing these dynamic changes are such commonplace activities as working at a desk, and reading where the required head position alters normal cervical lordosis. Local functional overload results, initiating the remodeling process.[3]

On a macroanatomic level, changes have been described in the bone marrow that can be seen on MR imaging. Modic et al classify them in two types. In type 1 changes, decreased signal intensity is seen on T1-weighted spin echo images (short TR and TE). Type 2 changes have an increased signal intensity on T1-weighted images, and are isointense or slightly increased intensity on T2-weighted images. Histopathologic study showed yellow marrow replacement in type 2 specimens studied. In type 1 MR changes, the end plates showed fissuring and vascular changes.[21] DeRoos et al also noted signal changes on MR in the vertebral marrow.[9] These changes occurred about 50% of the time when a degenerated disk was present. They concluded that normal marrow had undergone a change to fatty marrow. Although their study was done on the lumbar spine, there is good reason to believe that similar changes occur in the cervical region.

Ligaments

Ossification of the ligamentum flavum has been reported in conjunction with anterior osteophytes.[32] Most of the reported cases have been in Japanese although several cases have been observed in Caucasians.[13] Calcification occurs in the extracellular region and involves the collagen and elastic fibers, altering their response to stress and motion, which then induces change in their structures.[17] A more common problem involving the ligamentum flavum is hypertrophy. In its more severe form, this results in narrowing of the spinal canal and posterior compression, especially if degenerative changes are present anteriorly. A loss of elasticity in the ligament may result in an "infolding" which may cause posterior pressure on the cord, especially in extension.

Other Factors

The discussion so far has concentrated on the intrinsic components of the motion segment, since this is where the pathology of spondylosis is located. However, it is possible that factors extrinsic to these structures exert a modifying influence that may lead to changes. Syftestad et al showed that substances present in muscle can cause osteogenesis and chondrogenesis.[37] Activation of these factors in the spinal musculature may be a source of local degenerative changes that start a more widespread process.

Neurogenic factors may also be implicated. The resonant frequency of the human spine is 5 Hz, which is also the dominant frequency of many motor vehicles.[15,43] In the low back, several studies suggest that low frequencies such as this are a cause of disk herniation and pain.[20]

Two neuroactive peptides found in dorsal root ganglia were investigated as a possible cause of degenerative change.[29] Substance P has been associated with the development of degenerative arthritis through stimulation of synthesis of prostaglandin E2 and collagenase. Vasoactive intestinal peptide (VIP) increases bone resorption by altering c-AMP mechanisms. Both of these have been found in the outer portion of the annulus.[42] The course of events would involve (1) the dorsal root ganglia responding to low-grade irritation by long periods of repetitive firing which (2) in turn stimulates the synthesis and transport of these peptides leading (3) in turn, to further degenerative changes in the motion segment.

Pederini et al found that, when some damage to the disk was already present, low-grade trauma such as that produced by vibration caused degeneration of proteoglycans and collagen in the annulus.[29] The dorsal root ganglia mechanisms just described may be the source of the enzyme systems necessary for these degenerative changes. Although this work was done in animals, it indicates that neural factors may have a significant role in degenerative spondylosis.

Summary

The earliest observable change in spondylosis is fissuring of the cartilaginous end plate of the vertebral body. Although it occurs in normal aging, probably as a consequence of mineralization of the end plate seen with maturation, it is more severe in degenerative disease. A complex interplay of factors involving mechanical stresses and chemical changes that alter bone, ligament, cartilage, and disk occurs. Which of these is the initiating and which is the primary cause of these degenerative changes is unclear at present. All appear involved to a greater or lesser degree. Intriguingly, recent studies suggest that there may even be a neurogenic basis for some or all of the changes, but further work is required to confirm this.

References

1. Bernick S, Cailliet R. Vertebral end-plate changes with aging of human vertebrae. *Spine.* 1982;7:97-102.
2. Bishop PB. Proteoglycans and degenerative spondylosis. *J Manipulative Physiol Ther.* 1988;11:36-40.
3. Boni M, Denaro V. Anatomo-clinical correlations in cervical spondylosis. In: Kehr P, Weidner A, eds. *Cervical Spine I.* New York, NY: Springer-Verlag; 1987:3-20.
4. Brodin H. Paths of nutrition in articular cartilage and intervertebral discs. *Acta Orthop Scand.* 1954-55;24:171-183.
5. Brown MD, Tsaltas TT. Studies on the permeability of the intervertebral disc during skeletal maturation. *Spine.* 1976;1:240-244.
6. Bywaters EGL. The pathology of the spine. In: Sokoloff L, ed. *The Joints and Synovial Fluid, Vol II.* New York, NY: Academic Press; 1980:428-547.
7. Ceciliani L, Pedrotti L, Benazzo F, et al. Spondylosis of the cervical spine: formation of osteophytes. In: Louis R, Weidner A, eds. *Cervical Spine II.* New York, NY: Springer-Verlag; 1988:183-187.
8. Cherubino P, Benazzo F, Borromeo U, et al. Degenerative arthritis of the adjacent spinal joints following anterior cervical fusion: clinicoradiologic and statistical correlations. *Ital J Orthop Traumatol.* 1990;16:533-543.
9. DeRoos A, Kressel H, Spritzer C, et al. MR imaging of marrow changes adjacent to end plates in degenerative lumbar disc disease. *AJR.* 1987;149:531-534.
10. Frymoyer JW, Pope MH, Clements JH, et al. Risk factors in low-back pain. *J Bone Joint Surg.* 1983;65A:213-218.
11. Ghadially FN. Fine structure of joints. In: Sokoloff L, ed. *The Joints and Synovial Fluid, Vol 1.* New York, NY: Academic Press; 1978:105-176.
12. Gore DR, Sepic SB, Gardner GM, et al. Neck pain: a long-term follow-up of 205 patients. *Spine.* 1987;12:1-5.
13. Hankey GJ, Khangure MS. Cervical myelopathy due to calcification of the ligamentum flavum. *Aust N Z J Surg.* 1988;58:247-249.
14. Johnson EF, Chetty C, Moore IM, et al. The distribution and arrangement of elastic fibers in the intervertebral disc of the adult human. *J Anat.* 1982;135:301-309.
15. Kelsey JL, Hardy RJ. Driving of motor vehicles as a risk factor for acute herniated lumbar intervertebral disc. *Am J Epidemiol.* 1975;102:63-73.
16. Kempson GE, Tuke MA, Dingle JT, et al. The effects of proteolytic enzymes on the mechanical properties of adult human cartilage. *Biochem Biophys. ACTA.* 1987;428:741-760.
17. Kubota T, Kawano H, Yamashima , et al. Ultrastructural study of calcification process in the ligamentum flavum of the cervical spine. *Spine.* 1987;12:317-323.
18. Lacey DL, Bar-Shavit Z, Kahn AJ, et al. Bone resorption and the immune system. In: Sen A, Thornhill T, eds. *UCLA Symposium on Molecular and Cellular Biology, New Series.* New York, NY: Alan R Liss Inc; 1986;46:233-238.
19. Lestini WF, Wiesel SW. The pathogenesis of cervical spondylosis. *Clin Orthop.* 1989;239:69-93.
20. Miller EJ. The collagen joints. In: Sokoloff L, ed. *The Joints and Synovial Fluid, Vol. 1.* New York, NY: Academic Press; 1978:205-242.
21. Modic MT, Steinberg PM, Ross JS, et al. Degenerative disk disease: assessment of changes in vertebral body marrow with MR imaging. *Radiology.* 1988;166:193-199.
22. Mohr W, Beneke G, Mohing W. Proliferation of synovial lining cells and fibroblasts. *Ann Rheum Dis.* 1975;34:219-224.
23. Mundy GR. Bone resorption and turnover in health and disease. *Bone.* 1987;8(suppl 1):S9-S16.
24. Nakano N, Nakano T. Relationship between osteophyts and symptoms in the cervical spondylosis. In: Kehr P, Weidner A, eds. *Cervical Spine I.* New York, NY: Springer-Verlag; 1987:148-152.
25. Ng SCS, Weiss JB, Quennel R, et al. Abnormal connective tissue degrading enzyme patterns in prolapsed intervertebral discs. *Spine.* 1986;11:695-701.
26. Oda J, Tanaka H, Tsuzuki N. Intervertebral disc changes with aging of human cervical vertebra: from the neonate to the eighties. *Spine.* 1988;13:1205-1211.
27. Osdohy P, Oursler MG, Salino-Hugg T. et al. The cell surface and osteoclast development. In: Sen A, Thornhill T, eds. *UCLA Symposium on Molecular and Cellular Biology, New Series.* New York, NY: Alan R Liss Inc; 1986;46:221-231.
28. Palmer PES, Stadalnick R, Arnon S. The genetic factor in cervical spondylosis. *Skeletal Radiol.* 1984;11:178-182.
29. Pedrini-Mille A, Weinstein JN, Found EM, et al. Stimulation of dorsal root ganglia and degradation of rabbit annulus fibrosus. *Spine.* 1990;15:1252-1256.
30. Penning L. Functional anatomy of joints and discs. In: Cervical Spine Research Society Editorial Committee, ed. *The Cervical Spine.* 2nd ed. Philadelphia, Pa: JB Lippincott Co; 1989:33-56.
31. Raisy LG. Prostaglandins and other local factors regulating bone metabolism. In: Sen A, Thornhill T, eds. *UCLA Symposium on Mollecular and Cellular Biology, New Series.* New York, NY: Alan R Liss Inc; 1986;46:339-347.
32. Sato K, Hayashi M, Kubota T, et al. Symptomatic calcification and ossification of the cervical ligamentum flavum: clinical, radiological and pathological features. *Br J Neurosurg.* 1989;3:597-602.
33. Scher AT. Premature onset of degenerative disease of the cervical spine in rugby players. *S Afr Med J.* 1990;77:557-558.
34. Sedowofia KA, Tomlinson IW, Weiss JB, et al. Collagenolytic enzyme systems in human intervertebral disc: their control, mechanism, and their possible role in the initiation of biomechanical failure. *Spine.* 1982;7:213-222.
35. Shanfeld JL, Lally E, Lanese RR, et al. Osteoblastic and fibroblastic PGE: in vivo effects of indomethacin and mechanical force. In: *Normal and Abnormal Bone Growth: Basic Clinical Research.* New York, NY: Alan R Liss Inc; 1985:331-342.
36. *Stedman's Medical Dictionary.* 24th ed. Baltimore, Md: Williams and Wilkins; 1982:1322.

37. Syftestad GT, Lucas PA, Ohgushi H, et al. Chondrogenesis as an in vitro response to bioactive factors extracted from adult bone and non-skeletal tissues. In: Sen A, Thornhill T, eds. *UCLA Symposium on Molecular and Cellular Biology, New Series*. New York, NY: Alan R Liss Inc; 1986;46:187-199.
38. Ten Have HAMJ, Eulderink F. Degenerative changes in the cervical spine and their relationship to its mobility. *J Pathol*. 1980;132:133-159.
39. Ten Have HAMJ, Eulderink F. Mobility and degenerative changes of the aging cervical spine: a macroscopic and statistical study. *Gerontology*. 1981;27:42-50.
40. Teresi LM, Lufkin RB, Reicher MA, et al. Asymptomatic degenerative disc diseases and spondylosis of the cervical spine: MR imaging. *Radiology*. 1987;164:83-88.
41. Weidner N, Rice DT. Intervertebral disk material: criteria for determining probable prolapse. *Hum Pathol*. 1988;19:406-410.
42. Weinstein J, Claverie W, Gibson S. The pain of discography. *Spine*. 1988;13:1344-1348.
43. Wilder DG, Woodworth BB, Frymoyer JW, et al. Vibration and the human spine. *Spine*. 1982;7:243-254.

CHAPTER 3

Imaging and the Diagnosis of Degenerative Disease of the Cervical Spine

Andrew W. Litt, MD

Cervical spine degenerative disease is a common condition. While it is often symptomatic, many patients have varying degrees of degenerative disease without symptoms.[2,4-7,6,7,17,25,26,41] The bony, ligamentous, and disk changes usually are manifest as spondylosis, or as a discrete disk herniation, or a combination of the two. The evaluation of patients with symptoms of radiculopathy and/or myelopathy related to the cervical spine, and the selection of those patients who would benefit from surgical intervention rather than conservative therapy is a challenge to the neurologist and neurosurgeon.

Computed tomography (CT), either alone or in conjunction with myelography, as well as magnetic resonance imaging (MRI) significantly increase the ability of the radiologist to precisely define the anatomic disturbance produced by spondylosis or disk herniation and the resulting compression of neural structures. Our ability to define a functional correlate to this anatomic disturbance is often limited, however. In fact, the correlation of imaging findings with a patient's symptoms and signs is of increasing importance as newer techniques demonstrate abnormalities not previously appreciated.

Computed Tomography

Although the diagnosis of spondylosis and disk herniation by CT had been reported in the cervical spine as early as 1976-1977,[10,12] it was not until the development of third- and fourth-generation scanners in the late 1970s and early 1980s that a routine detailed examination of the cervical spine for these conditions was possible.

Technique

The patient is examined in the supine position. A lateral projection digital radiographic scout is obtained, followed by thin axial sections (usually 1.5 to 3.0 mm) at each disk space from C2-3 through C7-T1. The slices must be angled parallel to each disk space. Angulation should be continually adjusted by the technician to keep the slices parallel to the axis of the disk. Both "bone" and "soft-tissue" windows must be imaged for each slice. Reformatted images may be useful in individual cases, but need not be obtained in every patient. Intravenous contrast is not routinely administered at our institution.

Normal Anatomy

Regardless of the level of the section, the spinal canal is normally seen as a rounded triangle[27] with its transverse diameter greater than its anteroposterior one (Figure 1). Within the canal the spinal cord itself can

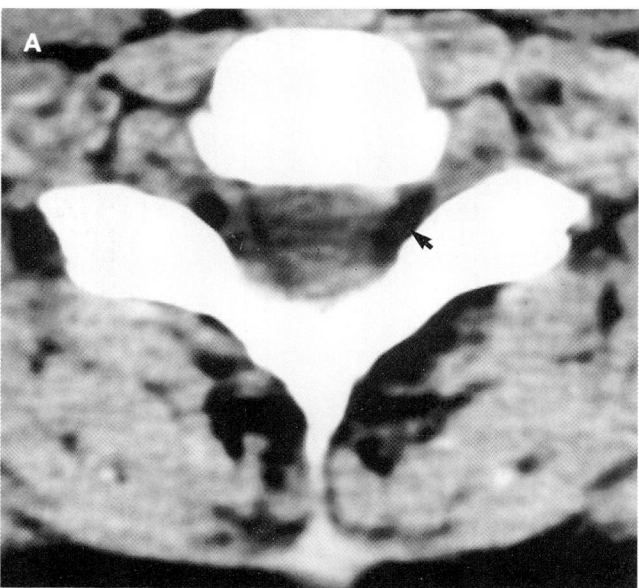

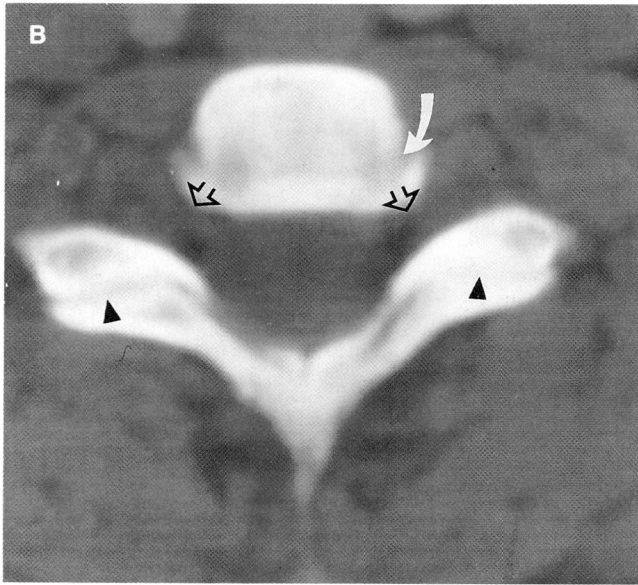

Figure 1. Normal cervical spine anatomy on CT. Soft-tissue and bone windows at the disk space **(A,B)** and at the center of the vertebral body **(C,D—opposite page)**. The neural foramina are not narrowed *(open arrows)*. There is a small amount of epidural fat lateral to the thecal sac *(small arrows)*. The facet joints are seen bilaterally *(arrowheads)*. The uncovertebral joints are seen at the level of the disk space *(curved arrow)*.

often be detected (usually down to the C4 level) as an area of slightly higher attenuation, relative to the surrounding cerebrospinal fluid (Figure 1). The extradural soft tissues, comprising both ligaments and venous plexus, may be seen as thin linear regions of increased attenuation bordering the subarachnoid space. Posteriorly, the ligamenta flava

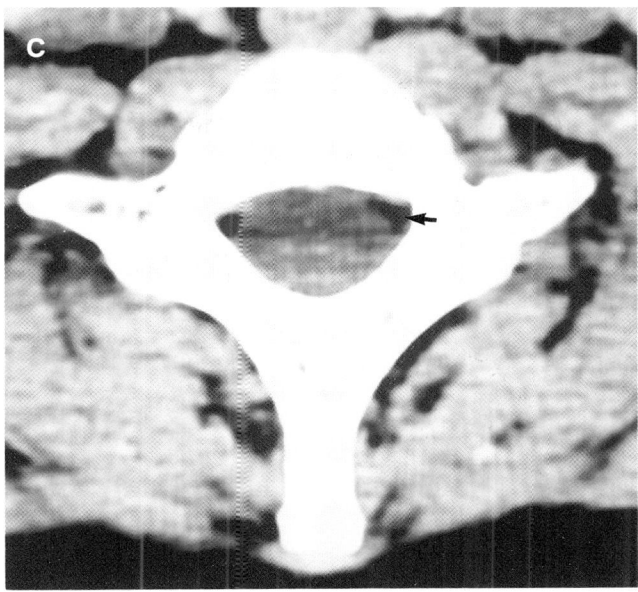

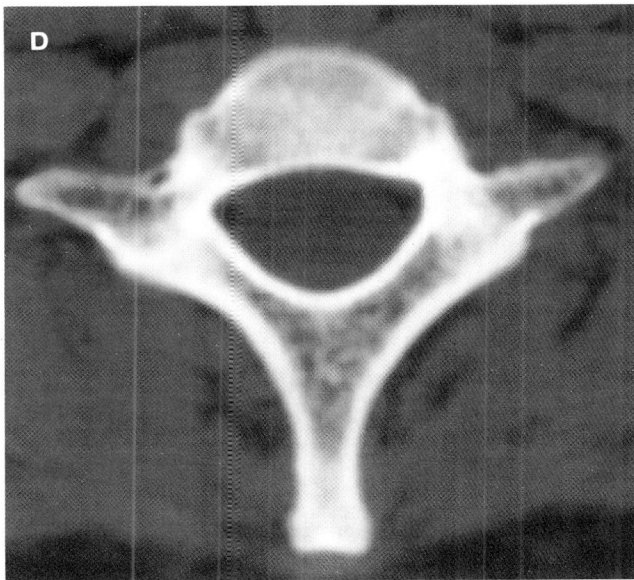

are barely seen along the anterior margin of the lamina.

The disk space level can be identified either by seeing the lower attenuation disk in place of the vertebral body or by noting the uncovertebral joints on either side (see Figures 1B,D). The neural foramina are also present at this level, and are usually filled with a fairly uniform soft-tissue density which represents both the exiting nerve root and the epidural venous plexus. In some cases, the nerve roots can be distinguished as linear areas of slightly increased attenuation in the decreased attenuation fat of the foramen.[31] The ganglion may be seen as a rounded area of increased attenuation laterally. The vertebral arteries can always be identified by their position within the foramen transversarium bilaterally, and as discrete round soft-tissue densities in the lateral and distal fat of the

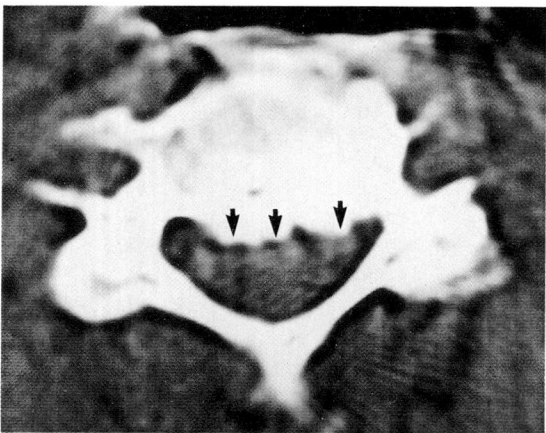

Figure 2. Central osteophytic ridges (arrows) with probable spinal cord compression.

neural foramen at the disk space level.

The facet joints on either side are comprised of the two semilunar appearing facets, with the superior articulating facet of the vertebral body below being anterior to the inferior articulating facet of the body above. The combined appearance of the two facets and the joints should approximate a circle or be slightly oval in shape without lateral or medial osteophyte extension.

Spondylotic Disease

Osteophytic ridges ("hard disks") are easily detected on routine CT as areas of irregular increased attenuation corresponding to bone projecting posteriorly from the vertebral body at the disk-space level. These are in continuity with the vertebral body itself. Osteophytes often are laterally placed, extending from the uncinate process as well as from the vertebral body itself (Figure 2). The osteophytes may be accompanied by abnormal soft-tissue density within the canal, with a higher attenuation than the cerebrospinal fluid. This most commonly represents fibrocartilage or a bulging annulus, and is directly related to the etiology of the spur.[27] A frank disk herniation may also be present.

If the spinal cord can be delineated, abnormalities in its size and shape can be defined. These may represent either compression by an osteophyte or atrophy of the spinal cord as a result of repeated trauma from the osteophyte. Even if the spinal cord is not discernible, the overall size of the canal should be assessed on the bone window images. If the anteroposterior diameter is less than 12 mm,[27] spinal stenosis is present.

Evaluation of the facet joints is important to detect any hypertrophic changes that may narrow the spinal canal at the lateral recess, causing nerve root or even lateral spinal cord compression. The ligamenta flava may also become prominent as a part of the spondylotic process. This is often not true thickening, but infolding as a result of foreshortening of the canal. Nonetheless, it further reduces the overall size of the spinal canal and may produce posterolateral compression of the spinal cord.[27] The ligaments may become calcified in long standing degenerative disease.

The disk space itself in spondylosis often shows decreased height on the digital scout radiograph which is not detected on the axial slices. There may be calcification within the disk, but this can be difficult to distinguish from degenerative changes at the endplates.[24] Vacuum phenomenon with gas in the intervertebral space is occasionally seen.

Herniated Disk

Frank disk herniations are seen as soft tissue with increased attenuation (Hounsfield units of approximately 100), surrounded by the normal epidural fat and cerebrospinal fluid, either centrally or laterally anterior to the thecal sac (Figure 3).[8,9] They are usually present at the disk-space level, and frequently extend inferiorly or superiorly by at least one slice. Herniated disks tend to be irregular or lobulated, and may be present independently or in association with spondylotic changes. Calcification within the disk fragment is not uncommon. This may be distinguished from osteophyte formation by its more punctate character, although this differentiation is not always possible.

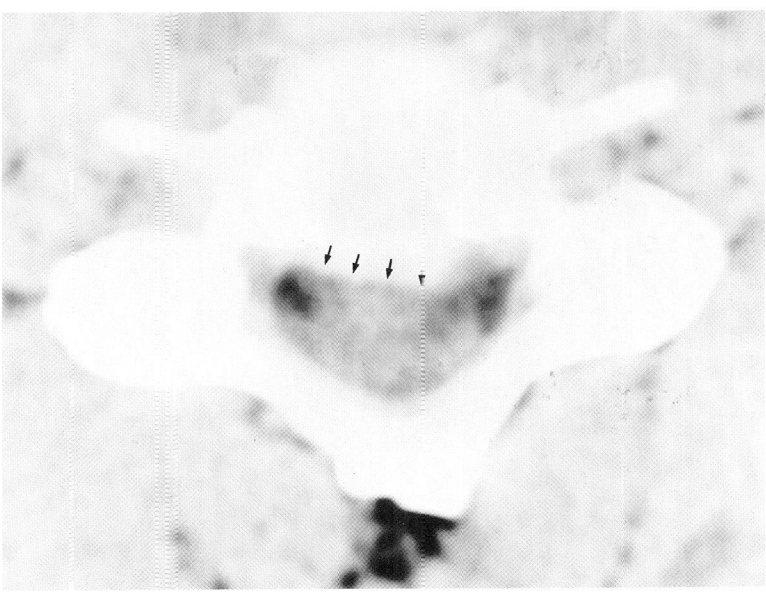

Figure 3. Diffuse herniated disk (arrows) extending across the midline on this soft-tissue window image. Although the cord is not well seen because of artifacts, it is likely to be compressed with this extensive herniation.

Computed Tomography with Intravenous Contrast

Because of the limited contrast difference between the soft-tissue density of a disk herniation and the cerebrospinal fluid and spinal cord within the spinal canal, and because of frequent artifacts overlying the cervical canal from the lateral facet joints and the shoulders, several authors have proposed using intravenous contrast to increase the sensitivity of CT for "soft" disk herniations in a relatively noninvasive manner.[3,34] The contrast enhances the normal basivertebral venous plexus against which the nonenhancing disk material is more easily identified.

At each cervical level, the venous drainage of the vertebral body is to the basivertebral vein, which drains into the retrocorporeal venous plexus just dorsal to the posterior longitudinal ligament.[34] This plexus is transversely oriented and communicates on each side with the paired, vertical anterior longitudinal epidural veins that lie just medial to the foramina. These communicate caudally with the level below and laterally with the foraminal veins which extend to the plexus surrounding the vertebral artery on each side.

In the normal individual, below the level of C2, the retrocorporeal plexus directly behind the vertebral body cannot be distinguished from the high attenuation of the cortex itself. The anterior longitudinal epidural veins can be seen in the lateral recess bilaterally, and the foraminal veins can be identified as linear enhancing structures within the foramina.

If the retrocorporeal plexus is visualized, this implies that it has been posteriorly displaced and is pathognomonic for a disk herniation.[34] In addition, disk fragments can usually be seen as irregular areas of soft-tissue attenuation within a rim of marginal enhancement (Figure 4). This enhancement represents the displaced plexus as well as local inflammatory reaction around the ruptured posterior longitudinal ligament caused by the herniation itself.[34]

The use of this technique is especially valuable in cases of localized radiculopathy in patients whose noncontrast CT has been equivocal. The limitation occurs in patients with extensive spondylotic disease where demonstration of the enhancing plexus may

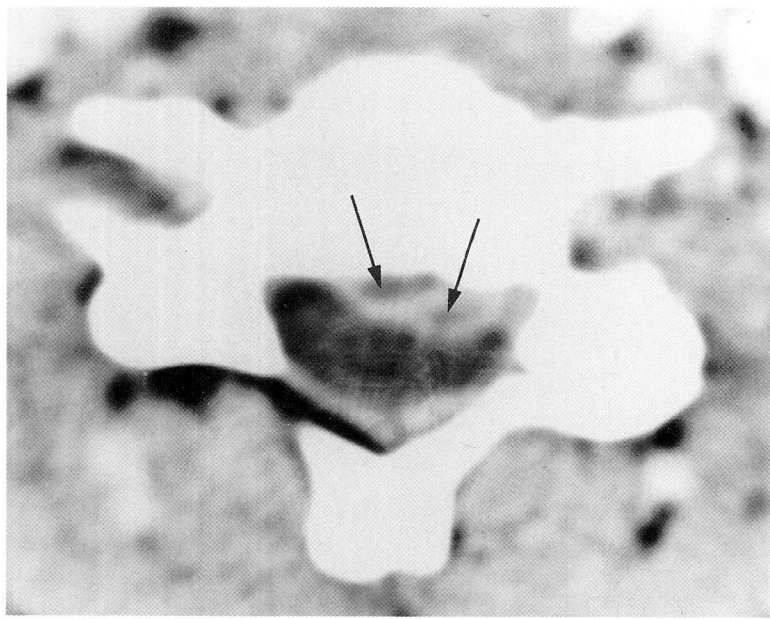

Figure 4. CT scan following intravenous contrast administration. The disk herniation is seen as areas of decreased attenuation with a rim of enhancement (arrows). (Figure courtesy of Eric Russell, MD)

be confused with ridges, both having high attenuation.[34]

Computed Tomography Following Myelography

Since its description by Di Chiro in 1976,[12] computed tomography following myelography (CTM) has become the "gold standard" for imaging the cervical spine for spondylosis and disk disease. Because of the increase in differential contrast provided by the intrathecal material (formerly metrizamide and now iopamidol or iohexol), better definition of a herniated disk or a spondylotic ridge is possible than with either plain CT or plain film myelography alone. In addition, intrathecal contrast provides an accurate assessment of the effect of the herniation or ridge on the spinal cord itself. Finally, the use of delayed CTM will often demonstrate pathology beyond the point of myelographic block and intramedullary changes of degeneration and syrinx formation secondary to spondylosis.

Technique

At our institution, CTM is performed after a complete cervical myelogram. Following the injection of nonionic contrast material in the lumbar subarachnoid space, routine myelographic images of the cervical spine are obtained and are used along with the clinical history in directing the CTM examination. Rather than obtaining a full cervical myelogram, some institutions merely instill 4-6 ml of contrast in the subarachnoid space and keep the patient in a decubitus position with the head slightly elevated for some time prior to scanning. While this method is effective in obtaining adequate contrast for CTM, it does not allow for tailoring of the examination.

If a myelographic block is noted on the plain film examination, CTM may be attempted shortly thereafter. Although a block may appear to be complete on the plain films, contrast will be seen often in the subarachnoid space on the CT beyond the block.[1] If this attempt is not successful, a C1-2 puncture with instillation of contrast can be em-

Imaging and the Diagnosis of Degenerative Disease of the Cervical Spine

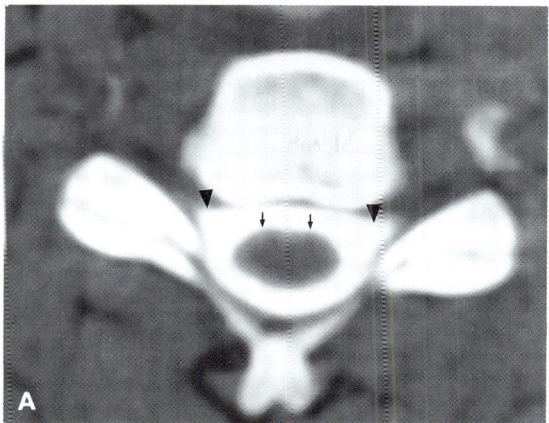

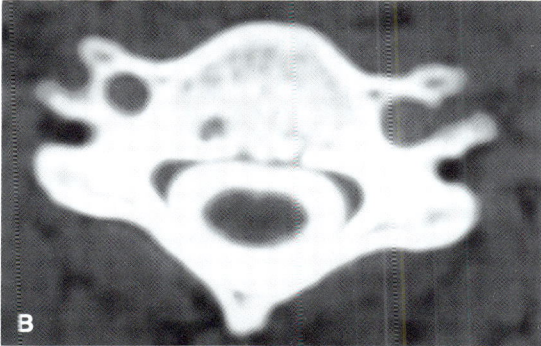

Figure 5. Normal CTM through (A) the disk space/vertebral endplate region, and (B) midvertebral body. The anterior margin of the spinal cord on both the left and the right has a rounded appearance (small arrows). The contrast-filled thecal sac extends into the lateral recess bilaterally (arrowheads). The sac is not deformed or flattened.

ployed, or a delayed (4-6 hour) study may show some contrast passing beyond the point of block.

In those cases where intramedullary degeneration or syrinx formation is suspected, either from the clinical history or the appearance of an expanded cord on either plain film myelography or initial CTM, a delayed (4-6 hour) study should be obtained to detect abnormal contrast uptake within the cord itself.

Normal Anatomy

The posterior surface of the vertebral body is separated from the opacified thecal sac by a 1-2 mm area of soft-tissue attenuation representing the posterior longitudinal ligament and the epidural venous plexus. The ligamenta flava are also seen as 1-2 mm curvilinear bands of soft-tissue attenuation between the lamina and the sac dorsally.

The spinal cord itself is well visualized as an ovoid or round structure; it is most ovoid at C4 and C5 and most round at T1 (Figure 5).[38] A very minimal anterior median indentation is often present, corresponding to the anterior median fissure. Nonetheless, the right and left anterior portions should remain rounded. There should be no anterior, posterior, or posterolateral flattening of the spinal cord. The anteroposterior diameter of the spinal cord is smallest at C4 and C5 and widens above and below, whereas the transverse diameter increases to a maximum at C4 and C5 and becomes smallest at T1.[38] The attenuation of the spinal cord should remain uniform and be similar to that of soft tissue.

The contrast-filled subarachnoid space is seen as a ring of increased attenuation around the spinal cord. It is usually reasonably symmetric and extends to the lateral recess adjacent to the medial portion of the facet joint. The dorsal and ventral roots may be seen as linear filling defects in the subarachnoid space. Unlike the lumbar spine, contrast is usually not seen extending into the lateral recess.

Spondylotic Changes

Ridges are seen as high-attenuation overgrowths adjacent to the vertebral endplate (Figures 6 and 7). They compress the dural sac and either narrow or obliterate the thin line of soft-tissue attenuation of the posterior longitudinal ligament. This process can be focal or diffuse, central or lateral. The dural sac itself may be deformed and posteriorly displaced. Minimal thinning of the anterior rim of the subarachnoid space relative to the posterior one is a subtle finding of small spurs.[1]

The spinal cord either may be flattened minimally or may demonstrate considerable

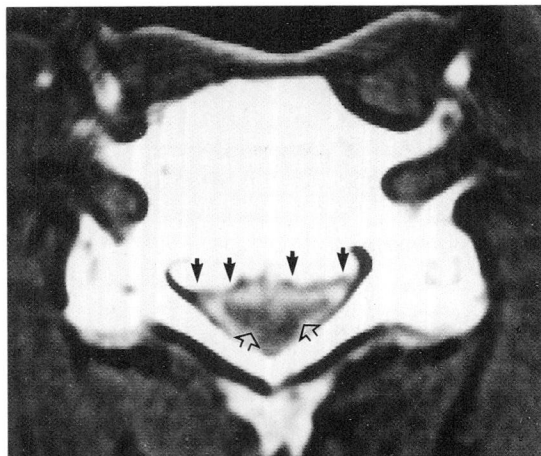

Figure 6. Large diffuse osteophyte (arrows) with narrowing of the thecal sac and an atrophic triangular spinal cord (open arrows).

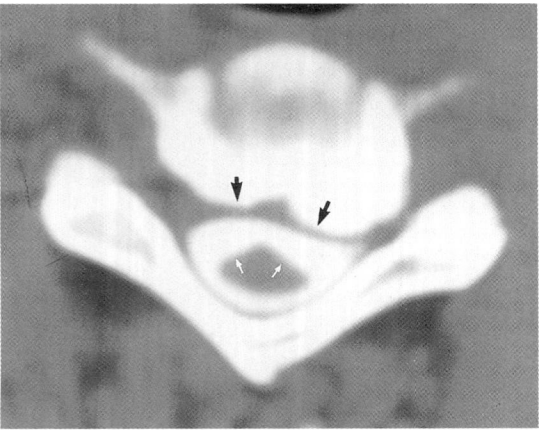

Figure 7. Bilateral osteophytes (black arrows) which have caused flattening of the spinal cord on both sides (small white arrows) despite a relatively normal thecal sac size.

loss of anteroposterior diameter (Figure 6). Any loss of the normal rounded margins of the anterolateral portions of the spinal cord should be considered significant. The spinal cord may be rotated and/or displaced posteriorly or posterolaterally by large osteophytes. Although the spinal cord itself may be small or flat, the subarachnoid space is often not significantly narrowed. This may be explained by one of two mechanisms: (1) the spinal cord is atrophied secondary to many years of compression, and/or (2) it is compressed only when the patient flexes or hyperextends the neck, yet it does not completely return to normal in the neutral position which is assumed during the CT examination (Figure 7).

This finding of a normal to increased ratio of the cross-sectional area of the cord-to-subarachnoid space may have some prognostic value. Badami et al found that in patients with a cord-to-subarachnoid space ratio of greater than 50% (a small subarachnoid space relative to spinal cord size), a good recovery of function was noted after surgical decompression. In those with a ratio less than 50% (a large subarachnoid space relative to spinal cord size), no recovery of function was noted.[1] This finding makes intuitive sense because one would not expect good recovery in patients with an atrophic spinal cord. However, the sample was small and the results have not been confirmed by other studies.

Intrinsic abnormalities of the spinal cord in the setting of spondylosis have also been demonstrated on delayed CTM. Repeat scans are obtained from 4-6 hours following myelography with water-soluble contrast. The presence of local or remote areas of contrast enhancement within the spinal cord has been documented.[19] It is not clear in all cases whether this abnormal enhancement represents a true syringomyelic cavity, similar to that seen in the post-traumatic state, or rather is an area of "cystic necrosis" or myelomalacia. Performing delayed CT scanning to search for these abnormalities is important in cases of spondylosis and clear-cut myelopathy, where the amount of spinal cord compression on the initial CT following the myelogram is not impressive. It is also useful when there appears to be expansion of the spinal cord.

Lateral spurring from the uncovertebral joints, causing either spinal cord or nerve root compression, is readily demonstrated on CTM. Plain film myelography may miss these laterally placed ridges.[16] Degenerative changes of the facet joints lateral to the dural sac as well as thickening of the ligamenta flava posterolaterally can also be well appreciated on the CTM. Flattening of the spinal cord from these posterior and lateral masses can be clinically significant.

Imaging and the Diagnosis of Degenerative Disease of the Cervical Spine

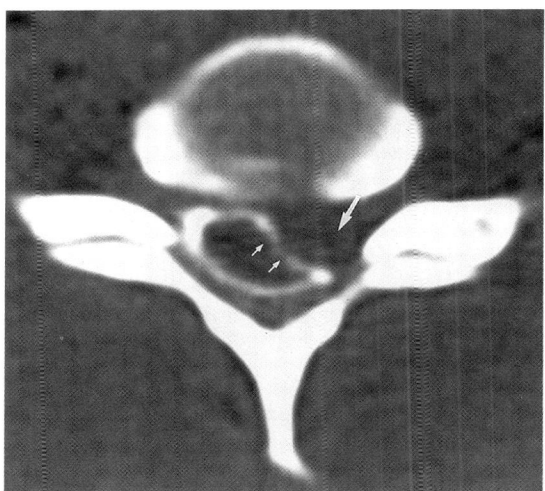

Figure 8. CT scan following the myelogram at the disk-space level. A large disk herniation (large arrow) is present. The cord is rotated and flattened on the left side (small arrows).

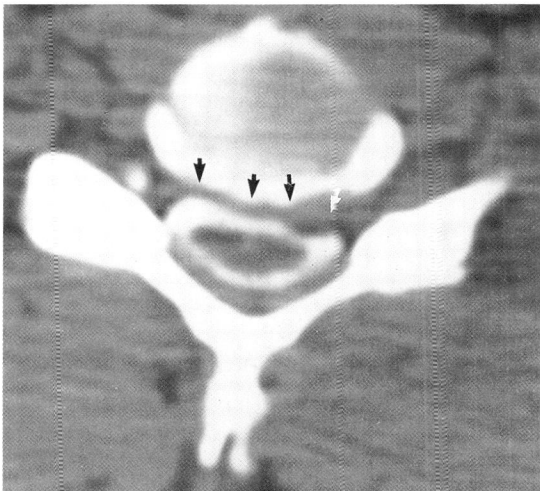

Figure 9. Postmyelographic CT at the level of the disk space. A small diffuse osteophytic ridge (black arrows) is causing spinal cord compression. A small herniated disk (white arrow) on the left is causing focal thecal sac narrowing and cord flattening.

Herniated Disk

The high contrast and spatial resolution of CTM is ideal for the detection and characterization of small fragments of herniated disk (Figures 8, 9), some of which may be missed on plain film myelography,[20] and on plain CT.[25] This is especially true for central disk herniations, which were considered rare until the advent of CTM.[30]

The distinction between "soft" or noncalcified disk material and osteophytic spur is easily made on CTM. The high-density subarachnoid space will be deformed by a soft-tissue density mass in the former and by a high-density mass in the latter. One may not see the disk fragment as a discrete entity; however, if the thecal sac is compressed or displaced and there is no osteophyte present at that level or at the levels above and below, one may assume the compression is due to a soft-disk herniation.[35]

Lateral disk herniations are also well shown on CTM. Detection of these lesions, especially in the setting of spondylotic changes at the same level, is important information for the surgeon. In the anterior approach, the surgeon's field of view is limited, especially on the side of entry, making knowledge of isolated lateral fragments extremely important.

Magnetic Resonance Imaging

The advent of MRI raised the possibility that patients could be examined for cervical spine disk and spondylotic disease without either ionizing radiation or the invasive myelogram. Although MRI has become the initial screening examination for these patients, it is still often not the definitive preoperative study. There are institutions where the surgeons will operate on patients with myelopathy and spondylotic cord compression visualized on MR; however, many still request the CTM for confirmation prior to surgery. In patients with radiculopathy, CTM is preferred often over MR because of better contrast, spatial resolution, and overall signal-to-noise ratio. In addition, CTM may better determine whether the pathology is a disk or a ridge. As the quality of MR imaging techniques improves, with new hardware and new scan sequences, increasingly it will become the definitive study.

Technique

The utility of MR lies in the combination of its multiplanar capability combined with its unique capacity to visualize the contrast between different tissues in multiple ways. Therefore, the complete MR examination in a patient with myelopathy or radiculopathy should include a multiplanar as well as multi-contrast evaluation.

Sagittal T1-weighted images are used for a preliminary overview of the cervical spine and canal. Thin sections (3 mm or 4 mm) should be used for the sagittal examination with a small (10% to 20%) interslice gap, and it is useful to have one slice positioned precisely through the middle of the spinal cord. The precise scan parameters (TR, TE, number of acquisitions, field-of-view, etc.) will depend on the specific MR imaging device used.

It is then often useful to obtain a T2-weighted (spin-echo) or T2*-weighted (gradient-echo) sequence in the sagittal plane. This will provide a "white CSF" appearance that will mimic the myelogram.[13,14,18,40] Although the T1-weighted sagittal study is ideal for anatomic resolution, there is minimal contrast between osteophytes, which are largely cortical bone and appear as low signal, and the CSF, which is also of low signal. This contrast is improved in the T2-weighted study where ridges causing anterior epidural impression on the thecal sac are more easily visualized. The T2-weighted study also allows for better detection of intrinsic spinal cord abnormalities that are related to the osteophyte formation or are independent, as seen in multiple sclerosis.

For further evaluation of findings on the sagittal studies, and for complete examination of the nerve roots in patients with radiculopathy, axial high-resolution T1-weighted and/or gradient echo images are required. The precise TR/TE and other sequence factors will depend on the machine used; in general, the slices should be thin enough (preferably 3-5 mm), and sufficient acquisitions should be used to clearly delineate the structures within the spinal canal as well as the nerve roots in the lateral recesses and foramina. Interslice gaps of 20% to 40% are acceptable, and the slices should be oriented parallel to the disk spaces. Axial slices should be acquired through those levels that appear abnormal on the sagittal images; in patients with radiculopathy, axial slices should also be obtained through the levels that correspond to the clinical abnormality.

Other MR techniques for evaluating the cervical spine in radiculopathy include postcontrast (gadolinium-DTPA) T1-weighted images,[32,33] oblique imaging,[11,15,28] where the plane of section is perpendicular to the neural foramina of interest, and thin section 3DFT imaging where multiple (40-60) contiguous 3D gradient echo axial slices are obtained covering the entire cervical canal.[39] The advantages of the 3DFT technique are thinner slices (1.5-2.0 mm) with resolution similar to that obtained in CT scanning, increased signal-to-noise ratio, better depiction of the neural foramina, and enhanced CSF signal intensity due to the short TR employed.

The exact MR protocol used for cervical spine imaging depends not only on the preferences of the individual radiologist and referring clinician, but also on the capabilities of the available scanner.

Normal Anatomy

On sagittal T1-weighted images the vertebrae should be of fairly uniform mid-intensity (Figure 10A). Small areas of increased and/or decreased signal within the bodies, especially adjacent to the endplates, may represent areas of degenerative change. The alignment should be examined and the presence or absence of subluxations noted. The disk spaces have a moderately high-signal inner region surrounded by a low-signal rim that represents the annulus along with the adjacent bony cortex. The posterior margin of the vertebral bodies also appears as a rim of low signal that merges with that of the posterior longitudinal ligament. Behind this is the higher signal "stripe" of the epidural venous plexus, which often appears thinner or even discon-

Imaging and the Diagnosis of Degenerative Disease of the Cervical Spine

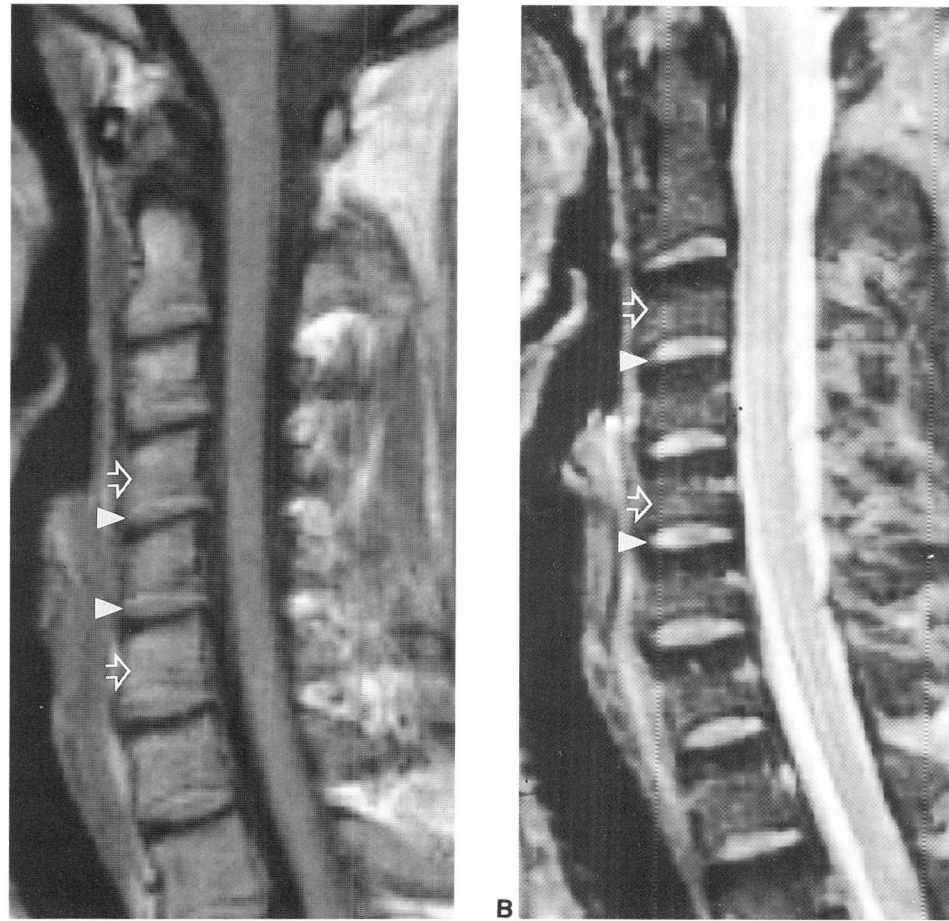

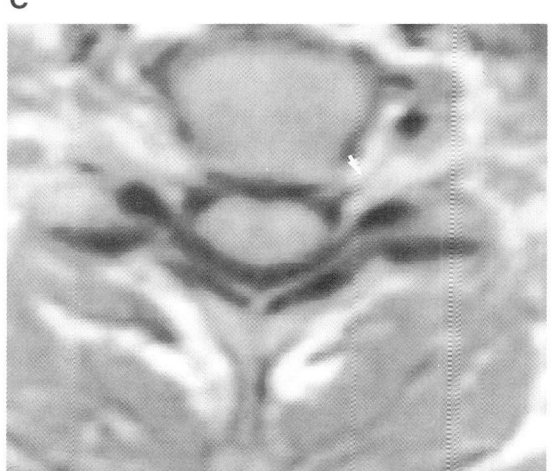
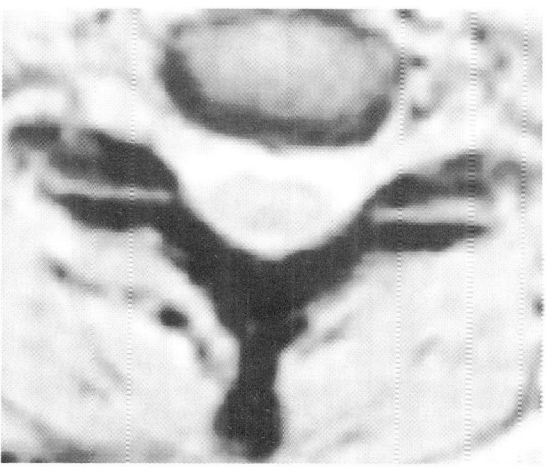

Figure 10. Normal anatomy on MR: **(A)** Midline sagittal T1-weighted image; **(B)** midline sagittal T2-weighted image; **(C)** axial T1-weighted through the disk space; **(D)** axial gradient-echo (T2-weighted) image through the disk space. Note the uniform signal intensity of the vertebral bodies (open arrows) and disk spaces (arrowheads) on the sagittal images. On the axial T1-weighted image **(C)** the nerve root may be seen in the foramen (white arrow).

tinuous at the disk space level. The overall thickness of this plexus in the sagittal plane is variable; on the midline sagittal image, it may not be clearly delineated.

Posterior to the vertebral column is the spinal canal; on T1-weighted images the CSF is low signal and the cord is moderate signal. It is often difficult to precisely define the interface between the posterior vertebral body cortex, posterior longitudinal ligament, and CSF. The posterior elements and associated fat and ligaments are situated behind the canal, and also may be difficult to evaluate on sagittal images.

Sagittal T2-weighted images are similar to T1-weighted ones, except that the vertebral bodies have decreased signal, the disks often have increased signal, and the CSF has significantly increased signal (Figure 10B). The cord remains of moderate signal intensity. These signal characteristics are usually present whether the T2-weighted study is of the spin-echo or gradient-echo type. The epidural venous plexus is not well seen and the interface between the CSF and the posterior longitudinal ligament/posterior cortex is better delineated. In the lumbar spine, the presence of decreased signal in the disk spaces on T2-weighted images is correlated with degenerative changes; however, in the cervical region this correlation is not as significant, and decreased signal is often noted in young patients without other evidence of disk disease.

Axial sections will mimic sagittal sections with regard to signal intensity, depending on the relative T1- or T2-weighting. On high-resolution examinations, the ventral and dorsal nerve roots can be seen exiting the spinal cord and heading toward the neural foramina (Figure 10C). These roots are often better seen on short TR/short TE gradient-echo sequences or gadolinium-DTPA enhanced T1-weighted sequences in which the epidural venous plexus can be seen anterior and posterior to the nerve roots in the lateral recess and in the foramen itself.

Although not routinely performed in most institutions, oblique sections parallel to the foramen may provide good visualizaton of the nerve root exiting the spinal cord and extending into the neural foramen.[11] Images obtained perpendicular to the foramen are similar to lateral sagittal images in the lumbar spine, and show the ventral and dorsal portions of the nerve root arranged in a vertical orientation in the inferior portion of the foramen. The superior foraminal canal is filled with high-intensity fat and the epidural veins.

Spondylotic Changes

Both Sagittal T1- and T2-weighted images depict degenerative changes of the vertebral bodies and disk spaces. The disk spaces are usually narrowed, often with decreased signal and a poorly defined margin between the inner higher-signal region and the annulus.[37] As mentioned before, increased or decreased signal changes in the vertebral body adjacent to the endplates are also consistent with degenerative disease. Subluxations that result from degenerative disease of the facets and ligamentous laxity are occasionally present (Figure 11).

Osteophyte formation is seen on the sagittal images as extensions of the vertebral body cortex, in a triangular configuration, either anteriorly or posteriorly.[37] On T1-weighted images these ridges have a low signal margin representing cortex, which may be difficult to differentiate from the low signal of CSF, depending on the exact scan parameters selected. If the osteophyte is small, only the low-signal cortex will be present. The larger the osteophyte grows, however, the more likely it is to have higher-signal marrow within it as an extension of the normal vertebral body marrow. This higher-signal marrow provides a better contrast with the CSF on T1-weighted study.

A T2-weighted study better delineates the margin between the osteophytic ridge and the CSF (see Figure 11). This may be particularly useful in cases where the amount of epidural compression is small and the spinal cord is not deformed. Because of the magnetic susceptibility effect produced at the

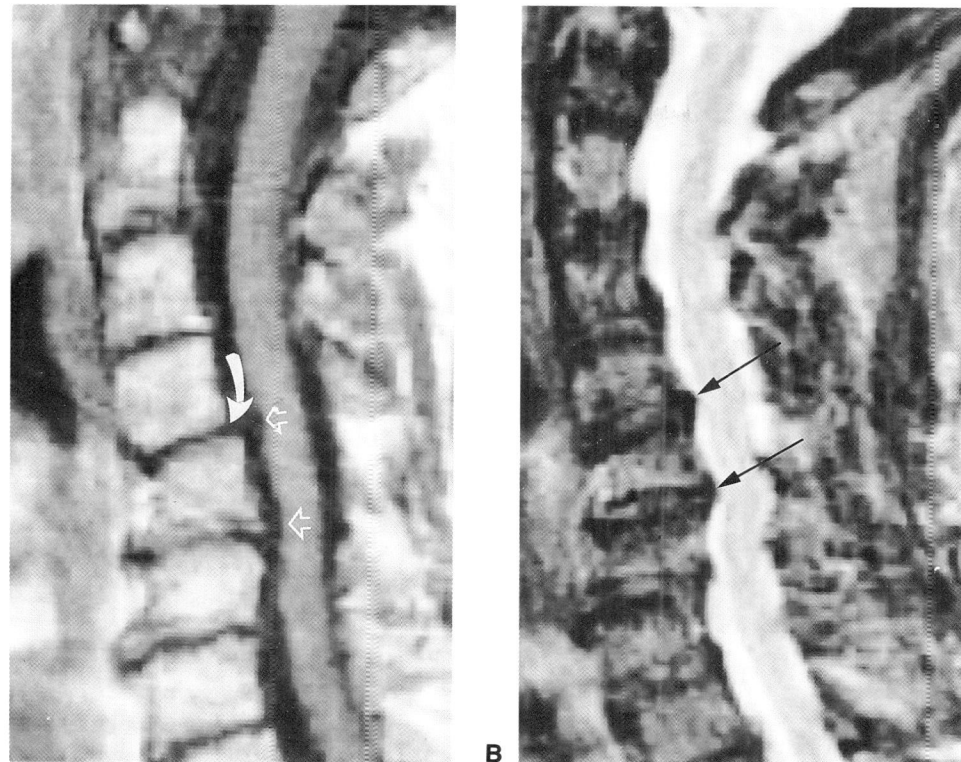

Figure 11. (A) Sagittal T1-weighted, *(B)* sagittal T2-weighted and *(C)* axial T1-weighted images of a patient with degenerative spondylosis affecting primarily C4-5 and C5-6. Note the anterior subluxation of C4 on C5 (curved arrow). The anterior epidural compressions of the thecal sac at C4-5 and C5-6 are best seen on the T2-weighted sagittal image (long arrows), but the compression of the spinal cord can be visualized on the T1-weighted sagittal and axial studies (open arrows). However, on the sagittal T1-weighted studies the osteophyte cannot be clearly distinguished from the CSF.

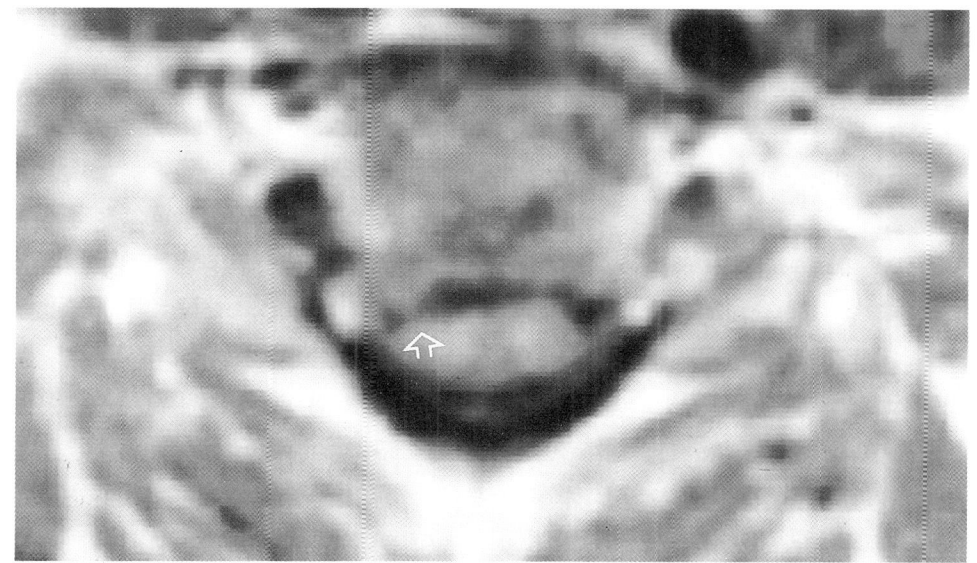

cortex-CSF interface, the size of the ridge and the amount of epidural compression may be exaggerated when gradient-echo sequences are used.

Depending on severity, spinal cord deformity or compression can be seen on the sagittal images, whether T1- or T2-weighted (see Figure 11). The cord can be seen to be locally indented by the extradural osteophyte and may often be displaced laterally over a longer segment. T1-weighted images better define the degree of indentation because of higher signal-to-noise. However, subtle changes are more conspicuous on T2-weighted images.

It is important to examine laterally placed sagittal images for osteophytes extending into the neural foramina from the uncovertebral joints. Although these ridges are often present in association with a central osteophyte, they may be also present independently. The axial images will serve to confirm the presence of foraminal narrowing.

Ossification of the posterior longitudinal ligament is occasionally difficult to detect with MR.[42] The band of ossification will appear as low signal on both T1-weighted and T2-weighted studies. This may merge with the posterior margin of the vertebral bodies and only become apparent when there is spinal cord compression. (See also Chapter 12.)

High signal may be noted within the spinal cord on T2-weighted images in the area of compression. It is important to distinguish among three causes of increased signal. The first is artifact-related, to truncation or to CSF pulsation, which in either case will be linear and extend along the entire length of the cord. These artifacts are usually not associated with corresponding areas of low-signal abnormality on the T1-weighted study, and often can be eliminated from the T2-weighted study by adjusting the scan parameters.

The second cause for increased intramedullary signal on T2-weighted images is syrinx formation. The formation of a syrinx in association with spondylotic changes and osteophytes is probably due to repetitive trauma of the ridge hitting the spinal cord, and is

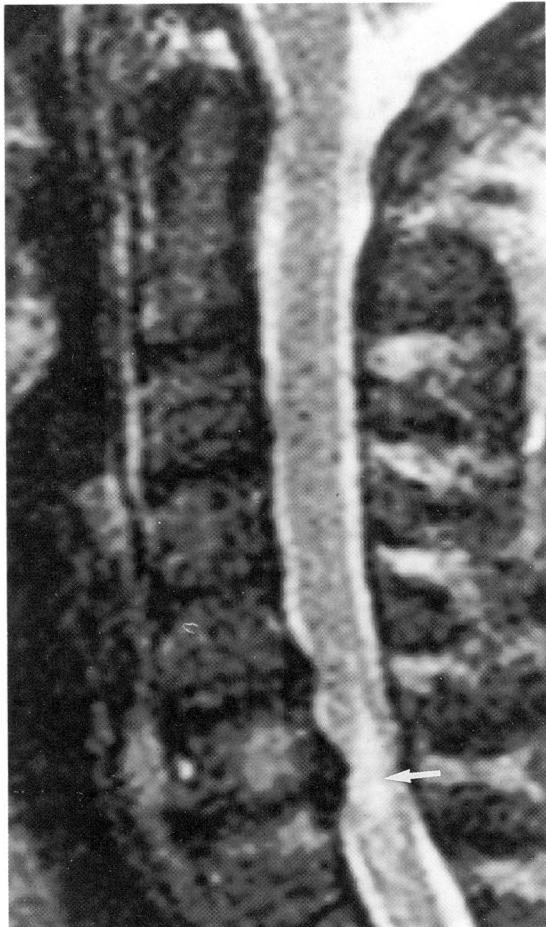

Figure 12. Sagittal T2-weighted image in a patient with anterior osteophytes at C5-6 and C6-7 causing spinal cord compression. There is patchy increased signal in the spinal cord at C6-7 (arrow).

rare. The syrinx is usually centered on the area of ridge formation and is also present on T1-weighted studies, both axial and sagittal, as an area of decreased signal. Septations may be present within the syrinx, but are usually not anatomically complete. The signal characteristics of the fluid within should match that of CSF on all pulse sequences.

The final cause for increased signal intensity within the spinal cord in patients with spondylosis has not been confirmed, but is suspected to represent demyelination or myelomalacia secondary to chronic compression (Figure 12).[23,36] T1-weighted images may show

Imaging and the Diagnosis of Degenerative Disease of the Cervical Spine

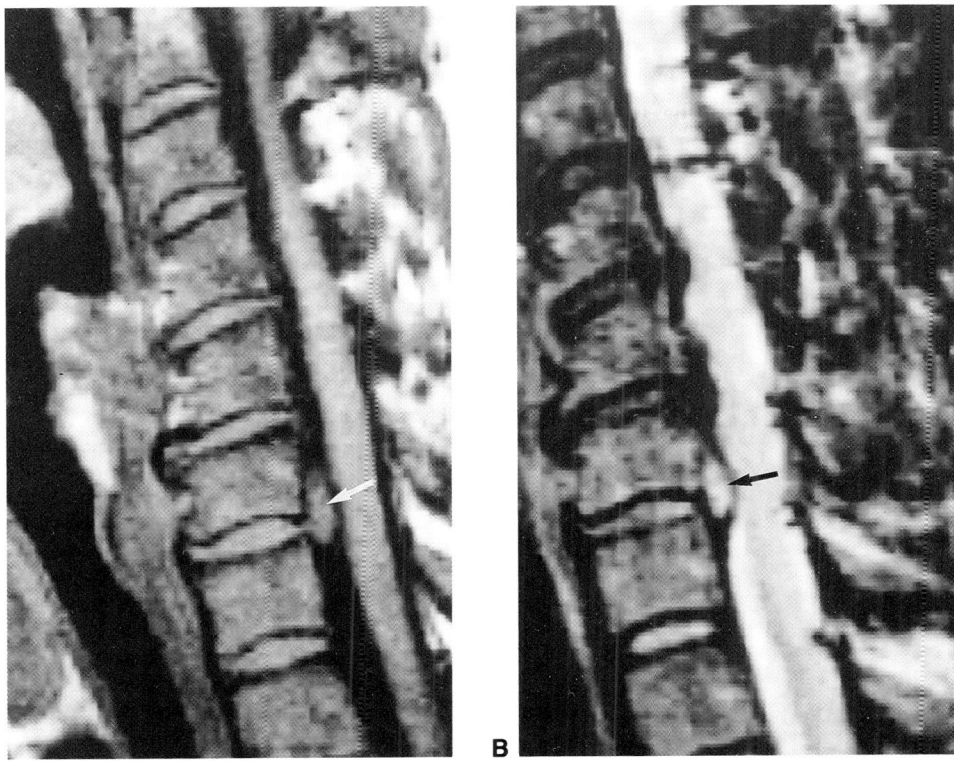

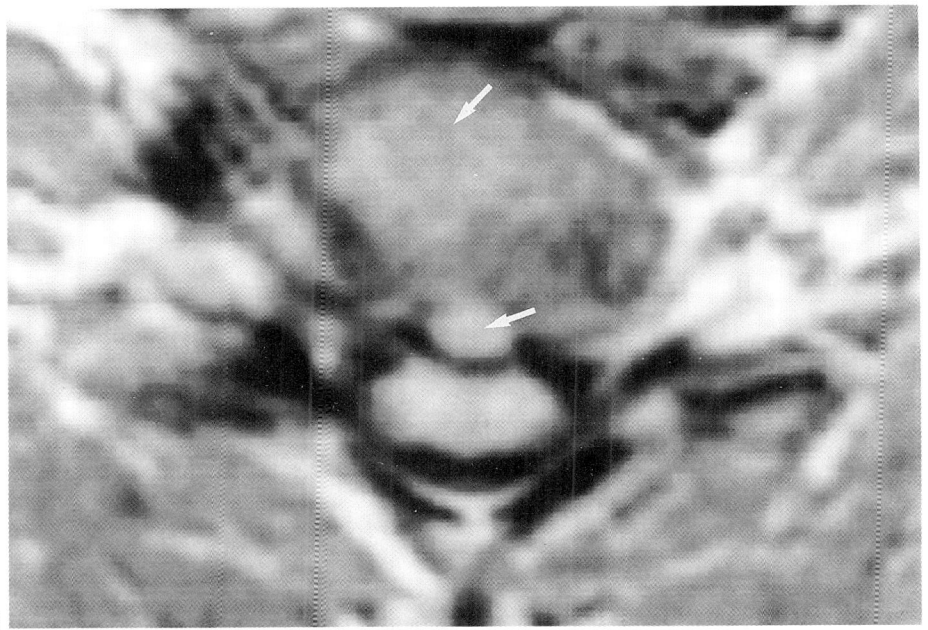

Figure 13. See text on next page. (A) Sagittal T1-weighted, (B) sagittal T2-weighted and (C) axial T1-weighted images of a patient with a focal disk herniation at C6-7 with spinal cord compression. Disk material extends superior to the disk space itself behind the vertebral body (arrow). On the axial T1-weighted image (C), the disk appears to have the same signal intensity as the "parent" disk space (arrows).

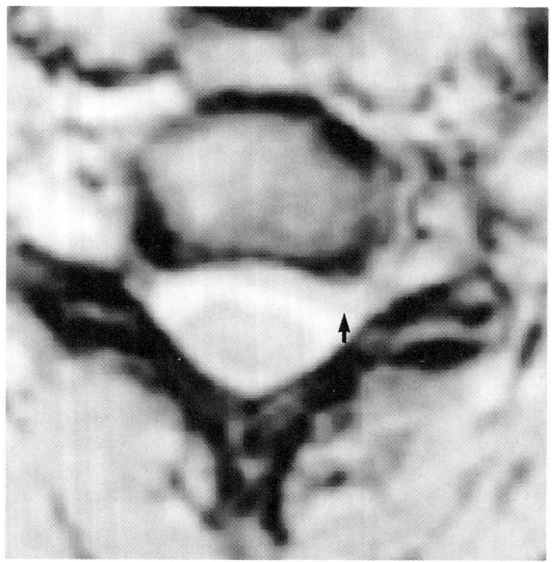

Figure 14. Axial gradient-echo image with a small foraminal disk herniation on the left side (arrow).

slightly decreased or normal signal intensity in these areas. This high signal on T2-weighted images may be similar to the cavitation or "cystic necrosis" seen on delayed postmyelogram CT.

A study of more than 600 patients with chronic spinal cord compression found this increased signal in 14.8%.[36] The presence of the finding was correlated with the severity of clinical myelopathy and the degree of spinal cord compression. Moreover, in 56% of patients with a high-signal area, there was little or no improvement following decompression surgery, compared with failure to improve in only 15% of patients with no abnormal signal. Interestingly, in the three patients with increased T2-weighted cord signal, who improved following surgery and were studied with repeat MR, the high signal was not present on the postoperative examination.

Herniated Disk

Some amount of disk material always accompanies the osteophytic ridges. In some cases, there is a frank disk herniation independent of other spondylotic changes. When the herniation is central or paracentral, it can be recognized often on sagittal images by an area of medium-intensity signal posterior to the disk space causing epidural compression. (Figure 13). Lateral herniations are more difficult to visualize on sagittal images and to separate from osteophytic ridges. On gradient-echo or T1-weighted sequences, disk material often has a higher signal than the dense cortical bone of a ridge, (Figure 14) although as previously mentioned higher-signal marrow is present in many osteophytes. Often the distinction between ridge, ridge with accompanying disk, and disk herniation alone is difficult. Some authors believe that this distinction may be easier on gradient-echo sequences.[18,39]

Much of the soft tissue within the epidural space may not represent disk material itself, but rather may be related to the inflammatory response to disk herniation. This can be demonstrated in some patients by performing T1-weighted scans after the administration of gadolinium-DTPA (Figure 15).

Comparative Studies

The question of which study—computed tomography, computed tomography following myelography, or magnetic resonance imaging—should be performed for the evaluation of patients with suspected cervical spine degenerative disease has not been fully answered. The rapid evolution of MR imaging techniques makes a study to examine this issue problematic. Experience, evaluation of the literature, and assessment of current state-of-the-art techniques allow for some conclusions to be drawn.

Myelopathy

An early study of body-coil MR of the cervical spine in patients with myelopathy found that MR was equal to, or more informative than, myelography in 75% of extradural lesions.[22] The majority of these patients had degenerative disk disease and spondylosis. It was suggested that the ability of MR to

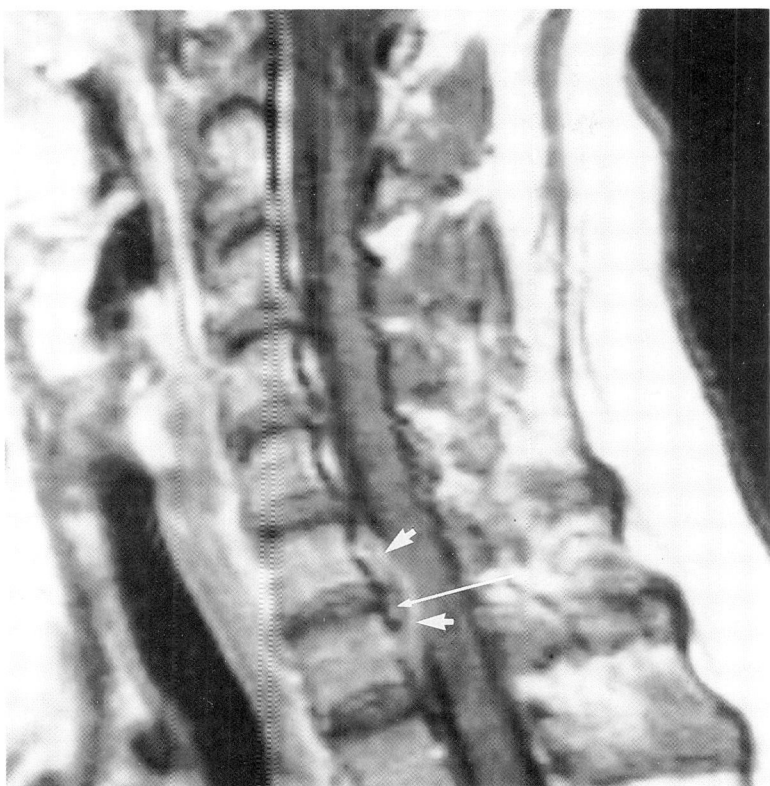

Figure 15. Sagittal postgadolinium-DTPA T1-weighted images in a patient with an acute disk herniation. Note the extensive enhancing material representing granulation tissue (small arrows) as well as the disk fragment that shows minimal central enhancement (long arrow).

accurately define the dimensions of the spinal canal as well as the spinal cord itself may have significant value. The ability of MR to detect other causes of myelopathy, such as intrinsic cord disease, syringohydromyelia, etc., was considered an additional benefit. In some cases, the T2-weighted image failed to accurately depict the epidural space narrowing at the site of osteophytes.

A more recent study of 26 patients, 8 of whom had myelopathic symptoms, demonstrated equivalent findings of cord compression on the CTM and the MR study.[21] Of 32 disk-space levels examined overall for degree of narrowing, there was agreement between CTM and MR in all but 2 levels. This report did corroborate previous studies in stating that MR is less able to distinguish disk herniation from osteophyte, but again, this is of limited clinical significance.

We believe that MR is indicated as the initial screening examination for myelopathy, with CTM reserved for those difficult cases where slightly better resolution is important for presurgical assessment.

Radiculopathy

Another early study of CTM versus MR, using surface-coil technology, showed that in patients with radiculopathy the correlation between surgical findings and the MR was 74%, and 85% for surgical findings and CTM.[29] In general, CTM was not more sensitive than MR, but provided better information as to the type of disease (disk versus ridge). The higher resolution possible with

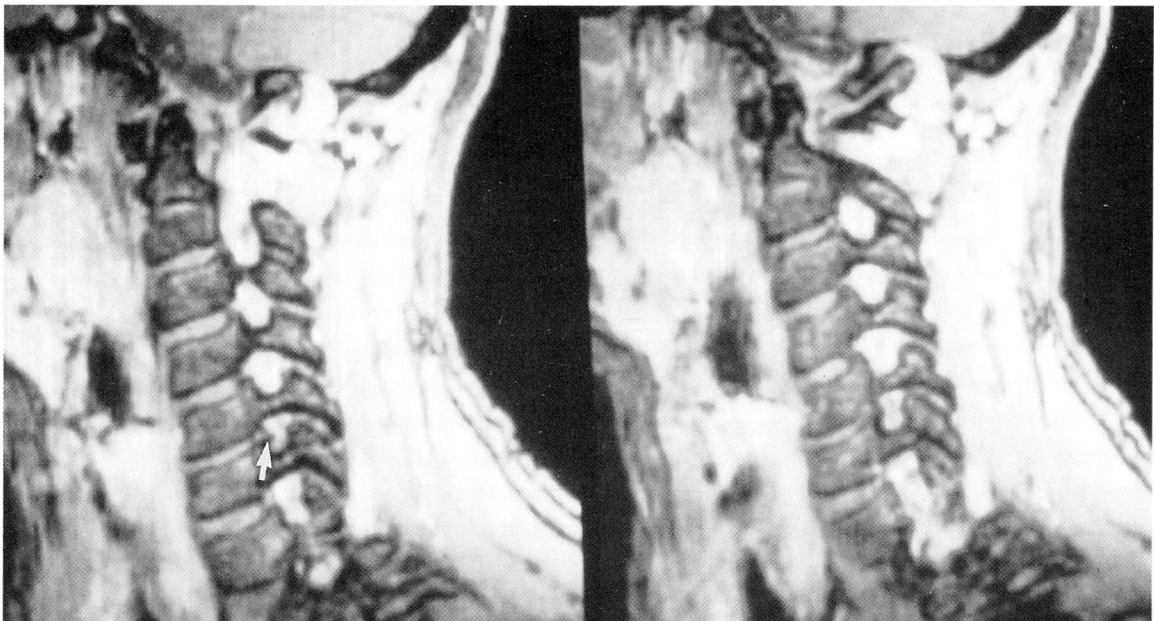

Figure 16. Oblique images through the left and right neural foramina reconstructed from three-dimensional imaging of the cervical spine. Note the herniated disk (left photo arrow) at C5-6 compressing the intraforaminal fat. (Figure courtesy of Jeffrey S. Ross, MD)

thin-section CTM also aided diagnostic accuracy. CTM provided a more accurate depiction of the nerve roots themselves, showing the effect of compressive lesions better. Laterally placed disease was better seen with CTM.

A more recent, although limited, study reported different results.[21] It found the accuracy of CTM and MR to be 73% and 77% respectively, using a dedicated cervical spine surface coil in the detection of nerve root sheath deformity. The authors also pointed out the difficulty of getting thin MR axial sections, and the problems associated with the gap between slices. The future widespread use of 3DFT gradient-echo contiguous axial images with slice thickness of 1.5-2.0 mm may obviate some of these concerns.[39]

The evaluation of patients with radiculopathy is still somewhat difficult. MR is probably the best screening study available, particularly if one has a good 3DFT gradient-echo capability (Figure 16). Nonetheless, high-resolution CT may be preferable to thick-section MR in some cases. CTM often remains the study of choice in patients with radiculopathy, particularly prior to surgery.

References

1. Badami JP, Norman D, Barbaro NM, et al. Metrizamide CT myelography in cervical myelopathy and radiculopathy: correlation with conventional myelography and surgical findings. *AJR*. 1985;144: 675-680.
2. Bailey P, Casamajor L. Osteo-arthritis of the spine as a cause of compression of the spinal cord and its roots. *J Nerv Ment Dis*. 1911;38:588-609.
3. Balériaux D, Noterman J, Ticket L. Recognition of cervical soft disk herniation by contrast-enhanced CT. *AJNR*. 1983;4:607-608.
4. Boden SD, McCowin PR, Davis DO, et al. Abnormal magnetic-resonance scans of the cervical spine in asymptomatic subjects. *J Bone Joint Surg Am*. 1990; 72A:1178-1184.
5. Brain WR. Some unsolved problems of cervical spondylosis. *Br Med J*. 1963;1:771-777.
6. Brain WR, Northfield D, Wilkinson M. The neurological manifestations of cervical spondylosis. *Brain*. 1952;75:187-225.
7. Brain WR, Wilkinson M, eds. *Cervical Spondylosis and Other Disorders of the Cervical Spine*. Philadelphia, Pa: WB Saunders Company; 1967.
8. Con CG. Cervical disk degeneration and herniation: diagnosis by computerized tomography. *South Med J*. 1984;77:979-982.
9. Coin CG, Coin JT. Computed tomography of cervical disk disease: technical considerations with representative case reports. *J Comput Assist Tomogr*. 1981;5:275-280.
10. Coin CG, Chan YS, Keranen V, et al. Computer assisted myelography in disk disease. *J Comput Assist Tomogr*. 1977;1:398-404.

11. Czervionke LF, Daniels DL, Ho PSP, et al. Cervical neural foramina: correlative anatomic and MR imaging study. *Radiology*. 1988;169:753-759.
12. Di Chiro G, Schellinger D. Computed tomography of spinal cord after lumbar intrathecal introduction of metrizamide (computer assisted myelography). *Radiology*. 1976;120:101-104.
13. Enzmann DR, Rubin JB. Cervical spine: MR imaging with a partial flip angle, gradient-refocused pulse sequence, part I: general considerations and disk disease. *Radiology*. 1988;166:467-472.
14. Enzmann DR, Rubin JB, Wright A. Cervical spine MR imaging: generating high-signal CSF in sagittal and axial images. *Radiology*. 1987;163:233-238.
15. Flannigan BD, Lufkin RB, McGlade CH, et al. MR imaging of the cervical spine: neurovascular anatomy. *AJR*. 1987;148:785-790.
16. Fox AJ, Lin JP, Pinto RS, et al. Myelographic cervical nerve root deformities. *Radiology*. 1975;116:355-361.
17. Friedenberg ZR, Miller WT. Degenerative disc disease of the cervical spine. *J Bone Joint Surg Am*. 1963;45A:1171-1178.
18. Hedberg MC, Drayer BP, Flom RA, et al. Gradient echo (GRASS) MR imaging in cervical radiculopathy. *AJR*. 1988;150:683-689.
19. Jinkins JR, Bashir R, Al-Mefty O, et al. Cystic necrosis of the spinal cord in compressive cervical myelopathy: demonstration by iopamidol CT-myelography. *AJR*. 1986;147:767-775.
20. Landman JA, Hoffman JC Jr, Braun IF, et al. Value of computed tomographic myelography in the recognition of cervical herniated disk. *AJNR*. 1984;5:391-394.
21. Larsson E-M, Holtås S, Cronqvist S, et al. Comparison of myelography, CT myelography and magnetic resonance imaging in cervical spondylosis and disk herniation: pre- and postoperative findings. *Acta Radiol*. 1989;30:233-239.
22. Masaryk TJ, Modic MT, Geisinger MA, et al. Cervical myelopathy: comparison of magnetic resonance and myelography. *J Comput Assist Tomogr*. 1986;10:184-194.
23. Matsuda Y, Miyazaki K, Kenji T, et al. Increased MR signal intensity due to cervical myelopathy: analysis of 29 surgical cases. *J Neurosurg*. 1991;74:887-892.
24. Matsuda T, Takahashi S. Latest developments in the evaluation of the spine with the Toshiba Transaxial Tomographic Unit. In: Post MJD, ed. *Radiographic Evaluation of the Spine. Current Advances with Emphasis on Computed Tomography*. New York, NY: Masson; 1980;491-507.
25. McRae DL. Bony abnormalities in the region of the foramen magnum: correlation of the anatomic and neurologic finding. *Acta Radiol*. 1953;40:335-355.
26. McRae DL. The significance of abnormalities of the cervical spine. *AJR*. 1960;84:3-25.
27. Miyasaka K, Isu T, Iwasaki Y, et al. High resolution computed tomography in the diagnosis of cervical disc disease. *Neuroradiology*. 1983;24:253-257.
28. Modic MT, Masaryk TJ, Ross JS, et al. Cervical radiculopathy: value of oblique MR imaging. *Radiology*. 1987;163:227-231.
29. Modic MT, Masaryk TJ, Mulopulos GP, et al. Cervical radiculopathy: prospective evaluation with surface coil MR imaging, CT with metrizamide and metrizamide myelography. *Radiology*. 1986;161:753-759.
30. Nakagawa H, Okumura T, Sugiyama T, et al. Discrepency between metrizamide CT and myelography in diagnosis of cervical disk protrusions. *AJNR*. 1983;4:604-606.
31. Pech P, Daniels DL, Williams AL, et al. The cervical neural foramina: correlation of microtome and CT anatomy. *Radiology*. 1985;155:143-146.
32. Ross JS, Modic MT, Masaryk TJ, et al. Assessment of extradural degenerative disease with Gd-DTPA-enhanced MR imaging: correlation with surgical and pathologic findings. *AJNR*. 1989;10:1243-1249.
33. Ross JS, Modic MT, Masaryk TJ. Tears of the annulus fibrosus: assessment with Gd-DTPA-enhanced MR imaging. *AJNR*. 1989;10:1251-1254.
34. Russell EJ, D'Angelo CM, Zimmerman RD, et al. Cervical disk herniation: CT demonstration after contrast enhancement. *Radiology*. 1984;152:703-712.
35. Scotti G, Scialfa G, Pieralli S, et al. Myelopathy and radiculopathy due to cervical spondylosis: myelographic-CT correlations. *AJNR*. 1983;4:601-603.
36. Takahashi M, Yamashita Y, Sakamoto Y, et al. Chronic cervical cord compression: clinical significance of increased signal intensity on MR images. *Radiology*. 1989;173:219-224.
37. Teresi LM, Lufkin RB, Reicher MA, et al. Asymptomatic degenerative disk disease and spondylosis of the cervical spine: MR imaging. *Radiology*. 1987;164:83-88.
38. Thijssen HOM, Keyser A, Horstink MWM, et al. Morphology of the cervical spinal cord on computed myelography. *Neuroradiology*. 1979;18:57-62.
39. Tsuruda JS, Norman D, Dillon W, et al. Three-dimensional gradient-recalled MR imaging as a screening tool for the diagnosis of cervical radiculopathy. *AJNR*. 1989;10:1263-1271.
40. VanDyke C, Ross JS, Tkach J, et al. Gradient-echo MR imaging of the cervical spine: evaluation of extradural disease. *AJR*. 1989;153:393-398.
41. Wilkinson HA, LeMay ML, Ferris EJ. Clinical-radiographic correlations in cervical spondylosis. *J Neurosurg*. 1969;30:213-218.
42. Yamashita Y, Takahasi M, Matsuno Y, et al. Spinal cord compression due to ossification of ligaments: MR imaging. *Radiology*. 1990;175:843-848.

CHAPTER 4

Diseases that Mimic Degenerative Disease of the Cervical Spine

E. Wayne Massey, MD

Patients frequently complain of nonspecific arm weakness, grip loss (hand weakness), or numbness. Other individuals have no symptomatology, yet on physical examination abnormalities are discovered. Interosseous muscle wasting is common in the elderly due to subcutaneous tissue loss, but focal atrophy or localized weakness should alert the physician to a possible underlying pathologic process. Some of these patients have cervical spine disease, others an alternate diagnosis.

The upper extremity is a synchronized amalgam of joints, nerves, muscles, and vascular structures in which dysfunction in any one element may lead to impairment. Joint disease with pain and subsequent weakness is common among the elderly and should not be difficult to diagnose. Likewise, vascular disease producing coolness and cyanosis of the hand does not usually present diagnostic difficulty. The complexities of innervation and function of muscles often lead to difficulties in localization, however. Various levels of dysfunction—brain, spinal cord, nerve root, brachial plexus, or peripheral nerve—give specific patterns of neurologic dysfunction. To facilitate the diagnosis and therapy of arm weakness, an anatomic approach should be used to differentiate various syndromes. Table 1 represents a useful anatomic approach to the patient and will serve as an outline for this review.

Signs and Symptoms

Cervical spine disease may produce spinal cord involvement with upper motor neuron signs such as myelopathy, root involvement with lower motor signs, or both. Sensory systems can likewise be due to spinal cord disease or local root compression; therefore, the differential diagnosis varies with the type of presentation of symptoms and signs. Upper motor neuron involvement is usually associated with weakness in the arm and increased reflexes; in lower motor neuron dysfunction, muscle atrophy and sensory loss predominate. If individual nerves are compromised, the deficit occurs in that specific distribution. Brachial plexus injuries usually produce a more diffuse pattern of loss. Anterior horn cell disease produces characteristic changes and is usually bilateral.

Upper Motor Neuron Dysfunction

Cerebral and Spinal Cord

Isolated weakness in the hand or arm originating from upper motor neuron (UMN) dysfunction is unusual. The somatotopic representation of the hand on the cortex and in descending corticospinal systems is such that pathologic processes that produce hand weakness generally also produce arm/face and/or

TABLE 1
Approach to Evaluation of Upper Extremity Weakness

I. Upper Motor Neuron:
  A. Signs: myelopathy (with paraparesis); monoparesis; hemiparesis
  B. Diseases:
  1. demyelinating diseases
     multiple sclerosis
     AIDS myelopathy
     Tropical spastic paraparesis (HTLV-1)
     Lupus myelopathy
     A Beta lipoproteinemia (hypo)
  2. Metabolic/nutritional
     B-12 deficiency
  3. Tumors (mass)
     (a) intrinsic - gliomas
     (b) extrinsic - neurofibromas
                    meningiomas
                    (i.e. foramen magnum)
  4. Syringomyelia
  5. Congenital malformations
     Chiari
  6. Primary lateral sclerosis

II. Lower Motor Neuron:
  A. Peripheral neuropathy
     B-12, DM, tomaculous, porphyria, distal muscular atrophies
  B. Peripheral nerve: mononeuropathy
     1. median
     2. ulnar
     3. radial
     4. brachial plexus
  C. Cervical spondylosis/radiculopathy (see chapter 1)
     1. double crush syndrome
  D. Motor neuron disease (anterior horn cell)
     1. Monomelic
     2. Primary lateral sclerosis
     3. GM-1, GA-1 ganglioside

leg weakness. Increased tone (spasticity) is found with a characteristic posturing of the upper extremity: the shoulder is adducted, the elbow flexed, with pronation of the hand and flexion of the fingers. Lower extremity posturing may also be found with increased tone, and adduction of the hip with extension of the leg and foot. Facial paresis is characterized by weakness of the seventh cranial nerve of a central type. Deep tendon reflexes are increased and, if sensory loss is present, generally not confined to the hand.

In the elderly patient, the most common cause of upper motor dysfunction in the hand is ischemic cerebrovascular disease (CVA). Other structural considerations also are in order when an elderly patient has a history inconsistent with a CVA but with signs of UMN dysfunction of the arm and hand. Both traumatic and spontaneous subdural hematomas occur in the elderly, as do central nervous system (CNS) tumors.

Diseases that Mimic Degenerative Disease of the Cervical Spine

Diseases Involving Cervical Cord

In younger patients, demyelinating disease such as multiple sclerosis causes upper extremity and hand symptoms. This may occur as an initial symptom or as the result of an exacerbation of known diseases and may be unilateral or bilateral. Usually these symptoms are simple paresthesias and it is unusual for them to be solely unilateral involving the upper extremity. When unilateral, they more often involve the entire one half of the body and are quite fleeting.

When these symptoms are accompanied by a L'Hermitte's sign in young persons—an electric-shock feeling down the back of the spine when the head is bent ("barber chair" sign)—this is very suggestive of cervical spinal cord irritation in multiple sclerosis. When the same phenomenon occurs in older individuals, it can be due to cervical stenosis. Symptoms and signs occurring in multiple locations over multiple time periods, with waxing and waning, are hallmarks of demyelinating disease.

Severe sensory ataxia with loss of finger movement is the exception on joint position sense testing, and suggests the "useless hand syndrome of Burdach." Other symptoms helpful in making the diagnosis include incontinence or difficulty with urination, episodes of diplopia or optic neuritis, history of trigeminal neuralgia, ataxia, and paresthesias. Visual loss associated with overheating (Ughtoff's sign) should always alert the clinician to the possibility of demyelinating disease.

Physical examination abnormalities can be confirmed by laboratory studies, including visual evoked responses and somatosensory evoked responses. Spinal fluid examination should include protein and cell count, immunoelectrophoresis, oligoclonal bands, and myelin basic protein. Magnetic resonance imaging (MRI) is a useful recent addition to laboratory studies and is frequently quite helpful in confirming the clinical diagnosis of demyelinating disease. Multiple T2-weighted image abnormalities can often be detected in the periaquaductal gray and periventricular regions, even in patients who have minimal symptoms.

The prognostic significance of these laboratory studies is unclear. The course of the disease in any one patient is difficult to predict, unless repeated severe attacks occur in rapid succession, which usually heralds a poor prognosis. Patients with vague (nonspecific) sensory symptoms in one or both upper extremities may have these symptoms for many years before definite signs of demyelinating disease are manifest.

Lupus erythematosis myelopathy, AIDS myelopathy, and HTLV-I-II-III can all produce cervical spinal cord involvement that may result in significant symptoms in the upper extremities. However, these are accompanied by lower extremity symptoms, suggesting a spinal cord problem in most situations. Spinal fluid examination is essential and is usually abnormal. A myelopathy due to AIDS or lupus erythematosis is usually not the presenting sign of these illnesses, but are usually manifest in patients whose diagnoses are already established. Familial spastic paraparesis associated with HTLV infections can have upper extremity symptoms, but always begins with lower extremity problems.

Syringomyelia produces gradual sensory and motor symptoms involving both upper extremities, sometimes asymmetrically. There are no pains or paresthesias, but there is loss of pain and temperature perception despite retention of light touch (dissociated anesthesia), sometimes in a cape-like fashion involving the arms, chest, shoulders. Sometimes painless burns are present (syndrome of Morvan). Reflexes are preserved or decreased. Spinal cord cysts occurring after trauma or in association with intramedullary spinal cord tumors may mimic the manifestations of syringomyelia.

Tumors, both intrinsic and extrinsic, produce upper-extremity weakness. Extrinsic neurofibromas or meningiomas at the foramen magnum can produce myelopathy. Interestingly, stocking-glove sensory loss may be present with high cervical lesions, yet

TABLE 2
Peripheral Neuropathies: Etiology

1. **Neuropathy Associated with Toxic/Metabolic States**
    A. Vitamin deficiency (B1, B12, B6, nicotinic acid, pantothenic acid and folic acid)
    B. Diabetic
    C. Uremic
    D. Hepatic
    E. Thyroid disease
    F. Dysproteinemia & paraproteinemia
    G. Ethanol use
    H. Amyloid

2. **Inherited Peripheral Neuropathy**
    A. Charcot-Marie-Tooth disease
    B. Déjerine-Sottas (hypertrophic)
    C. Roussy-Levy disease
    D. Refsum's disease
    E. Tangier disease and a-beta-lipoproteinemia (Bassen-Kornzweig's disease)
    F. Neuropathy associated with the leukodystrophies (metachromatic leukodystrophy, Krabbe's disease, adrenoleukodystrophy)
    G. Fabry's disease
    H. Porphyric neuropathy
    I. Tomaculous

3. **Infectious, Inflammatory and Postinfectious Neuropathy**
    A. Guillain-Barré syndrome, inflammatory polyradiculoneuropathy
    B. Diptheria
    C. Leprosy
    D. Sarcoid
    E. Chronic inflammatory demyelinating polyneuropathy (CIDP)
    F. AIDS

4. **Neuropathies Associated with Malignancy**
    A. Neuropathy associated with lymphoma and Hodgkin's disease
        1. Sensory
        2. Motor
        3. Sensory/motor (P.O.E.M.S.)

5. **Toxic Neuropathies**
    A. Heavy metals
        1. Lead
        2. Arsenic
        3. Mercury
        4. Thallium
    B. Toxins
        1. Acrylamide
        2. Trichloroethylene
        3. Benzene
        4. Carbon Tetrachloride
        5. Triorthocresyl phosphate (TOCP)

6. **Drugs**
    1. Vincristine, vinblastine
    2. Chloroquine
    3. Nitrofurantoin
    4. Phenytoin
    5. Disulfiram
    6. Isoniazid
    7. Thalidomide
    8. Excessive B6 administration

reflexes are brisk (or at least preserved) and Babinski reflexes are present.

The most serious myelopathy of metabolic origin is due to vitamin B^{12} deficiency, although diabetes mellitus and hypothyroidism may also produce spinal cord disease. A screen should include thyroid profile (including TSH), fasting blood sugar (two-hour postprandial blood sugar is needed), and complete blood count (CBC). If the mean corpuscular volume on the CBC is increased, a bone marrow examination or Schilling's test may be needed after checking a B^{12} level.

Lower Motor Neuron Dysfunction

Peripheral Neuropathy

Diffuse peripheral neuropathy (see Table 2) usually begins with symptoms involving the lower extremities. In fact, the upper extremity often remains asymptomatic even in the presence of severe lower extremity symptoms. However, there are several situations where upper extremity symptoms predominate.

Amyloidosis may begin in familial cases with median neuropathy before more diffuse symptoms occur. Acromegaly may cause carpal-tunnel symptoms only, and hypothyroidism can produce hand paresthesias from median nerve compression without diffuse neuropathic symptoms. Sensory symptoms involving the fingers, specifically a digital neuropathy, would be suggestive of rheumatoid arthritis, which may also present with carpal tunnel syndrome.

Another pitfall in evaluating patients with upper extremity neuropathic symptoms is the presence of diffuse subclinical peripheral neuropathy in patients who present with a superimposed entrapment (pressure) mononeuropathy. Patients with diabetes mellitus, chronic ethanol abuse, past history of Guillain-Barré syndrome, or tomaculous neuropathy, may develop median neuropathy at the carpal tunnel, ulnar neuropathy at the elbow, radial neuropathy from upper arm pressure, or any combination thereof.

Peripheral Nerves (Mononeuropathy)

Median Nerve

This nerve is derived from the fifth to eighth cervical roots and is formed by the union of the lateral and medial cords of the brachial plexus. It supplies both extrinsic and intrinsic hand muscles. The anterior interosseus nerve, a purely motor branch of the median nerve, supplies the extrinsic long and short flexors of the first two digits and the long flexor of the thumb. The terminal portion of the median nerve supplies four intrinsic hand muscles, including the short abductor and flexor of the thumb, the opponens of the thumb, and the first two lumbricals. The sensory distribution of the median nerve involves the radial two-thirds of the palmar aspect of the hand and the distal phalanges of the index and third fingers over the dorsum.

The anatomic course of the median nerve gives rise to two distinct syndromes. The first, by far the most common, is compression of the median nerve in the carpal tunnel.[1] Patients describe tingling, burning, and painful dysesthesias in the hand, often worse at night. They may be awakened repeatedly by hand paresthesias. They will often shake or massage the hand. They may arise from bed and walk around wringing their hands in order to get relief. Sometimes a deep aching pain extends into the forearm and even to the shoulder.[10]

Sensory symptoms engender the most complaints. Motor complaints are usually nonspecific and consist of decreased grip and hand weakness.

Examination may demonstrate sensory loss in the median distribution. Motor deficit, if present, is most commonly found in the abductor pollicis brevis and opponens muscles of the thumb. Tapping over the wrist may cause proximal or distal tingling (Tinel's sign). Hyperextension of the wrists may produce symptoms of pain and paresthesias (Phalan's sign).

The potential causes of this disorder are quite extensive (Table 3). Any increase in the contents of the carpal tunnel may produce median nerve compression. In the elderly, bony spurs arising within the carpal tunnel secondary to degenerative joint disease, rheumatoid arthritis, or old wrist fractures should be considered. Increased contents of soft tissue, either idiopathic or secondary to hypothyroidism, can produce carpal tunnel syndrome. Isolated carpal tunnel syndrome can be the first sign of systemic vasculitis.

Compression of the anterior interosseous nerve at the point where the median nerve passes into the forearm between the heads of the pronator teres produces elbow pain with radiation into the median nerve sensory area and forearm cramping pain. Examination shows minimal signs in the hand, with the exception of paralysis of the long finger flexors leading to difficulty pinching the first digit to the thumb. No sensory signs are present.

TABLE 3
Entrapment Neuropathies which May Cause Arm Weakness

Median	Carpal tunnel syndrome
	"Pseudo-carpal tunnel" (sublimis)
	Digital nerve
	Anterior interosseous nerve
	Pronator teres syndrome
	Ligament of Struthers
	"Double-crush" syndrome
Ulnar	Guyon's canal
	Digital nerve
	Cubital canal
	"Tardy ulnar palsy"
	"Double-crush"
Radial	Saturday night palsy
	Posterior interosseous nerve
	"Tennis elbow"
	Superficial radial nerve (cheiralgia paresthetica)
Brachial Plexus	Thoracic outlet syndrome
	Scalenus anticus
	Cervical rib
	Costoclavicular
	Hyperabduction

The usual "syndrome" arises secondary to occupations involving pronation and separation of the forearm ("arm wrestlers").[10]

Ulnar Nerve

The ulnar nerve is derived from the eighth cervical and first thoracic roots and is formed entirely from the medial cord of the brachial plexus. It innervates the ulnar half of the deep finger flexors, the dorsal and palmar interossei, adductor of the thumb, and the abductor, opponens and flexor of the small finger in the hand. Sensory distribution involves the fifth finger, ulnar aspect of the fourth finger, and the ventral and dorsal aspects of the ulnar border of the palm proximally to the wrist. Lesions may occur distally at the wrist or proximally at the elbow, creating distinct syndromes.[14]

Distal lesions of the ulnar nerve generally produce pure motor syndromes involving the intrinsic hand muscles. Nerve compression in the palm produces weakness of the interossei (Figure 1), the adductor of the thumb and the medial two lumbricals with sparing of the hypothenar muscles. Compression at or proximal to the pisohamate tunnel (Guyon's canal) produces weakness of all ulnar intrinsic hand muscles and variable sensory loss over the distal palmar and volar surface of the fourth and fifth fingers. In the elderly, recurrent pressure to the deep ulnar branch may occur through the inappropriate gripping of a cane or crutch. Alteration of the carpal bones secondary to fractures or inflammatory processes may also produce these problems.

A lesion of the ulnar nerve at the elbow produces both motor and sensory findings. Pain and parathesias occur in the ulnar innervated area. Motor loss includes all intrinsic hand muscles supplied by the ulnar nerve. Wasting of the hypothenar eminence appears as hollowing between the metacarpal bones.

Lesions of the ulnar nerve at the elbow are common. They arise secondary to fractures or local bone disease about the elbow. In the elderly, who may be confined to wheelchairs, beds, or spend much of their day sitting, compression of the ulnar nerve at the elbow can lead to a "tardy ulnar palsy". Ulnar nerve injury may also occur following surgery in the region of the elbow.[5]

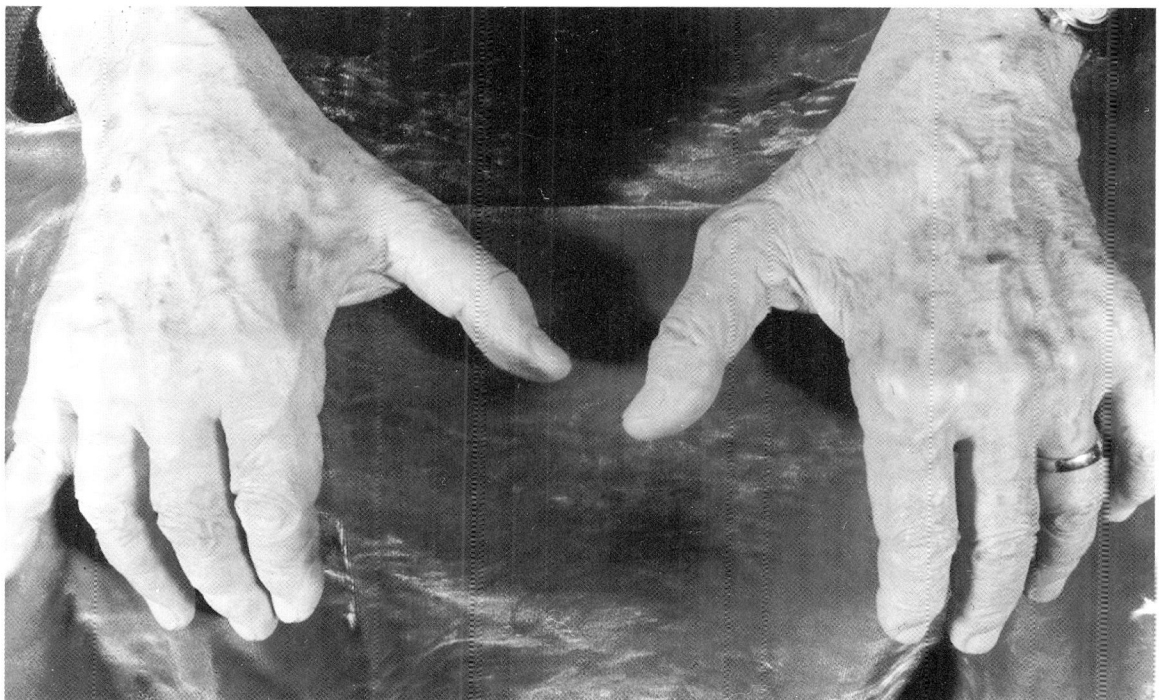

Figure 1. Hands of a patient with interosseous muscle atrophy secondary to bilateral ulnar neuropathy.

Radial Nerve

The radial nerve is derived from the fifth to eighth cervical root and is the termination of the posterior cord of the brachial plexus. It does not supply any intrinsic hand muscles, but does supply the extrinsic muscles necessary for finger extension. Sensory distribution of the radial nerve is variable, usually supplying the radial aspect of the dorsum of the hand, including the thumb and web space between the thumb and first digit. If the nerve is compressed proximally, the triceps muscle and brachioradialis muscle may be weak.

Isolated weakness of finger extension secondary to radial nerve dysfunction is rare. Most commonly, the nerve is injured as it winds around the humerous, leading not only to weakness of finger extension but weakness of forearm flexion in supination and forearm extension ("wrist drop"). Examination of the hand after a radial nerve lesion at this level may give the false impression of total hand weakness, since the full action of the intrinsic hand muscles cannot be accomplished with the wrist in flexion. If the wrist is supported and placed in a position of function, it becomes clear that there is no true weakness of the intrinsic hand muscles.[10]

Radial nerve injury usually arises secondary to compression occurring from hanging an arm over the back of a chair for extended periods of time ("Saturday night palsy," "Honeymooner's Palsy").[3] Injury also may arise from improper positioning of the arm during sleep, usually in the setting of alcohol or hypnotic drug use. Irritation and compression of the nerve by callous may be a late complication of fractures of the shaft of the humerous. Improper injections in the arm can also cause this injury.

Brachial Plexus

Brachial plexus lesions are most often incomplete and are characterized by a combi-

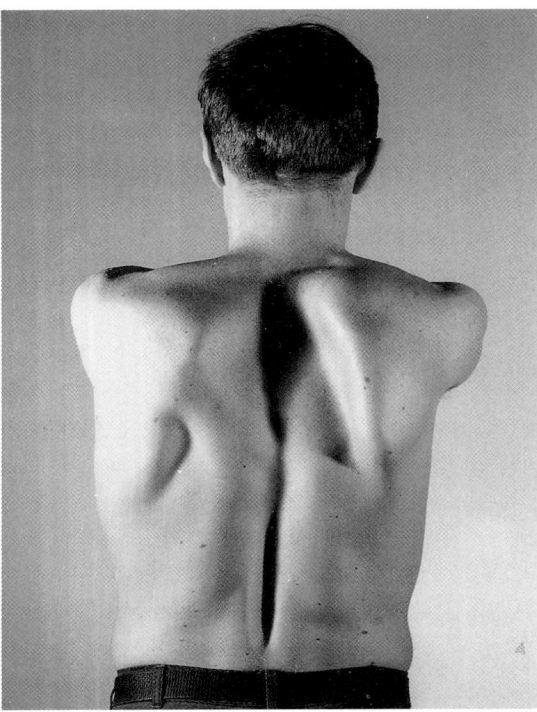

Figure 2. Winging of the right scapula secondary to a right brachial plexus injury.

nation of weakness and muscle atrophy. Less often, sensory changes, abnormalities of stretch reflexes, and sympathetic dysfunction are present. Lesions of the medial cord of the medial plexus, which contain the eighth cervical and first thoracic roots, produce profound deficits of intrinsic hand muscles simulating a combined median and ulnar nerve lesion. Sensory loss, if present, is not confined to the hand alone, but occurs along the ulnar aspect of the arm, forearm, and hand.

Idiopathic brachial plexus involvement (brachial plexopathy/plexitis; neuralgic amyotrophy; Parsonage-Turner syndrome) usually involves the upper plexus and sometimes only the proximal upper trunk, causing scapular winging (Figure 2). This is most common in young people and is usually associated with shoulder pain at the onset.[8]

The causes of brachial plexus lesions are numerous. Trauma from a sudden upward pull on the shoulder, or as a consequence of being dragged by the arm, may produce damage. Apical lung lesions such as Pancoast tumor frequently present with intrinsic hand muscle weakness in association with an ipsilateral Horner's syndrome secondary to compression of the lower trunk of the plexus and the exiting sympathic fibers. Direct invasion of the plexus by cancer can cause isolated hand weakness and arm pain.

Direct invasion of the plexus by breast cancer is a common cause of brachial plexopathy. Radiation therapy to the upper chest or shoulder in cancer patients may produce a plexus syndrome that is difficult to differentiate from direct invasion. Upper plexus involvement is more often secondary to radiation therapy than to direct tumor invasion.

Compression of the lower trunk or cord of the plexus at the thoracic outlet (thoracic outlet syndrome), produces both neurological and vascular signs, the latter being the most common. Patients complain of pain following use of the extremity. Paresthesias, especially nocturnal, are rare, a helpful sign in differentiating this entity from carpal tunnel syndrome. Examination of the extremity may reveal fingertip ulcers. When symptomatic, patients may experience mild weakness of the intrinsic hand muscles with altered sensation in the C8 and T1 dermatomal distribution. The etiology of this syndrome is believed to be trapping of the neurovascular bundle at the thoracic outlet by fixed anatomic structures such as muscle, callous formation from old fractures, or cervical ribs (see Table 3).

Double Crush Syndrome

Some patients with cervical radiculopathy, often at C5-6 level, may have concomitant carpal tunnel syndrome or, less often, ulnar compression. This may simply be two common problems occurring at the same time, but case histories often suggest simultaneous onset. If an upper extremity therapy fails, the clinician should consider that two neuropathic processes may be occurring simultaneously.

Anterior Horn Cell (Motor Neuron Disease)

Motor neuron disease or amyotrophic lateral sclerosis (ALS; "Lou Gehrig's disease") is among the most common primary neuromuscular diseases, with a peak incidence occuring in the sixth decade.[12] Symptoms result from degeneration of anterior horn cells throughout the nervous system One-third of patients present with upper extremity weakness, usually in the hand, unilaterally or bilaterally. Since only the motor system is affected, no sensory symptoms occur. Examination may reveal marked wasting and fasciculations of the hands not confined to any specific peripheral nerve or root distribution, with normal sensation. When these findings are present in association with abnormalities in other extremities or in the facial musculature, motor neuron disease should be strongly considered. Tongue fasciculations or fibrillations with atrophy suggest that the bulbar musculature is involved. Lower extremity atrophy and fasciculations suggest lower motor neuron involvement, although isolated fasciculations in the lower extremity without muscle weakness have been reported in cervical myelopathy as well.

The distinction between motor neuron disease and cervical stenosis with myelopathy can be a considerable diagnostic challenge.[13] Because both occur in individuals in the sixth decade of life and older, patients often have some amount of cervical stenosis, even though the underlying diagnosis is motor neuron disease.

Diagnosis of motor neuron disease at an early stage can be quite difficult. Diffuse muscle wasting and atrophy with or without fasciculations, often asymptomatic, and hyperreflexia or Babinski signs may be present. Therefore, the diagnosis must be made by confirmation of widespread motor neuron involvement. Electromyography is essential for making the diagnosis and can assist in confirming the diagnosis and preventing unwarranted surgical procedures in the cervical area.[7]

Although motor neuron disease has a poor prognosis, particularly when it involves the bulbar musculature, there is a small subcategory of patients with primary motor nerve involvement, including anterior horn cells, who seem to run a more benign course. These patients have slower progression of deficit, and weakness which is asymmetrical. The proximal weakness is often greater than distal weakness, with conduction block on electroneuromyography. Some of these patients may respond to cyclophosphamide.[11] Patients may have elevation of GM-1 and GA-1 antibody titers, but the exact characterization of this subcategory has not yet been established.[6] The major questions appear to be whether this antibody is a reaction to nerve cell loss or whether it is somehow causative.

On rare occasions, myotonic muscular dystrophy in a younger patient can resemble motor neuron disease and cause muscle wasting and hand weakness. This is almost always associated with myotonia in the hands; electromyographic studies will help to differentiate the entity from motor neuron disease. Patients with spinal muscular atrophy in later decades usually have proximal weakness, as also seen in inclusion body myositis, but these are not limited to the upper extremities in most situations. Paraneoplastic syndromes may also be associated with motor neuron disease.

Evaluation and Therapy

Since arm symptoms may arise from different nervous system lesions and multiple etiologies, the first step in evaluation should be the history and physical examination in order to distinguish the various syndromes in Table 1.

For peripheral nerve, brachial plexus, root and anterior horn cell disease, electromyography with nerve conductions is valuable in pinpointing the exact location of the neurological dysfunction.[3] In the median, ulnar, and radial nerves distal motor latencies, conduction velocities and sensory potentials may be recorded. Electromyography, may reliably assist in the distinguishing plexus from root lesions (Table 4).

Electrophysiologic tests must be performed to rule out diffuse neuropathy in patients who may present with an isolated mononeu-

TABLE 4
Electroneuromyography
Upper Extremity Weakness

	Spinal Cord	Nerve Root			Peripheral Nerve
	Anterior Horn Cell	Anterior Motor Root	Dorsal Ganglion Pre	Dorsal Ganglion Post	
Motor nerve conduction velocity	N	N	N	N	+
Sensory nerve action potential	N	N	N	±	+
Electromyography	+	+	N	N	+
F wave	+	+	N	N	+
H reflex	+	+	+	+	+

N = normal
+ = abnormal
± = sometimes abnormal

ropathy involving the upper extremity. Any patients with underlying neuropathy may develop a superimposed compression neuropathy. Electrical studies of other nerves always must be performed and should be requested by the physician asking for the electrophysiologic help. Patients with underlying neuropathy from diabetes or chronic alcohol use are particularly susceptible. Patients with tomaculous neuropathy or any other neuropathy are also prone to compression.

As stated earlier, electromyography is particularly important when evaluating for motor neuron disease or any form of isolated myopathy involving the upper extremities. Conduction blocks may alter work-up.[7] The exact location of the muscles involved will help in differentiating a peripheral nerve lesion from a more diffuse process. Similarly, involvement of other extremities or cranial nerve involvement would suggest a widespread involvement such as that seen in motor neuron disease.[4]

Although idiopathic compression is the most common etiology of peripheral nerve lesions, diabetes mellitus, hypothyroidism, vasculitis, rheumatoid arthritis, amyloid, acromegaly, and paraproteinemias must all be considered. Therapy should be directed toward the underlying disease process.

If idiopathic median neuropathy is found, surgical decompression, for relief of persistent numbness, pain, and weakness if present, is indicated. Local steroid injection or a wrist splint may give relief of symptoms in some.[14]

Lower trunk or medial cord symptoms accompanied by a Horner's sign should raise the suspicion of an apical lung lesion. Chest x-ray with special views should be obtained. Computerized tomography (CT) or MRI may also be helpful. In cervical radiculopathy, cervical spine films followed by myelography may be indicated. Conservative measures with bed rest and cervical traction are usually employed if no myelopathy exists.

No proven therapy is available for anterior horn cell disease. This diagnosis should be one of exclusion, the major differential being cervical spondylosis with myelopathy. Electromyography has definite value in most cases (see Table 4). Denervation, beyond a specific root distribution which includes the lower extremities, supports the diagnosis. Myelography should be performed if doubt remains.

An upper motor neuron lesion producing weakness of the hand is not usually difficult to diagnose. Accompanying signs suggest a suprasegmental deficit. If no etiology is apparent from the history, MRI, CT scan with contrast, or myelography should be undertaken if a high cervical lesion is suspected. An MRI of the brain will be useful if intracranial signs are present. MRI of the brachial plexus may sometimes be of value.

Spinal fluid examination is a less important part of the neurological evaluation than it was in the past. However, it is still helpful for the diagnosis of demyelinating disease. CSF protein, cell count and special studies for IgG, oligoclonal bands, and myelin basic protein will assist in the diagnosis. Abnormalities in protein or cell count may be present in patients with diseases of infectious etiology such as AIDS; protein and cell counts are often abnormal in collagen vascular myelopathies such as lupus erythematosis.

Some patients with malignancy present with upper cervical symptoms, either from epidural extension of a paravertebral malignancy or as a systemic effect of a cancer. Leptomeningeal involvement can be diagnosed by evaluating the spinal fluid cytology.

References

1. Bleecker ML, Bohlman M, Moreland R, et al. Carpal tunnel syndrome: role of carpal canal size. *Neurology*. 1985;35:1599-1604.
2. Dawson DM, Hallett M, Millender LH. *Entrapment Neuropathies*. Boston, Mass: Little Brown; 1983.
3. Donofrio PD, Albers JW. AAEE minimonograph #34: polyneuropathy, classification by nerve conduction studies and electromyography. *Muscle Nerve*. 1990;13:889-903.
4. Drachman DB, Kuncl RW. Amyotrophic lateral sclerosis: an unconventional autoimmune disease? *Ann Neurol*. 1989;26:269-274.
5. Kincaid JC. AAEE minimonograph #31: the electrodiagnosis of ulnar neuropathy at the elbow. *Muscle Nerve*. 1988;11:1005-1015.
6. Latov N. Antibodies to glycoconjugates in neurologic disease. *Clin Aspects Autoimmunity*. 1990; 4:18-29.
7. Lewis RA, Sumner AJ, Brown MJ, et al. Multifocal demyelinating neuropathy with persistent conduction block. *Neurology*. 1982;32:958-964.
8. Massey EW. Nontraumatic brachial plexopathy. In: Wilkins RH, Rengachary SS, eds. *Neurosurgery*. New York, NY: McGraw Hill; 1985;2:1909-1912.
9. Mitsumoto H, Wilbourn AJ, Goren H. Perineurioma as the cause of localized hypertrophic neuropathy. *Muscle Nerve*. 1980;3:403-412.
10. Nakano KK. The entrapment neuropathies. *Muscle Nerve*. 1978;1:264-279.
11. Pestronk A. Invited review: motor neuropathies, motor neuron disorders, and antiglycolipid antibodies. *Muscle Nerve*. 1991;14:927-936.
12. Rowland LP, ed. *Advances in Neurology Vol. 36: Human Motor Neuron Diseases*. New York, NY: Raven Press; 1982.
13. Stevens JC. AAEE minimonograph #26: the electrodiagnosis of carpel tunnel syndrome. *Muscle Nerve*. 1987;10:99-113.
14. Stewart JD. The variable clinical manifestations of ulnar neuropathies at the elbow. *J Neurol Neurosurg Psychiatry*. 1987;50:252-258.

CHAPTER 5

Somatosensory Evoked Potential Monitoring in Cervical Spine Surgery

Nancy E. Epstein, MD

Somatosensory evoked potentials (SSEPs) are elicited by electrical stimulation of median, ulnar, peroneal, or posterior tibial nerve fibers at the wrist and ankles and recorded over the postcentral gyrus of the cortex. Employed intraoperatively by electrophysiologists, anesthesiologists, orthopedists, and neurosurgeons, SSEPs help document that the spinal cord has not been injured during spinal operations.

Neuroanatomy

Stimulation of the three classes of cutaneous receptors—the mechanoreceptors, thermoreceptors, and nociceptors—produces afferent volleys which are recorded from the postcentral gyrus (Figure 1).[36] These potentials travel from the peripheral receptors via dorsal nerve roots to cell bodies in the spinal ganglia,

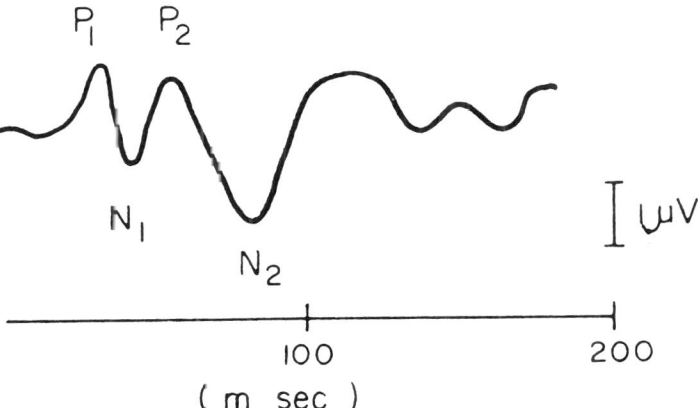

Figure 1. Typical somatosensory evoked potentials. The first upward deflection (P1) usually appears between 33 and 36 milliseconds after the stimulus, while P2 usually appears at between 54 and 58 milliseconds. The amplitude varies with the stimulation voltage and level of anesthesia. In this tracing P1 was approximately 1 microvolt and occurred at 34.5 milliseconds, while P2 was approximately 0.8 microvolt and occurred at 56.5 milliseconds. (Reference 13: Figure 1, Page 530.)

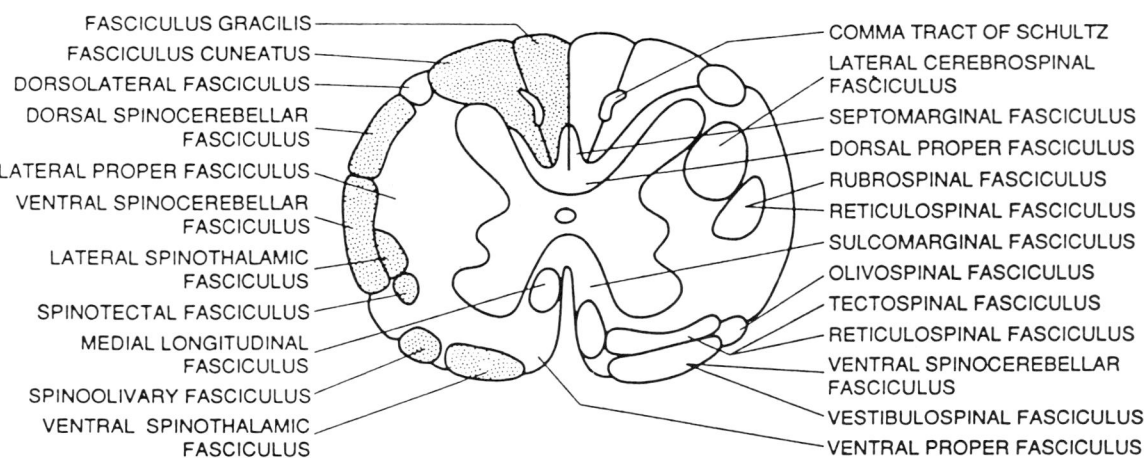

Figure 2. For clarity, ascending pathways are shown only in the left half of the drawing, and descending pathways only in the right half. (Reference 36: Figure 2.69, Page 283.)

through the dorsal root entry zones of the spinal cord, to the thalamus, and ultimately, the cerebral cortex.

The ascending pathways of the spinal cord include the ipsilateral posterior columns, contralateral spinotectal tracts, bilateral ventral spinothalamic, and bilateral ventral spinoreticular pathways (Figures 2, 3).[36] Transmission of high frequency (>60 Hz) vibration occurs in the ipsilateral posterior columns, whereas position appreciation travels through ipsilateral dorsal and ventral quadrants. Flutter or low-frequency vibration (5-40 Hz), touch, pressure, and visceral potentials utilize unilateral dorsal but bilateral ventral pathways, while pain traverses ipsilateral dorsal but contralateral ventral quadrants (Figure 3).[36]

Both unilateral and bilateral somatosensory pathways project to the thalamus and then to six separate topographic body projections in the somatosensory cortex (see Figure 4 on flipside of opposite page).[36]

Four purely contralateral inputs project to the postcentral SI somatosensory cortex in a medial to lateral and caudal to cephalic fashion. The stimuli to the fifth topographic SII region, located deep in the lateral sulcus, and to the sixth area 7B, found in the retroinsular cortex, are bilateral in nature.

Physiology

In the monkey, Cusik et al demonstrated that SSEPs were conducted in the dorsal columns as selective section of the posterior columns produced a complete obliteration of the SSEP response. Conversely, SSEPs remained normal if the dorsal columns were preserved and adjacent ventral and lateral tracts were ablated.[8] Additionally, in the cat, Cohen, Young, and Ransohoff confirmed that the posterior columns were both necessary and sufficient for the preservation of SSEP responses, and that the removal of contiguous ventral and lateral tracts did not affect SSEP recordings.[7]

On the other hand, Powers, Bolger, and Edwards demonstrated that SSEP transmission occurred in all three ventral, lateral, and posterior quadrants.[34] Lesion experiments, performed in cats, established that the ipsilateral dorsal posterior columns, dorsal spinocerebellar tracts, and contralateral ventrolateral pathways participated in the cortically evoked somatosensory responses. The ability to record SSEPs from all three columns was attributed to the adoption of high-intensity peripheral nerve stimulation sufficient to activate C and Aδ fibers in addition to AB

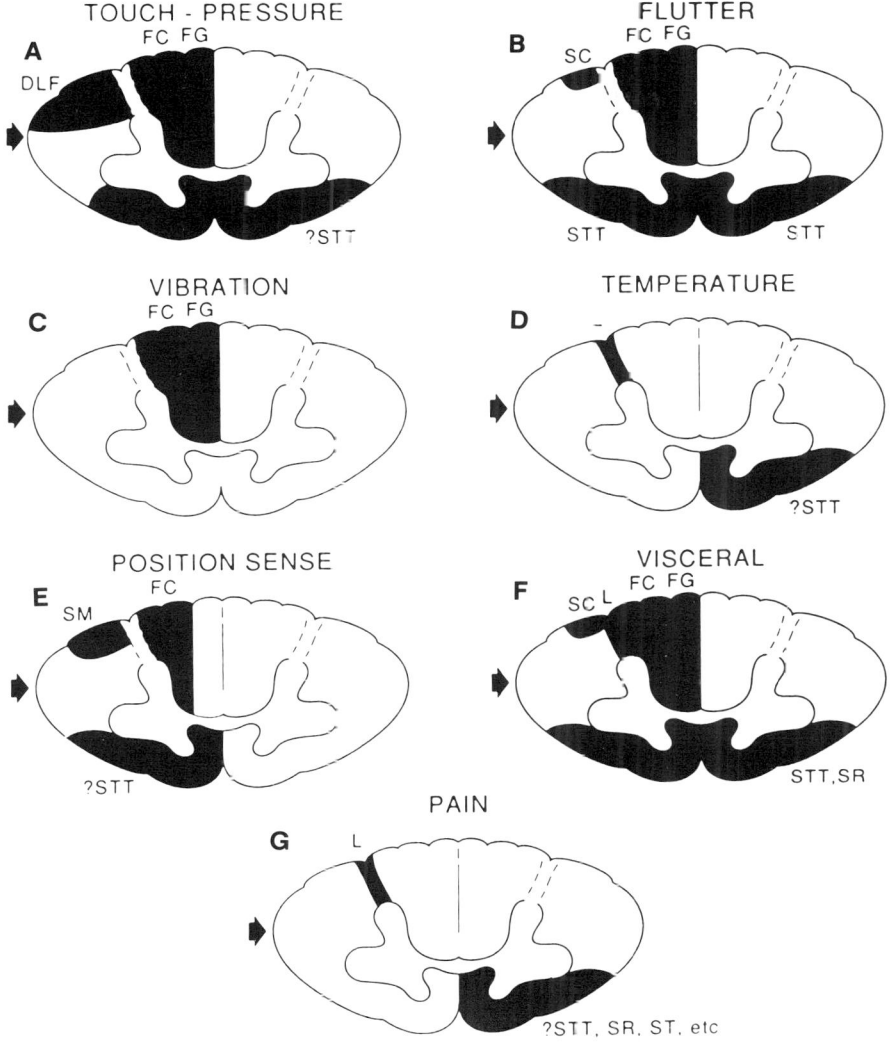

Figure 3. Spinal cord pathways. Blackened areas show the pathways that are thought to transmit touch pressure. **(A)** The arrow indicates the stimulated side. Pathways include the fasciculus cuneatus and fasciculus gracilis (FC, FG), the dorsolateral fasciculus (DLF), and possibly the spinothalamic tract (STT). **(B)** The pathways for flutter include FC and FG, spinocervical tract (SC) and STT. **(C)** The pathways for vibration are the dorsal column (FC and FG) **(D)** Pathways for thermal information include Lissauer's tract (L) and probably contralateral STT **(E)** Pathways for position sense include FC but not FG, the spinomedullothalamic pathway (SM), and a pathways in the ventral quadrant, possibly STT, all on the side stimulated. **(F)** Pathways carrying information from visceral receptors include FC and FG, L, and the spinocervical tract (SC) on the same side as the stimulus, and STT and spinoreticular tract (SR) bilaterally. **(G)** The major pain pathways are in L on the side stimulated and in the contralateral ventral quadrant, possibly including STT, SR and the spinotectal tract (ST). The arrows in panels *A - G* indicate the side stimulated. (Modified from Willis WD, Cogeshall RE: Sensory Mechanisms of the Spinal Cord, New York Plenum Press, 1978). (Reference 36: Figure 2.69, Page 283.)

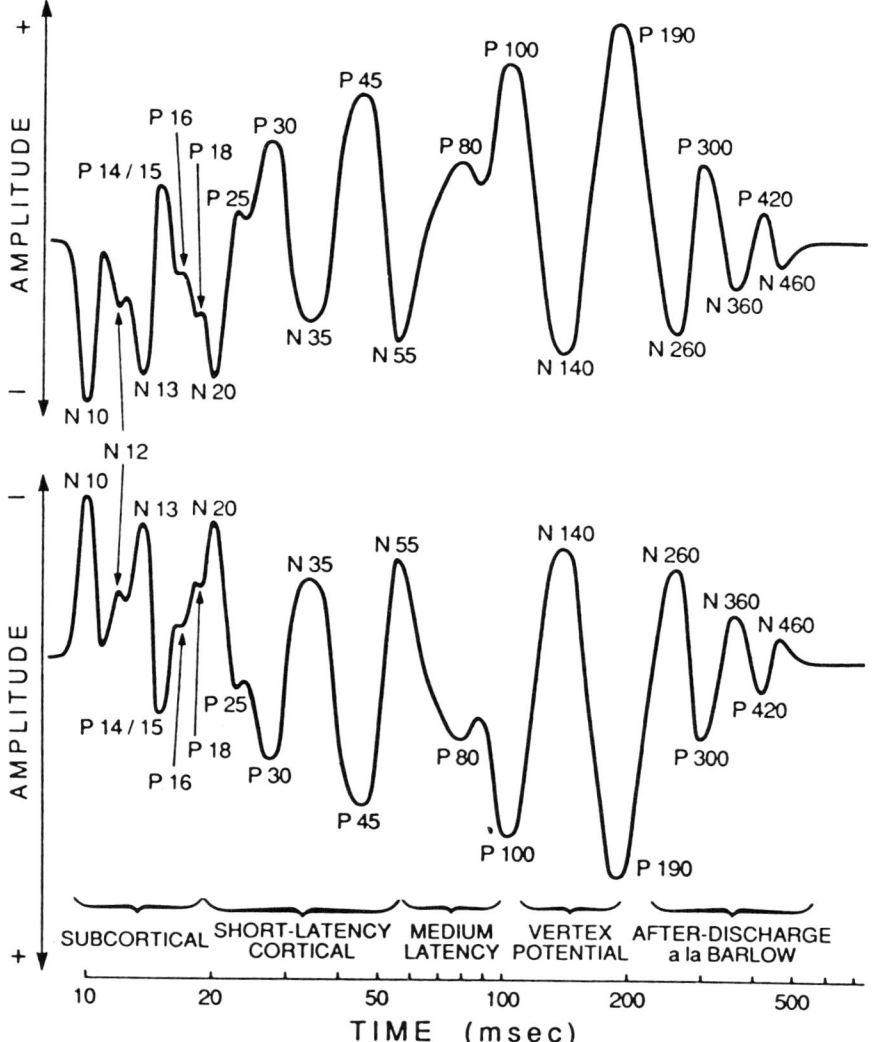

Figure 4. Schematic Nerve Somatosensory Evoked Potential. This figure illustrates the relationship of subcortical potentials, early cortical potentials, and the later cortical potentials with latencies greater than about 70 msec. The time axis is logarithmic. The ordinate is nonlinear to show both low-amplitude and high-amplitude potentials on the same plot. The waveform is a composite of potentials recorded from Erb's point (N10), neck (N12, N13), and parietal scalp (later waves) and is therefore not as logical as the log - log AEP plot of Figure 2.13 A. Additional peaks can be recorded from other scalp locations. (This sketch, kindly provided by T. Allison, is based on data reported by Goff et al and Allison et al.) (Reference 36: Figure 2.71, Page 289)

fibers more typically activated at lower stimulus intensities. To do so, they had to employ stimulus intensities 20 times the norm in anesthetized animals.

When considering these alternate hypotheses of SSEP transmission, it must be recalled that the twenty-fold stimulus intensity levels employed by Powers et al would not be tolerated in clinical situations. For this reason, the majority of clinical recordings most likely reflect posterior column function alone.

SSEPs and Spinal Cord Injury in Animal Models

Surgeons, using intraoperative SSEPs, assume that early corrective measures adopted in response to significant changes help avert the evolution of fixed neurologic deficits. Animal studies contributed to these assumptions.[10,3,19,23,24,32,34,36,37,39]

Schramm et al assured SSEP changes in cats in proportion to show graded spinal cord compression.[39] They noted that SSEPs only changed with greater than 80% compression in the antero-posterior canal diameter, and that slow graded compression was better tolerated than acute compromise. SSEP changes typically consisted of an initial reduction of amplitude, whereas latency changes occurred later and were smaller. The abrupt decreases or loss of amplitude better correlated with acute mechanical or focal vascular compromise than with chronic injury. Conversely, SSEP recovery was more rapid with the reversal of acute than with chronic compromise.

In monkeys, Larson et al determined that SSEP monitoring of amplitude proved more sensitive and reliable than latency changes in detecting spinal cord dysfunction during distractions and flexion maneuvers.[24] SSEPs showed a reversible reduction in amplitude when limited pathologic distractions and flexion were applied. Distraction caused SSEP amplitudes to diminish when the bodies were separated by more than 2 cm or when spinal cord length was increased by 15%. When distraction was released before the amplitude loss exceeded 50%, full recovery often followed. When further increases in distraction resulted in the precipitous deterioration (greater than 50%) or loss of amplitude, animals developed permanent neurologic sequelae. Flexion injuries produced similar outcomes depending on whether flexion was released before or after amplitude changes exceeded 50%. It is noteworthy that the amplitude changes observed in the study of Larson et al were attributed to traumatic mechanical axonal stretching occurring in both the dorsal and lateral columns in response to distraction and flexion injuries, rather than to anterolateral spinal cord ischemia.[8,15,23,24,46]

Laboratory and clinical investigations further established that neurologic deficits were reversible if present for less than 10-15 minutes, but were more likely to be permanent if they lasted more than 15 minutes.[9,22,32,33] Nuwer noted neurologic dysfunction in laboratory animals where compression, distraction, and mechanical injuries had been sufficient to produce significant amplitude and latency changes.[32] He found that significant SSEP changes were reversible when they were present for less than 15 minutes but permanent if they lasted longer. Acute rather than chronic injuries causing significant SSEP changes lasting for more than 15 minutes, were more likely to result in permanent sequelae.[9,22]

Brown and Nash, along with Larson et al further established that amplitude changes larger than 50% to 60% were more sensitive indicators of impending neurologic dysfunction than comparable changes in latency.[4,24] In particular, Larson et al determined that amplitude declines of less than 50%, lasting less than 15 minutes, were well tolerated, whereas amplitude losses exceeding 50% for more than 15 minutes were associated with permanent neurologic injury.[24]

Monitoring Techniques

A variety of monitoring techniques have been used during surgery. They include (1) the wake-up test, (2) motor evoked potentials (MEPs), (3) somatosensory spinal evoked potentials, (4) spinal evoked potentials, and (5) somatosensory cortical evoked potentials (SSEPs).[4]

Wake-Up Test

The wake-up test, introduced in 1973 to monitor spinal cord integrity during scoliosis surgery, is capable of confirming normal spinal cord function, but only at the time of the examination.[4] It provides no indication of the patient's subsequent neurologic status.

This examination relies on the full intraoperative cooperation of the patient, requires careful titration of anesthetic agents, and poses significant risks to the patient. Low-dose inhalation (halogenated) or balanced narcotic techniques, combined with reversible paralytic agents, allow patients to follow verbal commands and move the appropriate extremities during surgery. Risks include air embolism, inadvertent extubation, and self-induced neurologic injury. Although many surgeons continue to use both the wake-up test and intraoperative SSEP recordings, others now rely solely on SSEP monitoring.[9,13,31]

Motor Evoked Potentials

Motor evoked potentials (MEPs) allow for the direct assessment of the ventral motor pathways, using either transcranial electrical or magnetic stimulation techniques.[4,37] Electrical techniques rely on anodal stimulation and hyperpolarization of the pyramidal neurons and apical dendrites which induce indirect depolarization of axons in the deep gray subcortical layers. Magnetic motor evoked potentials (MMEPs), introduced in 1985, rely on the production of a magnetic field of sufficient intensity to produce similar depolarization of the underlying neural tissues.[37] Although experimental evidence suggests that MMEPs may be more sensitive and show earlier alterations compared with other monitoring modalities, direct stimulation of motor tracts remains, at present, the least useful technique for intraoperative monitoring. Shortcomings of electrical techniques include an increased risk of seizures or transient motor deficits.[39] General drawbacks of MMEPs include inadequate specificity, lack of applicability to patients with metallic implants (e.g. pacemakers), increased risks associated with strong magnetic fields in the operating room, and short-term problems such as transient memory loss, headaches, and altered sleep patterns.[4] Further improvement in MEP and MMEP monitoring techniques may lead to their more widespread use in the operating room.[37]

Spinal Evoked Potentials

With spinal evoked potentials (SEPs), stimulation and recording are directly obtained from the spinal cord itself. Subdural electrodes are typically placed in the upper cervical and lower cauda equina regions. Although this technique is more invasive than those described below, the polyphasic action potentials generated by these catheters are larger than those seen with cortical monitoring modalities.[4] Data are obtained with a better signal-to-noise ratio using higher stimulus frequencies (20-25 Hz), and simultaneous ascending and descending records are generated in shorter periods of time.

Shortcomings include the inability to monitor the patient prior to induction and through closing as electrodes must be placed intraoperatively. Electrode displacement and migration may occur during the operation, and produce inaccurate recording or neurologic injury.

Somatosensory Spinal Evoked Potentials

Somatosensory spinal evoked potentials (SSEPs), elicited from peripheral stimulation of median, ulnar, peroneal, or posterior tibial nerves, are recorded from electrodes placed in the spinous processes, interspinous ligaments, epidural, subdural, or subarachnoid spaces. Recording is obtained from the spinal cord itself rather than the cerebral cortex. Although somatosensory spinal evoked recordings may be used alone, they may also be readily combined with SSEPs.[3,4,9,28]

One major advantage of somatosensory *spinal* evoked potentials over somatosensory *cortical* evoked potentials is the generation of a high-amplitude, stable response which exhibits minimal fluctuation over shorter periods with different anesthetic techniques. Spinous process and interspinous ligament recordings can be acquired in 1-2 minutes, whereas the generation of extradural thoracic or subarachnoid thoracolumbar potentials

TABLE 1
Acquisition Parameters for SSEPs

Electrodes	Skin (cup) (subdermal, interspinous, epidural, subdural)
Measure	Latency milliseconds (msec) Amplitude microvolts (μV)
Nerves	Median Nerve Posterior Tibial Nerves
Side	Right/Left (alternate)
Intensity	>2-3 Times motor threshold
Repetition Rate	3.88-5.1/Second
Pulse Width	200 Microseconds (μsec)
Trials Averaged	200
Analysis Time	200 Milliseconds (msec)
Filter	10-500 Herz (Hz)
Recording Channels	E1-C2/Ez-FPz

(near the conus) may take from 10-230 seconds.[3,4,9]

The use of interspinous SEPs also allows monitoring above and below the level of surgery, ensuring more accurate detection of operative changes from the surgical site itself.[9] In the series of Dinner at al,[9] 70 of the 100 patients monitored with interspinous recordings underwent scoliosis procedures. Electrodes could be kept safely out of the operative field and did not contribute to neurologic injury. The potentials obtained also proved more reliable and reproducible than most SSEP recordings. Lueders et al similarly employed interspinous ligament recordings during 40 spinal operations, including 32 scoliosis procedures for the placement of Harrington rods, and 8 operations for the treatment of syrinxes, tumors, and AVMs.[28]

Somatosensory Evoked Cortical Potentials

The SSEP response is elicited by application of a short-duration electrical stimulus to a large mixed peripheral nerve such as the median, ulnar, peroneal, or posterior tibial complexes (Table 1).[1,36] The stimulus, typically two to three times the sensory threshold, excites the majority of large diameter Aα and Aβ fast-conducting peripheral nerve fibers, and is sufficiently above the motor threshold to produce a small muscle twitch.

Noninvasive skin or surface cup electrodes may be used to elicit the SSEP response.[4] With this noninvasive technique, monitoring may begin prior to induction and continue through closing, as the recording devices are outside of the operative field. These scalp recordings of SSEP potentials can be acquired in 1-2 minutes. However, due to inhalation anesthetics, these advantages must be weighed against the increased variability when compared with spinal potential.[14,32]

All somatosensory evoked responses are described by both amplitude and latency. Amplitudes are measured in microvolts (μV) as the height of the wave from the trough of the preceding negative potential (N) to the peak of the succeeding positive potential (P), or from the baseline to the positive peak (P). Latencies, measured in milliseconds (msec), are defined by the time span between the onset of the stimulus and the peak of the response. Latency responses, comprised of

TABLE 2
Components of Median and Posterior Tibial SSEP Responses

Median SSEPs	
N9	Medial Cord
	Brachial Plexus
N11	Dorsal Horn
N13	Nucleus Cuneatus
N14	Thalamus
N20	Cortical
Posterior Tibial SSEPs	
PV	Cauda Equina
	Gracile Tract
N22	Spine (T10-L1)
N22/P22	Dorsal Thoracolumbar Cord
N29	Cervical Spine
	Gracile Nucleus
N28/P31	Medial Lemniscus
N34	Thalamus/Stem
P38/N38	Cortical Potentials

positive (P) and negative (N) waveforms, are also routinely employed to describe median, ulnar, peroneal, and posterior tibial potentials, whereas amplitude recordings play no part in these short-hand references.

Median nerve potentials, generated at the wrists and measured at the postcentral cortical sulcus, are therefore described by the normal latency of the following major negative peaks (Table 2) (Figure 5).[36] According to Regan's scheme, N10 indicates the afferent volley at the level of the brachial plexus; N12a, activity within the segmental dorsal column; N13a, impulses in the dorsal horn; N12b, activity in the ascending dorsal column; N13b, SSEP transmission in the cuneate nucleus; N14, cephalad propagation through the medial lemniscus; and N20, activity in the somatosensory cortex.[36]

El Negamy and Sedgwick offered an alternate explanation involving four major negative peaks N9, N11, N13/N14, and N20.[12] Here, N9 signifies the afferent volley as it traverses the median cord of the brachial plexus, N11 indicates activity in the dorsal horn of the spinal cord, N13/N14 reflects the afferent volley at the nucleus cuneatus and thalamus, while N20 represents the first cortical response.[12] An abnormal N9 response reflects disease distal to the dorsal root ganglion at the C6-7 level in median or C8-T1 level in ulnar nerve recordings, while changes of N13/N14 with normal N9 responses are consistent with intrinsic cord disease.[49] The most important latency parameter for intraoperative recording is N20, the cortical potential.

Posterior tibial recordings, generated at the ankle and recorded over the cortex, are also represented by a multiplicity of intervening negative and positive peaks.[36] Peak PV reflects transmission at the level of the cauda equina and gracile tract, N22/P22 denotes the response in the posterior horn and T10-L1 thoracolumbar cord, N29 indicates transmission in the cervical spinal cord at the level of the gracile nucleus, P31 denotes the SSEP at the level of the medial lemniscus, N34 is recorded from the thalamus and brain stem, while P38/N38 and P40 represent the cortical potentials (Table 2).[36] Here, too, the final cortical potentials (N38, P38, P40) are the most critical for intraoperative monitoring.

One monitoring option is to place cortical electrodes using the classical vertex array of the International Ten Twenty System (Figure 6).[32] With this system, positioning is based on measurements of the head circumference, interaural distance, and distance from the

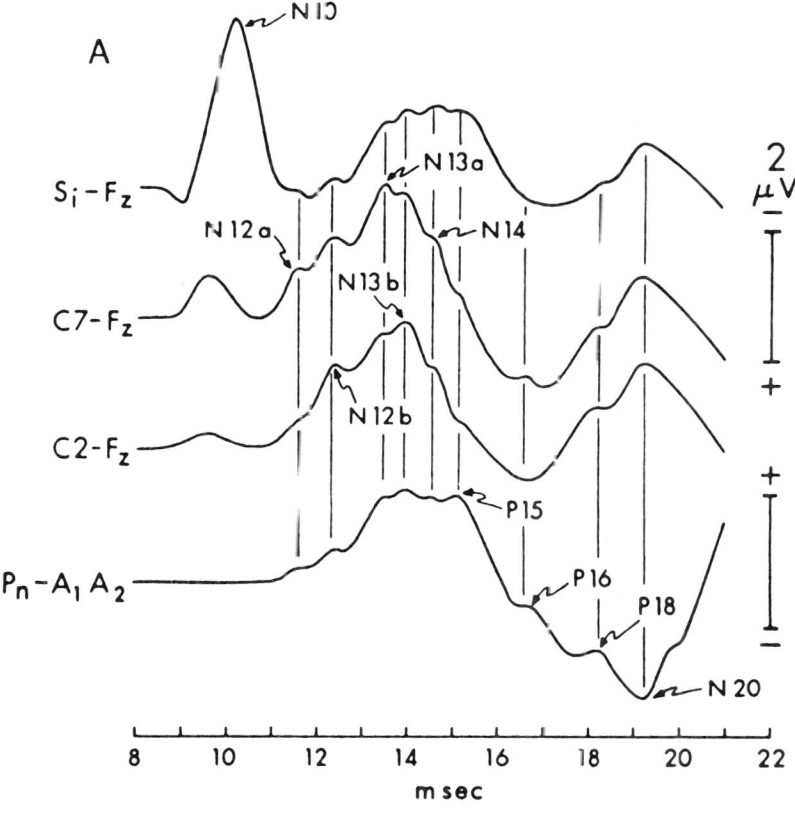

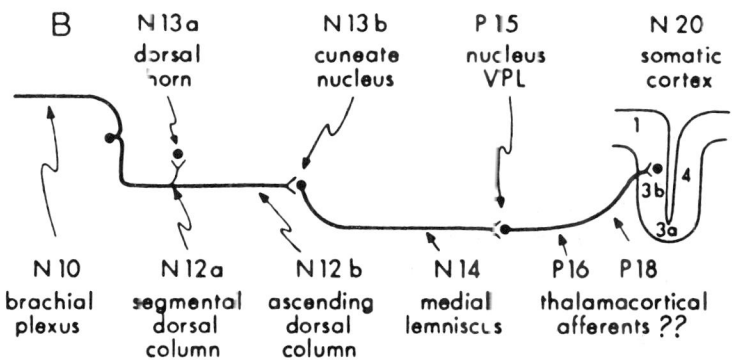

Figure 5. Early components of the somatosensory evoked potential. Panel A illustrates that the several components are differently emphasized at different recording sites. Panel B summarizes the New Haven group's views on the site of origin of early SEP components. (From Allison T: Developmental and aging changes in human evoked potentials, in Barber C, Blum T, Nodar R (eds): Evoked Potentials III. Boston, Butterworth 1987, pp 72-90. Figure kindly provided by T. Allison.) (Reference 16: Figure 2.73, Page 291.)

nasion to the inion. Cortical recording electrodes are typically applied at Cz^1 (large empty arrow), 2 cm posterior to Cz in the sagittal plane, with C3 and C4 being placed parasagitally for bilateral recording. Fz (small empty arrow) then serves as the anterior ref-

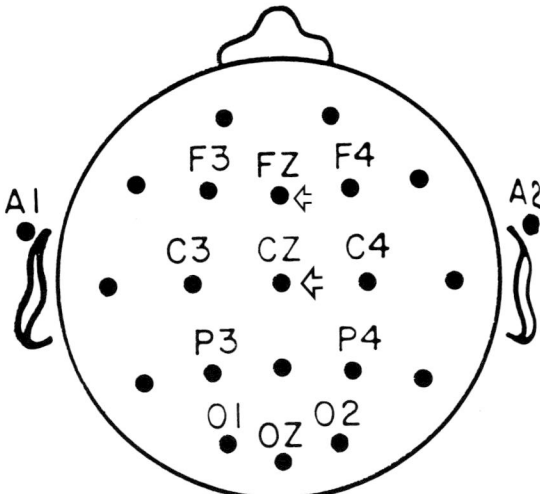

Figure 6. Electrode locations designated by the International Ten Twenty System. These positions are based on measurements of head circumference, interaural distance, and the distance from nasion to inion. Cz^1 = large open arrows, Fz^1 = small arrows. Arrows placed at sites along the midsagittal plane to approximate the placement of the two electrodes used to monitor cervical surgery in the author's series (arrows). Reproduced with permission.[19]

erence electrode. The technique described by the author for monitoring median and posterior tibial potentials employs only two cortical Cz and Fz electrodes applied in the midsagittal plane (Figure 6).[14]

SSEPs are small potentials relative to ongoing EEG activity and noise in the recording environment. By averaging hundreds of signals, the SSEP, which is time-locked to the stimulus, is enhanced while the ongoing EEG activity and random noise are averaged out.[1] One hundred to 200 microsecond pulses are delivered at rates of 3-5 per second for a total of 200 events per epoch, and are passed through band pass filters of 10-500 Hz. The technique which alternates stimulation of the right and left sides, produces waveforms that can be monitored on a pseudosplit screen array so that at any one time the responses from two extremities are visible—i.e. the upper extremity on one side and lower extremity on the other. Alternating stimulation sites provides data for 2 extremities in 50 seconds, and for all 4 extremities in 100 seconds.[14]

When conducting intraoperative SSEP monitoring, several critical assumptions are made.[10,13,14,23,24,32,34,36,37,39] First, normal intraoperative SSEPs must be presumed to reflect intact neurologic function. Second, SSEP changes are assumed to indicate impending neurologic injury.[10,23,24,32,34] Since deteriorating SSEPs typically fluctuate before being lost, we assume that emergency resuscitative measures allow these potentials to return to normal, thereby avoiding permanent neurologic deterioration.[32,37,39] Third, significant SSEP changes which do not revert to normal, signal irreversible neurologic dysfunction.[10,19,23,24,32,34] Fourth, SSEP improvement indicates recovery of function.[13,14,32,36,39]

Thus, essential to any SSEP monitoring protocol are the definitions of the magnitude of changes (significance criteria) that predict neurologic injury. The majority of studies employing intraoperative spinal cord monitoring consider a greater than 5% to 10% increase in latency and greater than 50% to 60% decline in amplitude as evidence of significant SSEP deterioration.[1,9,22-24,32,47] For example, Aminoff[1]; Wilber et al[47]; Keith et al[22]; and Dinner et al[9] all considered latency to be significantly prolonged when the mean was exceeded by 5% to 10%, with amplitude being significantly compromised when a decline of over 50% was observed.

Preoperative SSEPs

Although cervical spondylosis is a prominent radiographic abnormality, and is present in more than 50% of people over 50 years of age, few develop significant clinical disease.[33] However, in instances where radiculopathy and myelopathy become clinically evident, elective preoperative SSEP recordings may indicate the onset of pathological alterations in the large myelinated afferent fibers in the somatosensory pathways.[33] The majority of these changes, attributed to micromechanical and microvascular trauma, are found in the white matter of the posterior columns even when imaging studies indicate ventral or lateral compression predominates over posterior compression.[12,49]

Attempts to better correlate these anatomic changes and resulting SSEP abnormalities with radiculopathy or myelopathy have given rise to three different theories.[1,11,12,17,33,42,49] Firstly, SSEP responses equally reflect pathological severity in patients with either radiculopathy or myelopathy. Secondly, SSEPs more clearly distinguish radiculopathy from myelopathy. In the series of Perlik and Fisher, SSEP changes could be detected even in patients with radicular symptoms without neurologic signs.[33] Thirdly, median and posterior tibial SSEPs more accurately reflect myelopathy than radiculopathy.[1,11,12,17,35,42,49]

Most authorities believe that SSEPs are better indicators of myelopathy than radiculopathy. Using median potentials alone in 14 patients, El Negamy and Sedgwick readily differentiated patients with myelopathy from those with radiculopathy. The patients with myelopathy exhibited more severe N11-N13 changes, while those with radiculopathy showed only mild N9-N11 conduction delays.[12] Also using preoperative median SSEPs, Siivola et al[42] found that the most marked changes occurred in patients with myelopathy, milder SSEP findings in those with radiculopathy, and normal SSEPs in patients with minimal symptoms and no signs.

Yu and Jones, using preoperative median, ulnar, and posterior tibial recordings, found that significant SSEP changes in 34 spondylotic patients more closely correlated with myelopathy than with radiculopathy.[49] In particular, significant SSEP changes were seen in 83% of patients with myelopathy and radiculopathy, 87% of patients with myelopathy alone, 33% of patients with radiculopathy, and 29% of patients with only neck pain. Ganes also found that SSEP changes in 21 patients with cervical disease were most marked when myelopathy was present, were mild in those with radicular symptoms and signs, and were normal in patients with purely subjective complaints.[17]

Posterior tibial recordings, more sensitive to myelopathy, spinal cord compression, and intrinsic neurologic dysfunction when compared with median nerve recordings, also better differentiated the level, extent, and severity of myelopathy.[1,11,12,17,32,33,42,49] Posterior tibial potentials proved even more sensitive than median nerve recordings to intrinsic and extrinsic cord injury above the C5-6 level.[1,14,16,17,25] El Negamy and Sedgwick noted that posterior tibial responses more reliably predicted clinical and subclinical abnormalities in the somatosensory pathways than median nerve recordings.[12] Perlik and Fisher had 13 patients with cervical spondylotic myelopathy all with abnormal or absent posterior tibial SSEPs preoperatively, whereas only 9 median responses were abnormal.[33]

Yu and Jones similarly demonstrated that posterior tibial responses were more sensitive indicators of myelopathy than median or ulnar potentials as 56% of posterior tibial responses in 34 patients with cervical myelopathy were abnormal, compared with 41% of ulnar, and only 18% of median nerve recordings.[49] They attributed this greater sensitivity and specificity to the greater peripheral and central conduction distances posterior tibial potentials traversed.[49] Dorfman et al evaluated posterior tibial potentials in 23 patients with intramedullary, extramedullary, and traumatic disease above and below the C6 level, and also demonstrated that posterior tibial responses were more sensitive to myelopathy than median potentials: 8 of 46 possible posterior tibial responses were abnormal, compared with only 1 pathologic response out of 46 median nerve potentials.[11]

The origin of myelopathic complaints from intrinsic posterior column pathology, particularly in the medial gracile tracts, may also explain why some lower extremity complaints resolve following cervical decompression in patients with coexisting cervical and lumbar stenosis. The resolution of lumbar complaints in these tandem settings indicates that some "lumbar" symptoms originate not from cauda equina or root compression, but within the cervical somatosensory funiculi.

A vascular (arterial, venous) rather than mechanical etiology of injury better explains why time plays so critical a role in the production of irreversible neurologic deficits. Vascular compromise over longer segments may also account for the greater sensitivity of posterior tibial compared with median nerve potentials in detecting myelopathic disease.[25,49]

SSEPs as Predictors of Post-traumatic Outcome

Several studies have attempted to correlate SSEP changes with neurologic outcomes for patients following acute spinal cord trauma.[27,38,48] Li et al demonstrated that acute, and even delayed, SSEP changes could help predict long-term prognosis in 36 spine-injured patients with complete and incomplete neurologic deficits.[26] They found that patients with complete injuries and absent SSEPs were least likely to recover useful neurologic function, while those with absent SSEPs but incomplete injuries exhibited only slightly better outcomes. However, those with incomplete injuries but initially intact SSEP responses, or those for whom SSEPs reappeared in the first post-traumatic weeks, had a better prognosis. They also noted that combined ulnar and posterior tibial recordings better predicted outcome than either response alone.[26]

Intraoperative SSEP Monitoring Technique

Continuous SSEP monitoring, routinely employed during scoliosis surgery for over a decade, was adopted by the author during cervical procedures for treatment of disk disease, stenosis, spondylosis, and ossification of the posterior longitudinal ligament (OPPL).[14] This required the development of a complete SSEP monitoring and anesthesia protocol which will be presented below.

SSEP Monitoring Protocol

The amplitude and latency of both median (N20) and posterior tibial (N38) somatosensory evoked cortical potentials (SSEPs) are continuously monitored throughout cervical procedures. Median and posterior tibial nerve responses are elicited by skin surface or cup electrode stimulation over the wrists and ankles (Figure 7). By using surface cup electrodes monitoring may begin prior to inducing anesthesia and can be maintained through closing, without posing the risk of infection.[7,12,16] Erb's point, or the elbow, and the popliteal fossa serve as the peripheral reference sites, while cortical responses are measured using two electrodes placed at the vertex (Cz or Cz^1 and Fz) in the mid-sagittal plane.

Most abnormal or even initially absent median and posterior tibial potentials can be followed intraoperatively, as SSEP potentials are often enhanced by monitoring techniques. Even the most severely myelopathic individuals, particularly those with OPLL, diabetics with neuropathy, and persons with carpal tunnel disease can be monitored intra operatively. Monitoring is feasible since patients do not exhibit an absence of SSEP in all four extremities. In fact, potentials are rarely absent in more than one extremity. Of 24 patients recently evaluated with OPLL, 6 demonstrated absent preoperative amplitude and/or latency SSEP potentials. Two of the four patients with bilaterally absent posterior tibial potentials preoperatively demonstrated postoperative recovery. Similarly, absent median nerve potentials improved in 2 of 4 patients with OPLL.

Even when unilateral or bilateral posterior tibial or median nerve potentials are initially absent, half recover in the course of surgery. This recovery is in part due to the use of higher baseline stimulus intensities in sedated preoperative and anesthetized intraoperative patients, and to the elimination of muscle artifact following the induction of general anesthesia.[14] Baseline stimulus intensities, set at two to three times the motor threshold in awake patients receiving intravenous sedation (such as 1-5 mg of midazolam titrated to the desired effect), enhance this baseline SSEP acquisition. Patients therefore tolerate greater preoperative baseline stimulus intensities, which can be maintained throughout the

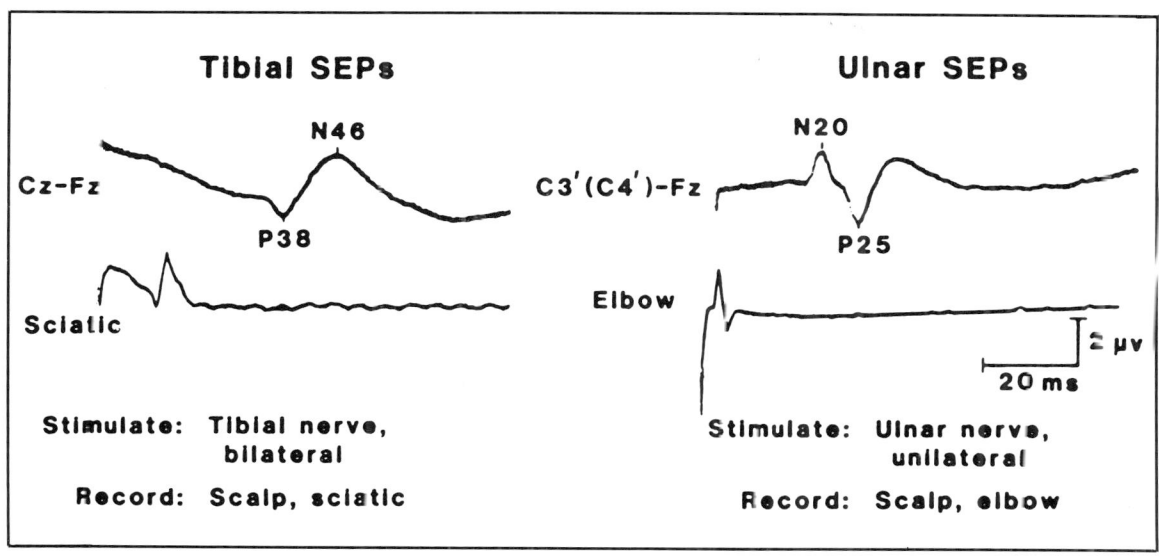

Figure 7. Intraoperative monitoring of tibial and ulnar cortical evoked potentials during operative procedure on cervical spine. Tibial somatosensory evoked potentials (SSEPs) were obtained after bilateral stimulation of tibial nerves at ankle and recording over scalp and sciatic nerve. Ulnar SSEPs were obtained after unilateral stimulation of ulnar nerve at wrist and recording at scalp and elbow sites. Latencies of tibial (P38) and ulnar (N20) cortical evoked potentials were measured by using an electronic cursor. P38 amplitude was measured from trough of P38 to next negative peak (N46), and N20 amplitude was measured from peak of N20 to next positive trough (P25). C3', C4', z, and Fz denote positions of scalp electrodes. (Reference 45: Figure 1, Page 258.)

surgery.[1,6,14,17,32] Paralytic agents such as vecuronium, employed during general anesthesia, further eliminate muscle artifact and facilitate SSEP acquisition.[16]

Baseline SSEPs are generated in the operating suite immediately prior to surgery. Significant SSEP changes in baseline and intraoperative recordings are defined as a 10% or greater increase in latency and/or a 50% or greater decrease in amplitude.[1,5,10,14,16,18,19,21,24] Our protocol dictates that immediate nonsurgical (i.e. anesthetic) and surgical measures be adopted as soon as significant SSEP changes are manifest on two averages.[1,5,10,14,16,24] Significant SSEP changes attributed to hypotension, hypothermia, and high levels of inhalation or intravenous anesthestics can be reversed by inducing hypertension, hyperthermia, wound hyperoxygenation (peroxide irrigation), the reduction or elimination of inhalation anesthestics, and elevation of inspired oxygen concentrations.[8,14-16,20] High doses of methylprednisolone (30 mg/kg as an initial bolus followed by 5.4 mg/kg/hr for 23 hours) can theoretically limit neurologic injury, particularly where significant SSEP changes persist.[2] Surgical maneuvers, including spinal cord or root manipulation, distraction, and graft placement are also immediately stopped if SSEP changes are noted. Early use of these resuscitative measures in response to significant SSEP changes can help avoid permanent neurologic injury, while rarely delaying surgery.[8,14]

Anesthesia Technique

A specific anesthesia protocol is needed to minimize the unique perioperative risks associated with intubation and positioning in patients with degenerative cervical disease.[14] Patients with cervical disk disease, stenosis, spondylosis, and OPLL with compromised cervical spinal canals are more susceptible to neurologic injury during intubation. In particular, hyperextension during intubation may result in spinal cord injury and quadriplegia. Furthermore, since SSEP monitoring is transiently compromised following bolus injections of barbiturates during anesthesia induction, SSEP monitoring during this critical intubation and positioning phase is often suboptimal. In order to minimize the risk of injury to the cervical spinal cord at the time of intubation and operative positioning, nasotracheal fiberoptic intubations are performed in awake patients, who are simultaneously immobilized in hard cervical collars.[14]

Continuous SSEP monitoring of awake patients throughout intubation and positioning requires a specified premedication regimen. Premedications include hydroxyzine 1mg/kg, meperidine 1mg/kg, and atropine (0.2-0.4 mg). After arriving in the induction suite, local nasopharyngeal anesthesia is initiated with 4% cocaine placed topically in the nasopharynx. Then 10 ml of 2% xylocaine jelly is then introduced directly into the nasopharyngeal passages with a 14 French nasotracheal aspiration catheter, accompanied by a transtracheal injection of 5 ml (100 mg) of 2% xylocaine. The fiberoptic bronchoscope then slips through a 7 or 8 mm metal reinforced Anode tube, which is introduced through a nasal passage and guided into the larynx and trachea where its location can be directly verified. Throughout this process, the patient receives 1-5 mg midazolam as needed.

For patients undergoing anterior surgical procedures, the final supine position is attained prior to intubation. No further alteration of position is performed once intubation has been completed. Baseline SSEP recordings and the neurologic examination are followed before, during, and after intubation. Once SSEPs are stable, induction ensues.

Similarly, patients undergoing posterior surgical procedures (laminectomy, hemilaminectomy, laminotomy) in the sitting position are kept awake during intubation and positioning. The Mayfield three-pin head piece is applied using a total of 15 ml of 1% xylocaine infiltrated at the three pin sites. Patients are then slowly raised to the sitting position, while their necks are maintained in a neutral posture with a hard collar. The collar is only removed once the final neck position is achieved, and the head holder is fixed to the table's Mayfield head rest. Shoulders, arms, and hands are next elevated over blanks and pillows to minimize intraoperative tension to the nerve roots, brachial plexus, and peripheral nerves. A simultaneous decline in latency and amplitude, frequently observed while raising patients to the sitting position, is attributed to "relative" cord hypotension—a relative drop in cord perfusion occurring in the presence of a normal systemic blood pressure measured with the arterial line set at neck level.[14] The induction of systemic hypertension causes these SSEP changes to immediately revert to normal.

The so-called neutral position frequently has to be modified if SSEP changes occur during positioning of the neck. These changes will usually resolve with slightly more flexion or extension. The immediate alteration of shoulder, arm, and/or wrist position(s) frequently reverse initial significant SSEP changes, a maneuver which is presumed to avert potential radicular damage.

Induction follows only after SSEPs are stable in supine or seated patients, as bolus injections of thiopental 2-3mg/kg or diprivan 1-2mg/kg usually produce transient (5-7 minutes) blunting of SSEP responses. To further avoid interfering with SSEP acquisition, inhalation anesthetics such as isoflurane are maintained at levels of 0.2% to 0.4%, while the nitrous oxide percentage is maintained between 60% and 70%. Intraoperative relaxation is provided by vecuronium, administered as a loading dose of 0.1 mg/kg and repeated as needed. Anterior and posterior cervical skin incisions are then infiltrated with 10-30 ml of 0.5% bupivicaine hydrochloride with epinephrine (1:200,000). The addition of local anesthesia allows the anesthesiologist to decrease inhalation and intravenous anesthetics earlier in the surgical course so that patients awaken immediately at the end of the procedure, and can be examined on the operating room table prior to transfer to the recovery room.

Factors Affecting SSEP Acquisition

Patient Factors

The most reliable SSEP recordings are obtained in patients between the ages of 8 and 80.[11,32] Patients in this age range exhibit longer and more stable SSEP latencies, although amplitude recordings prove more susceptible to changes in anesthetic technique.

Temperature

Intraoperative hypothermia, the reduction of core temperature by 1-2 degrees and an even greater temperature loss in the extremities, can contribute to the deterioration of intraoperative SSEP potentials.[18,19,23] Limb hypothermia can best be evaluated by the peripheral reference electrodes located at Erb's point in the upper extremities and the popliteal fossa in the lower extremities.[13,29,32,40] Profound systemic hypothermia produces early amplitude and later latency changes in posterior tibial recordings, which are less resistant to temperature changes than median responses.[32] Cold irrigating solutions applied directly to the cervical cord or upper brain stem also produce immediate, although reversible, decreases or losses in SSEP potentials.[14]

Hypotension

Hypotension, defined by depression of the mean systolic blood pressure to below 80 mm Hg, first produces a diminution or loss of amplitude followed by deterioration of latency.[32] Deliberate intraoperative hypotension to minimize blood loss can contribute to significant SSEP loss and mask neurologic injury associated with such critical operative maneuvers as Harrington rod placement and distraction. During these intervals, hypotension should be reversed in an attempt to restore SSEPs to baseline, so that changes in SSEP potentials can be correctly interpreted and appropriately addressed.

Hypotension is not always easily recognized. For example, during cervical spine surgery performed with the patient in the sitting position, systemic normotension did not prevent "relative hypotension" or underperfusion of the spinal cord. This relative hypotension is only recognized when raising patients to the seated position produces significant simultaneous declines in amplitude and latency recordings for both median and posterior tibial potentials. The return of potentials following the artificial induction of hypertension correctly identifies the etiology of the evolved potential changes. The rapidity with which relative hypotension is recognized and reversed determines how quickly SSEPs return to base line. Early detection and correction averts major neurologic injury, particularly in older patients with cervical stenosis about to undergo laminectomies, who account for the majority of quadriplegics in previous unmonitored series.[14]

Anesthesia

SSEPs may be more difficult to study intraoperatively in severely compromised (radiculopathic, myelopathic) individuals, either because potentials are initially absent, or because abnormal potentials are more susceptible to anesthetic compromise.[13,29,32,40] Anesthetic techniques may be responsible for the significant loss of the SSEP responses, as SSEP monitoring is uniquely sensitive to high levels of halogenated anesthetics. These agents, particularly in concentrations greater than 0.45%, decrease SSEP amplitudes while increasing latencies.[30,43,44] The depression or loss of SSEP responses when using volatile anesthetics is attributed to the anesthesia's inhibition of neuronal transmission and reduction in the number of innervated neurons. The fact that cortical potentials are even more affected than subcortical recordings is attributed to the greater number of synapses required for cortical transmission.

Sebel et al determined that enflurane interfered less than halothane ($>1.0\%$) with intraoperative SSEP recordings.[40] Although all halogenated anesthetics contribute to the loss of cortical potentials, the detrimental impact of some can be minimized by keeping concentrations, particularly of isoflurane, below 0.4%.[32,40]

Nitrous oxide (N_2O) employed with both low-dose halogenated agents and a balanced narcotic technique also reduces SSEP amplitudes.[32,45,46] Sloan and Koht evaluated the effect of 50% nitrous oxide on cortical SSEPs, and demonstrated that it produces a consistent decline in SSEP amplitude without affecting latency.[43] Reductions in amplitude approached 50% when N_2O concentrations exceeded 50%; the observed decreases in SSEP amplitude were immediately reversed when N_2O was discontinued. The negative impact of N_2O, narcotics, and inhalation agents on SSEP responses are also cumulative.

The sensitivity of surface SSEP monitoring techniques to inhalation, balanced narcotic, and other techniques is increased further when bolus injections of centrally acting barbiturates are used for induction. Bolus injection typically results in transient but profound SSEP changes, typically lasting for up to 10 minutes.[32] Maurette evaluated the impact of diprivan on posterior tibial responses in 20 patients undergoing spinal surgery.[30] Induction, using diprivan (2 mg/kg) was followed by an initial constant infusion of 6 mg/kg, and a subsequent dose of 3 mg/kg for the duration of the procedure. The significant depression of SSEPs, noted 10 minutes after induction and persisting into early recovery phases, cast some doubt on the value of diprivan's value in SSEP monitored cases.[29,32]

The 10-minute period following the initial bolus of centrally acting medications (e.g. diprivan, thiopental) during which monitoring is not possible, is a time during which critical spinal cord and/or root damage can occur. Although continuous drip, rather than bolus delivery, can minimize the impact of induction on SSEP acquisition, these difficulties can be circumvented with a protocol of awake intubation and positioning. SSEP acquisition can therefore continue throughout these critical maneuvers, and induction can follow once normal baselines are obtained after 5-10 minutes. This protocol lessens the risk that significant neurologic injury will occur during these critical maneuvers. The anticipated decrement or loss of the SSEP responses, which ensues for approximately 10 minutes after injection of barbiturates, poses a lesser risk of missing significant neurologic compromise.

Neuromuscular Blockade

At the time of induction, paralytic agents enhance SSEP acquisition by eliminating noise attributed to muscle artifact. Therefore, neuromuscular blockade improves the quality of SSEPs and often transforms poor responses into readable potentials.[14]

Manipulation

SSEP changes indicate when surgical maneuvers contribute to vascular and/or mechanical spinal cord compromise. Significant SSEP changes in the lumbar region, associated with manipulation, compression or distraction, can alter blood flow from the anterior spinal artery or artery of Adamkiewicz. Resulting ischemia to the posterior columns and adjacent tracts produces a diminution or loss in SSEP responses.[13] Distraction of the cervical spine can similarly result in SSEP loss, particularly in the more severely myelopathic patients with OPLL. The immediate release of distraction and rapid reappearance of potentials confirms that focal mechanical compression is at fault.[14]

Responses to SSEP Changes
False Positives

It is not clear how to interpret significant changes in SSEPs occurring intraoperatively in patients who remain neurologically intact. On the one hand, these may represent false positives, correctly attributed to noise, or to changes associated with increased levels of anesthesia and poor intraoperative SSEP acquisition in patients with severe pre-existing abnormalities in SSEP pathways. More recent experience, particularly in cervical surgery, indicates that some so-called false positives may actually represent significant SSEP changes which reflect impending neurologic injury which is successfully averted with timely resuscitative maneuvers.[14]

In almost any study, significant SSEP changes may be seen in patients who exhibit no new neurologic deficits. A certain number of these false positives should be anticipated, as they reflect the sensitivity of the significance criteria used in monitoring. Excessively liberal significance criteria may contribute to unacceptably high false-positive rates, unnecessary emotional strain, and an abundance of unwelcome operative delays. When the frequency of false positives is too high, more restricted significance criteria can be defined so that fewer SSEP changes are considered significant. Adjusting the significance criteria to reduce the false-positive rate increases the risk that unwanted false negatives, "misses," or devastating new neurologic deficits will occur in the absence of significant SSEP changes. Since the primary aim of SSEP monitoring is to avoid devastating neurologic injuries, significant criteria should err in the direction of creating more false positives in order to avoid the false negatives.

False Negatives

SSEP monitoring is employed during scoliosis surgery so that impending neurologic injury may be recognized and avoided. However, new neurologic deficits may occur even when normal intraoperative SSEPs have been maintained. These false negatives are attributable to a number of factors: (1) some neuroanatomic studies indicate that the ventral and lateral spinal cord is not involved in somatosensory potential transmission, and injury to these areas may go unnoticed[7,8,23,24] (2); preoperative posterior column dysfunction may either preclude monitoring entirely or make useful monitoring difficult; and, (3) other factors such as noise, anesthesia, hypotension, and monitoring method, including the time after monitoring leads are removed, may further limit SSEP accuracy.

False negatives may also reflect shortcomings, not in the monitoring technique itself, but rather a failure to adequately define and choose criteria of significance. On the one hand, overly liberal significance criteria may contribute to an intolerably high false-positive rate, but a very acceptable low incidence of false negatives. On the other hand, restricted significance criteria may reduce the number of false positives, but produce an unacceptable increase in false negatives. Since the aim of intraoperative SSEP monitoring is to minimize or eliminate false negatives, the risks versus benefits of altering significance criteria to minimize the frequency of both false positives and false negatives must be carefully weighed.

The choice of appropriate significance criteria for intraoperative SSEP monitoring during spinal procedures reduced the incidence of false negatives in most series, occasionally eliminating them entirely from others.[9,33] Monitoring of both median and posterior tibial potentials additionally reduced the incidence of false negatives.[1,14,32,33,49]

False Negatives or Negative Surgeons

One of the major limitations of SSEP monitoring is the surgeon's failure to appropriately modify technique when significant changes occur. Since delayed responses can result in irretrievable neurologic dysfunction, the operating surgeon must alter operative technique as soon as significant SSEP changes are replicated. Furthermore, SSEP changes rarely simply disappear. They typically fluctuate before being lost, indicating that neurologic compromise was impending over a period of time.[9,14,32] The neurologic deficits are, therefore, not solely attributable to a failure in electrophysiologic technique.[32]

False negatives may therefore reflect an intrinsic limitation of the monitoring technique, and consideration must be given to whether more timely responses from the surgeon to more liberal significance criteria may optimize results.

Significant Improvement

An added but unanticipated benefit of intraoperative SSEP monitoring is the appearance of significant intraoperative and postoperative improvement. Significant SSEP amplitude improvement was observed following the excision of extra-axial lesions in Nuwer's study, while Engler observed SSEP improvement in 42% of patients having scoliosis surgery.[13,32] A 12% to 18% frequency of significant SSEP improvement during cervical surgery for disk disease, stenosis, spondylosis, and OPLL was observed in the author's series.[14]

Timing of Resuscitative Measures

Significant SSEP changes lasting more than 15-20 minutes frequently correlate with a higher incidence of permanent neurologic dysfunction.[28] The adoption of resuscitative measures as soon as significant changes can be replicated over typical 100-second intervals is essential. In certain instances, these measures can be initiated even when reproducible changes have not yet reached significant levels.

Timely adoption of appropriate nonsurgical or surgical resuscitative maneuvers is important if SSEP monitoring is to reduce the incidence of permanent neurologic sequelae. Some nonsurgical measures include increasing inspired oxygen levels, elevating mean arterial blood pressures or central pressures, and discontinuation of inhalation anesthetics. Surgical modifications aimed at reducing deficits include irrigating wounds with warm saline or peroxide, cessation of manipulation or dissection, removal of instrumentation, or release of distraction.[31] In the series of Meyer et al, significant SSEP changes occurred in 6 of 150 monitored individuals.[31] Immediate resuscitative maneuvers reversed SSEP changes in 4 of the 6 patients and all four remained neurologically intact, while only 1 of the 2 remaining with persistent SSEP abnormalities (0.7%) exhibited new postoperative neurologic dysfunction.

Preoperative Prophylaxis

In an attempt to limit operative morbidity, some surgeons have recently given methyprednisolone prophylaxis, as described by Bracken et al, in high-risk elective cervical procedures.[2,14] The efficacy of this high-dose regimen in an elective setting is yet unproven.[14]

SSEPs in Cervical Surgery

Intraoperative SSEP monitoring, first used during scoliosis surgery in the 1970s, has more recently been adapted to cervical operations.[6,9,12,14,31,32,44,47] In 1986, Sloan et al, using median and posterior tibial SSEPs during anterior cervical spine fusions, detected SSEP changes when retractors produced ipsilateral carotid artery compression.[44] Intraoperative SSEP changes, consisting of prolonged latencies and reduced amplitudes, signalled the evolution of neurologic injuries that could be easily reversed with appropriate resuscitative measures. The immediate release and repositioning of retractors reversed cerebral ischemia, allowing potentials and neurologic function to return to normal.

Acknowledging that the risk of injury to the spinal cord had increased along with greater sophistication of cervical instrumentation techniques, Veilleux et al used SSEP monitoring for cervical spine surgery in 1987.[45] He conducted unilateral ulnar and bilateral posterior tibial recording every 20 minutes over a minimum of 3 hours in 81 patients, although data proved adequate for only 43. The operative protocol called for early SSEP changes to be rapidly addressed, with modification of surgical technique so that fixed deficits could be averted. Major reductions in intraoperative SSEPs were observed in 10 patients (Figure 7). Of these, 9 sustained a complete loss of SSEPs, attributed to the level of anaesthesia and severity of preoperative SSEP abnormalities. In the tenth patient, SSEP loss was directly correlated with wire tightening performed in the course of a posterior wiring and fusion for a C5-7 fracture/dislocation. Release of the wire correlated with the immediate return of normal SSEP responses, and the patient awakened neurologically intact.

SSEP Monitoring in 100 Cervical Operations

SSEP monitoring has contributed to the reduction of neurologic injury associated with scoliosis surgery from 4% to 6.9% to 0% to 0.7%.[9,31,33,47] We and others have reported median and posterior tibial SSEP monitoring during cervical surgery as a means of assessing spinal cord function.[6,9,12,14]

In order to assess whether SSEP monitoring would benefit patients with radiculopathy and myelopathy having cervical surgery for disk disease, stenosis, spondylosis, and OPLL, we compared the morbidity and mortality associated with 218 unmonitored cases performed between 1985-1989 to 100 consecutively SSEP-monitored procedures conducted from 1989-1990 (Table 3A, B, C).[14] We immediately altered anesthetic or surgical techniques in response to early, significant, but presumably still reversible SSEP abnormalities in order to limit postoperative neurologic dysfunction.

Evaluation of the clinical status of patients preoperative and postoperatively was based on Ranawat, O'Leary, and Edward's classification system.[14,28,37,43] Using Ranawat's criteria, similar clinical data were obtained for the two populations. This included nearly identical preoperative Ranawat neurologic classes—the better Classes I and II (46% and 44%) and more impaired IIIA and IIIB (54% and 56%), respectively. One prominent difference between the two populations was the shift away from posterior surgery in the unmonitored (67%) toward more anterior procedures (48%) for the SSEP monitored patients (Table 3A).[14,35]

Morbidity and mortality figures for patients having cervical surgery without and with SSEP monitoring markedly differed. Eight or 3.7% of the 218 patients having unmonitored cervical procedures were newly Class IIIB quadriplegic following surgery, and 1 of these 8 died. Alternatively, all 99 correctly-monitored patients remained intact and there were no deaths. One inadequately monitored patient did become quadriplegic. This incident was attributed to a technical error—the failure to follow posterior tibial potentials throughout a cervical laminectomy. When posterior tibial leads were reapplied and found to be absent, immediate reoperation resulted in a Class II recovery 3 months later.

SSEP monitoring also appeared to enhance postoperative neurologic outcomes. Seventy percent of unmonitored, compared with 85% of SSEP monitored patients, exhibited good to excellent (Class I/II) outcomes, with more monitored (56%) than unmonitored (35%) patients being found in the best Class I group. Patients were also assigned postoperative Ranawat grades based on comparison of preoperative and postoperative Ranawat classes. In order to assign these grades, patients who improved one class, as from IIIA to II, were assigned a positive one, while those who deteriorated, as from I to IIA, were given a negative one. Based on this grading system, the 218 unmonitored patients improved an average of one-half a Ranawat grade while the 100 SSEP monitored patients improved an average of one grade.

The improvement in postoperative Ranawat classes and grades for SSEP monitored patients could not be attributed to fewer high-risk cervical laminectomies being performed in SSEP monitored patients. The incidence of these procedures was nearly identical for the two groups: 38% of unmonitored cervical procedures were multilevel laminectomies compared with 35% of SSEP monitored patients. The switch from posterior to anterior surgical approaches occurred predominantly among the so-called lower risk diskectomy patients. While 29% of unmonitored patients had posterior cervical diskectomies, this figure decreased to 17% for the SSEP group. Conversely, the incidence of anterior diskectomies increased from 31% in unmonitored patients to 44% for SSEP monitored individuals. Multilevel anterior vertebrectomies also increased from 2% to 4% for the respective unmonitored and SSEP monitored categories.

Electrophysiology of Intraoperative SSEPs

To quantify SSEP changes, the most abnormal changes occurring in both latency and amplitude were compared to baseline measures in one of four operative periods: (1) preinduction (PRE) for establishing baseline SSEP cortical responses, (2) (ANES), the time from awake intubation and awake positioning to anesthesia induction, (3) manipulation (MAN) phase, and (4) closing (CLOSE). As anticipated, some changes occurred during the PRE and ANES periods associated with intubation and positioning, but the majority of abnormalities were encountered during the phase of maximal manipulation.

Latency and amplitude data were compared for both median and posterior tibial responses in all four extremities (100 patients). This was accomplished by normalizing data for each patient, which required dividing the maximal abnormal recorded values for each patient during each of the four periods by the patient's own preoperative (PRE) baseline latency and amplitude (Figures 8, 9). preamplitude) (Figures 8, 9).

Significant latency and amplitude changes were then divided into those lasting under 15 minutes and those lasting over 15 minutes. The 46 changes which lasted less than 15 minutes ranged from 2-4 minutes in duration, and were therefore extremely transient. The 19 which persisted for more than 15 minutes were of greater significance, as these more prolonged changes were thought to be associated with potentially irreversible deficits. Almost all persistent SSEP changes occurred in the most severely myelopathic patients, two-thirds of whom had anterior operations. SSEP latency and amplitude data for all 100 patients also proved both reliable and reproducible, despite the fact that 65 significant SSEP changes had occurred.

Each of 65 patients demonstrated significant SSEP deterioration in at least one of eight possible SSEP recordings of latency or amplitude for median or posterior tibial responses in either of four extremities (Table 4). Significant abnormalities were observed among 28% of 520 total responses. These significant changes occurred equally on the right and left sides, in nearly identical numbers for amplitude and latency recordings, with similar numbers of changes being detected in posterior tibial and median nerve potentials.

SSEP deterioration occurred with an almost equal frequency among patients undergoing anterior or posterior surgical procedures. SSEP changes were also observed with nearly the same overall frequency in patients with radiculopathy versus myelopathy, regardless of whether diskectomy or decompression for stenosis was being performed. Comparable frequencies of significant SSEP deterioration in patients undergoing the latter diskectomy and stenosis procedures indicated that all patients should be monitored, and that no one group could be considered less vulnerable to developing significant SSEP deterioration and therefore neurologic injury.

An unanticipated 12% to 18% incidence of significant intraoperative SSEP involvement was also observed among monitored patients. The greater 18% frequency of improvement occurred among the 35 patients without evidence of SSEP deterioration compared to the 65 patients with coincident evidence of significant intraoperative SSEP deterioration. Favorable changes, more likely to be noted in latency than amplitude recordings for posterior tibial (60%) than median

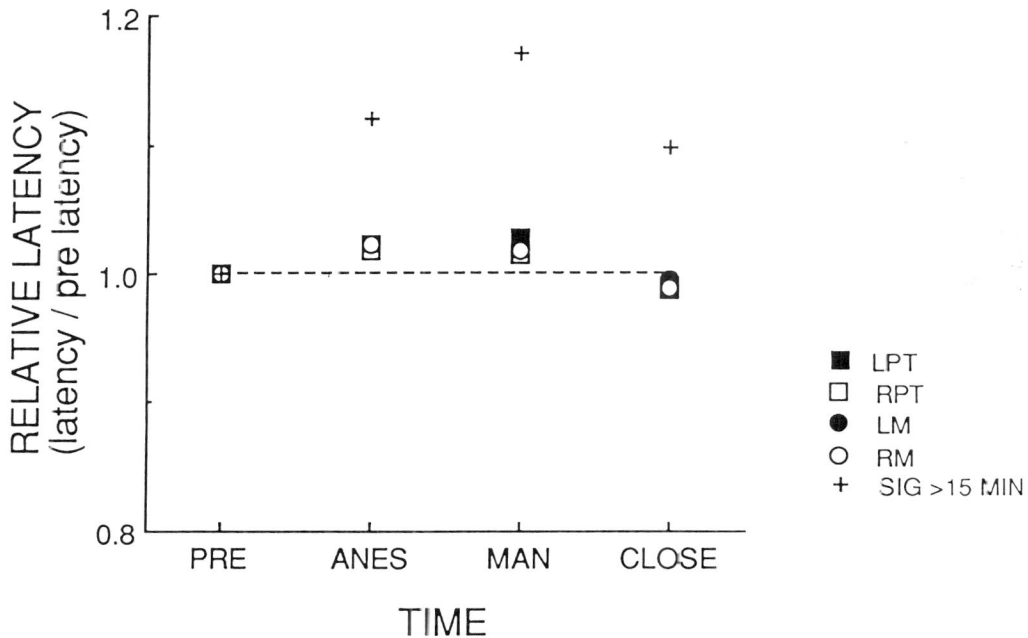

Figure 8. The horizontal axis shows the time of surgery artificially divided into four intervals: **Pre**—preoperative, **Anes** — period of operative positioning and induction of anesthesia, **Man** — operative manipulation, and **Close** — closing. The vertical axis represents the normalized or relative latency for each individual (latency/prelatency). Right and left median and posterior tibial recordings of latency are represented for all 100 patients by the opened and closed squares and circles: LPT-left posterior tibial, RPT-right posterior tibial, LM-left median, RM-right median. The SSEP recordings for 19 patients with persistent changes lasting over 15 inutes are separately represented by the crosses(+).

responses (40%), did not differentially forecast improved outcome.

Conclusion

Using continuous intraoperative SSEP recording during 100 consecutive cervical operations for cervical disk disease, stenosis, spondylosis, and OPLL, we attempted to assess whether SSEPs would warn of and help prevent permanent neurologic injury. Neuroanatomic review and pathophysiologic assessment further indicated that SSEP potentials should reflect complete spinal cord rather than isolated posterior column dysfunction.

Intraoperative SSEP monitoring does benefit patients having cervical surgery. No new neurologic complications occurred among patients having cervical surgery with intraoperative SSEP monitoring. The absence of devastating neurologic injury in this series sharply contrasted with the 3.7% incidence of quadriplegia and one death (0.5%) encountered among the 218 unmonitored individuals.

Our experience with continuous intraoperative SSEP monitoring also taught us that: (1) simultaneous monitoring of posterior tibial and median nerve potentials is

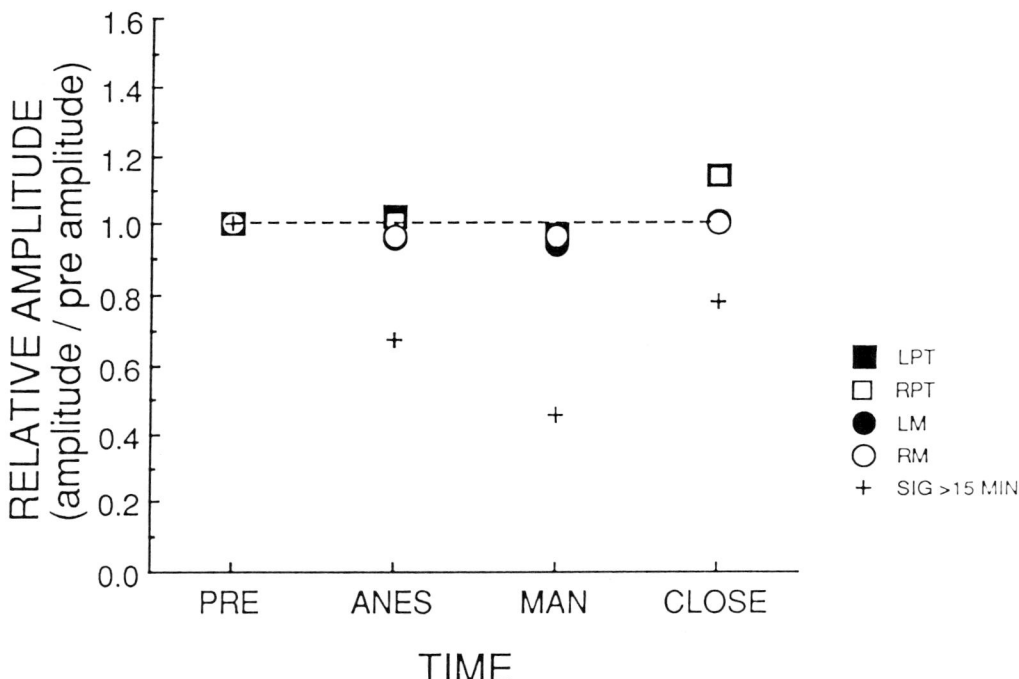

Figure 9. The horizontal axis in this figure shows the four periods of surgery: **Pre**—preoperative, **Anes** — period of operative positioning and induction of anesthesia, **Man** — operative manipulation, and **Close**—closing. The vertical axis indicates the normalized or relative amplitudes for each individual (amplitude/ preamplitude). Right and left median and posterior tibial recordings of amplitude are represented for all 100 patients by the opened and closed squares and circles: LPT-left posterior tibial, RPT-right posterior tibial, LM-left median, RM-right median. The SSEP recordings for 19 patients with persistent changes lasting over 15 minutes are separately represented by the crosses(+).

essential to minimize the risk of false negatives; (2) the significance criteria we chose appear to be adequate, as correct SSEP monitoring did not result in the introduction of any false negatives; and (3) these significance criteria carry a high incidence of false positives. We prefer to consider some of these significant SSEP changes in patients who remain neurologically intact as "mini" true positives, which allowed us to successfully avert neurologic injury where monitoring changes prompted the immediate adoption of appropriate resuscitative measures. Evoked potential monitoring was reliable and reproducible, and did not significantly delay surgery.

References

1. Aminoff MJ. The use of somatosensory evoked potentials in the evaluation of the central nervous system. *Neurol Clin.* 1988;6:809-823.
2. Bracken MB, Shepard MJ, Collins WF, et al. A randomized controlled trial of methylprednisolone or nalaxone in the treatment of acute spinal-cord injury: results of the Second National Acute Spinal Cord Injury Study. *N Eng J Med.* 1990;322:1405-1411.
3. Brown RH, Nash CL Jr. Current status of spinal cord monitoring. *Spine.* 1979;4:466-470.
4. Brown RH, Nash CL Jr. Intra-operative spinal cord monitoring. In: Frymoyer JW, ed. *The Adult Spine: Principles and Practice.* New York, NY: Raven Press; 1991;1:549-564.
5. Chabot R, York DH, Watts C, et al. Somatosensory evoked potentials evaluated in normal subjects and spinal cord-injured patients. *J Neurosurg.* 1985;63:544-551.

6. Chatrian G-E, Berger MS, Wirch AL. Discrepancy between intraoperative SSEP's and postoperative function: case report. *J Neurosurg.* 1988;69:450-454.
7. Cohen AR, Young W, Ransohoff J. Intraspinal localization of the somatosensory evoked potential. *Neurosurgery.* 1981;9:157-162.
8. Cusick JF, Myklebust J, Larson SJ, et al. Spinal evoked potentials in the primate: neural substrate. *J Neurosurg.* 1978;49:551-557.
9. Dinner DS, Lüders H, Lesser RP, et al. Intraoperative spinal somatosensory evoked potential monitoring. *J Neurosurg.* 1986;65:807-814.
10. Dolan EJ, Transfeldt EE, Tator CH. et al. The effect of spinal distraction on regional spinal cord blood flow in cats. *J Neurosurg.* 1980;53:756-764.
11. Dorfman LJ, Perkash I, Bosley TM, et al. Use of cerebral evoked potentials to evaluate spinal somatosensory function in patients with traumatic and surgical myelopathies. *J Neurosurg.* 1980;52:654-660.
12. El Negamy E, Sedgwick EM. Delayed cervical somatosensory potentials in cervical spondylosis. *J Neurol Neurosurg Psychiatry.* 1979;42:238-241.
13. Engler GL, Spielholz NI, Bernhard WN, et al. Somatosensory evoked potentials during Harrington instrumentation for scoliosis. *J Bone Joint Surg Am.* 1978;60A:528-532.
14. Epstein NE, Danto J, Nardi D. Evaluation of intraoperative somatosensory evoked potential monitoring in 100 cervical operations. **Spine.** In press. 1993.
15. Feinsod M, Selhorst JB, Hoyt WF, et al. Monitoring optic nerve function during craniotomy. *J Neurosurg.* 1976;44:29-31.
16. Frymoyer JW, ed. *The Adult Spine: Principles and Practice: Volumes I, II.* New York, NY: Raven Press, 1991.
17. Ganes T. Somatosensory conduction times and peripheral, cervical and cortical evoked potentials in patients with cervical spondylosis. *J Neurol Neurosurg Psychiatry.* 1980;43:683-689.
18. Grundy BL. Monitoring of sensory evoked potentials during neurosurgical operations: methods and applications. *Neurosurgery.* 1982;11:556-575.
19. Grundy BL. Intraoperative monitoring of sensory-evoked potentials. *Anesthesiology.* 1983;58:72-87.
20. Harding GFA, Bland JDP, Smith VH. Visual evoked potential monitoring of optic nerve function during surgery. *J Neurol Neurosurg Psychiatry.* 1990;53:890-895.
21. Jacobson GP, Tew JM Jr. Intraoperative evoked potential monitoring. *J Clin Neurophysiol.* 1987;4:145-176.
22. Keith RW, Stambough JL, Awender SH. Somatosensory cortical evoked potentials: a review of 100 cases of intraoperative spinal surgery monitoring. *J Spinal Disord.* 1990;3:220-226.
23. Larson SJ, Sances A Jr, Christenson PC. Evoked somatosensory potentials in man. *Arch Neurol.* 1966;15:88-93.
24. Larson SJ, Walsh PR, Sances A Jr, et al. Evoked potentials in experimental myelopathy. *Spine.* 1980;5:299-302.
25. Lesser RP, Raudzens P, Lüders H, et al. Postoperative neurological deficits may occur despite unchanged intraoperative somatosensory evoked potentials. *Ann Neurol.* 1986;19:22-25.
26. Li C, Houlden DA, Rowed DW. Somatosensory evoked potentials and neurological grades as predictors of outcome in acute spinal cord injury. *J Neurosurg.* 1990;72:600-609.
27. Lucas JT, Ducker TB. Motor classification of spinal cord injuries with mobility, morbidity and recovery indices. *Am Surg.* 1979;45:151-158.
28. Lueders H, Gurd A, Hahn J, et al. A new technique for intraoperative monitoring of spinal cord function: multichannel recording of spinal cord and subcortical evoked potentials. *Spine.* 1982;7:110-115.
29. McPherson RW, Mahla M, Johnson R, et al. Effects of enflurane, isoflurane and nitrous oxides in somatosensory evoked potentials during spinal surgery.
30. Maurette P, Simeon F, Castagnera L, et al. Propofol anaesthesia alters somatosensory evoked cortical potentials. *Anaesthesia.* 1988;43(suppl):44-45.
31. Meyer PR Jr, Cotler BH, Gireesan GT. Operative neurological complications resulting from thoracic and lumbar spine internal fixation. *Clin Orthop.* 1988;237:125-131.
32. Nuwer MR. Use of somatosensory evoked potentials for intraoperative monitoring of cerebral and spinal cord function. *Neurol Clin.* 1988;6:881-897.
33. Perlik SJ, Fisher MA. Somatosensory evoked response evaluation of cervical spondylotic myelopathy. *Muscle Nerve.* 1987;10:481-489.
34. Powers SK, Bolger CA, Edwards MSB. Spinal cord pathways mediating somatosensory evoked potentials. *J Neurosurg.* 1982;57:472-482.
35. Ranawat CS, O'Leary P, Pellicci P, et al. Cervical spine fusion in rheumatoid arthritis. *J Bone Joint Surg Am.* 1979;61A:1003-1010.
36. Regan D. The somatosensory pathway. In: *Human Brain Electrophysiology. Evoked Potentials and Evoked Magnetic Fields in Science and Medicine.* New York, NY: Elsevier Science Publishing Co; 1989:281-288.
37. Rossini PM. The anatomic and physiologic bases of motor-evoked potentials. *Neurol Clin.* 1988;6:751-769.
38. Rowed DW, McLean JAG, Tator CH. Somatosensory evoked potentials in acute spinal cord injury: prognostic value. *Surg Neurol.* 1978;9:203-210.
39. Schramm J, Hashizume K, Fukushima T, et al. Experimental spinal cord injury produced by slow, graded compression: alterations of cortical and spinal evoked potentials. *J Neurosurg.* 1979;50:48-57.
40. Sebel PS, Erwin CW, Neville WK. Effects of halothane and enflurane on far and near field somatosensory evoked potentials. *Br J Anaesth.* 1987;59:1492-1496.
41. Sedgwick EM, El Negamy E, Frankel H. Spinal cord potentials in traumatic paraplegia and quadriplegia. *J Neurol Neurosurg Psychiatry.* 1980;43:823-830.
42. Siivola J, Sulg I, Heiskari M. Somatosensory evoked potentials in diagnostics of cervical spondylosis and herniated disc. *Electroencephalogr Clin Neurophysiol.* 1981;52:276-282.
43. Sloan TB, Koht A. Depression of cortical somatosensory evoked potentials by nitrous oxide. *Br J Anaesth.* 1985;57:849-852.
44. Sloan TB, Ronai AK, Koht A. Reversible loss of somatosensory evoked potentials during anterior

cervical spine fusion. *Anesth Analg.* 1986;65:96-99.
45. Veilleux M, Daube JR, Cucchiara RF. Monitoring of cortical evoked potentials during surgical procedures on the cervical spine. *Mayo Clin Proc.* 1987; 62:256-264.
46. Whittle IR, Johnston IH, Besser M. Recording of spinal somatosensory evoked potentials for intraoperative spinal cord monitoring. *J Neurosurg.* 1986;64:601-612.
47. Wilber RG, Thompson GH, Shaffer JW, et al. Postoperative neurological deficits in segmental spinal instrumentation: a study using spinal cord monitoring. *J Bone Joint Surg Am.* 1984;66A:1178-1187.
48. York DH, Watts C, Raffensberger M, et al. Utilization of somatosensory evoked cortical potentials in spinal cord injury: prognostic limitations. *Spine.* 1983;8:832-839.
49. Yu YL, Jones SJ. Somatosensory evoked potentials in cervical spondylosis: correlation of median, ulnar and posterior tibial nerve responses with clinical and radiological findings. *Brain.* 1985;108:273-300.

CHAPTER 6

Cervical Spondylotic Myelopathy: Management with Anterior Operation

Paul R. Cooper, MD

Cervical spondylotic myelopathy is said to be "the most common spinal cord disorder in persons over 55"[40] and anterior cervical decompression and fusion probably is the most frequently performed surgical procedure for the treatment of this condition. Although anterior decompression for the treatment of cervical spondylotic myelopathy is believed to be superior to laminectomy,[53] the patient characteristics that will lead to a satisfactory outcome are not well defined. Moreover, technical factors such as the necessity for fusion and the extent of bone removal required to optimize outcome remain sources of considerable debate. This may explain, in part, a certain pessimism that exists among neurosurgeons regarding the effectiveness of this procedure in reversing neurologic deficit.

This author believes that in a high percentage of patients, the operation is incorrectly tailored to the extent of the patient's pathology and decompression is insufficient to result in amelioration or stabilization of neurologic function. In the postoperative period, unsatisfactory neurologic results frequently are attributed to the disease process rather than to failure of adequate decompression, and imaging studies are not performed to determine the reasons for the patient's failure to improve neurologically. Meticulous attention to operative detail and adapting the operation to the anatomic configuration of the patient's pathology will optimize results of operation.

This chapter is divided into three parts. In the first section, the techniques for achieving safe and successful decompression of the spinal cord from an anterior approach are detailed. In the subsequent section, complications and means for avoiding them are discussed. Finally, a critical analysis of results reported in the literature is undertaken.

Operative Technique
Perioperative Preparation

Preoperative use of corticosteroids are not employed. In a patient with severe neurologic deficit it is possible that preoperative treatment with corticosteroids may improve neurologic function and protect the spinal cord during operation, but no data support the efficacy of this policy.

Operation with the neck in extension facilitates exposure, particularly in operations on the upper cervical spine. However, in a patient with severe spinal cord compression, operation with the neck in an extended position may result in enhancement of compression by osteophytes or hypertrophied ligaments with exacerbation of neurologic deficit. For this reason, in the preoperative period, we place the patient in bed with the neck in the degree of extension similar to the anticipated position during operation.[6] If the patient can maintain this position for one-half hour without producing weakness or paresthesias, operation with the neck in extension can be performed safely. If symptoms are produced during this maneuver, the neck must be kept in a neutral position during operation. In such a patient, awake fiberoptic intubation with the neck in a neutral position also is indicated.

Intraoperative evoked potential monitoring in all patients undergoing anterior cervical decompression has been advocated in Chapter 5 in this volume as a means of identifying dangerous intraoperative maneuvers that may compromise neurologic function. For similar reasons, it has been advocated during intubation and positioning. Epstein, in Chapter 5, contends that there was a significant difference in outcome when patients who were managed with intraoperative evoked potential monitoring were compared with those who had no such monitoring. The study was not controlled and for this reason any conclusions as to the efficacy of monitoring must be regarded skeptically. Moreover, neurologic deterioration is so unusual with anterior operation for spondylotic myelopathy that one must question whether the additional time and expense entailed with monitoring justify its routine use.

Intubation and Operative Positioning

In the patient who does not develop neurologic symptoms during preoperative neck extension, routine oral endotracheal intubation is safe provided that the neck is moved slowly and gently. In patients with short necks and those who develop paresthesias or L'Hermitte's Sign with the neck in extension, an awake fiberoptic intubation should be performed.

After the neck is positioned, but before the patient is draped, wide adhesive tape is placed over the patient's shoulders and fixed to the end of the operating table to pull the shoulders down. This maneuver is particularly useful in patients with short necks and those who are to undergo decompression at C5-6 or C6-7 to allow visualization of this region when a localizing x-ray is taken.

Operative Incision

We usually empoy a transverse incision made in a skin crease to minimize the prominence of the scar in the postoperative period. The incision is begun just lateral to the midline and carried to the medial border of the sternocleidomastoid muscle. The precise level is determined by a localizing x-ray taken before the incision is made. It is not uncommon to incorrectly estimate the level of the incision by a distance of several centimeters, and an x-ray taken before the incision is made minimizes the chances of this happening.

A vertical incision along the medial border of the sternocleidomastoid muscle leaves a more obvious scar and therefore is less desirable than a transverse incision. A vertical incision sometimes is necessary in patients with short necks, when very high exposure is needed (e.g. C2-3) or a two-level vertebrectomy is contemplated. For the most part, however, a transverse incision provides adequate exposure for two- or even three-level osteophyte removal.

A right-sided incision is easier for a right-handed surgeon and the approach usually is made from this side regardless of the orientation of the incision. In the lower cervical spine, a left-sided incision sometimes is preferred because it is less likely to cause injury to the recurrent laryngeal nerve. However, recurrent laryngeal nerve injury is so infrequent that we do not believe that this is a sufficient reason for a left-sided incision. When osteophytes are predominantly right-sided, the left-sided approach has the advantage of directing the surgeon's line of vision to the right.

Soft-Tissue Dissection

The subcutaneous tissue is incised and a plane is dissected both rostrally and caudally for several centimeters between the subcutaneous tissue and the platysma muscle to facilitate rostral and caudal exposure. We prefer to cut the platysma perpendicular to its fibers although it also may be split parallel to its fibers. The latter technique is said to produce a cosmetically superior result. However, cutting the muscle produces better exposure and there is little or no difference in the prominence of the incision. Using a combination of blunt and sharp dissection, a plane then is developed between the sternocleidomastoid muscle and carotid artery laterally and the trachea and esophagus medially. The pulsation of the carotid artery should be palpated beneath the operator's finger and the vessel then may be retracted laterally under a hand-held retractor. A second hand-held retractor directs the esophagus medially. Both retractors are pressed posteriorly at the same time, which has the effect of clearing the midline of soft tissue. The prevertebral fascia is opened sharply. Midline orientation is obtained by observing the longus coli muscles on either side of the midline. The midline is marked, a needle is placed in the disk space, and an x-ray is taken to confirm the correct level. The medial borders of the longus coli muscles are cauterized and are freed from their attachment to the vertebral bodies using scissors or small periosteal elevators at least 2—3 cm above and below the area of intended bone and disk resection. In a medial-lateral direction, the muscles should be freed for a distance of 3 cm to permit adequate bone resection.

Sharp self-retaining retractor blades are placed beneath the medial aspect of the longus coli muscles and the retractor is spread to gain medial-lateral exposure. We prefer to use the retractors designed by Caspar[12] for this purpose, for they are strong and will not pull out of the muscle as is often the case with the Cloward retractors. A second set of dull-bladed retractors is placed to gain rostral-caudal exposure.

Bone Removal

Bone, disk, and osteophyte removal may be undertaken using the instruments developed by Cloward[13] or a variant of the operation originally described by Robinson and Smith[41] and subsequently adapted by others.[1] We prefer the Smith-Robinson operation, for it allows the bone removal to be tailored to the existing pathology better than the technique described by Cloward.[13]

The disk space is identified, and using a sharp knife blade the anterior longitudinal ligament and anterior annulus are incised and excised. Additional disk is removed using curettes. Bone from the adjacent vertebral bodies is removed using the high-speed air drill. Adequate bone removal appropriate to the location of the osteophytic compression is essential to achieving satisfactory decompression of the spinal cord. Careful examination of the bone windows on the computed tomography (CT) scan is important to define the location and extent of bone removal that will be necessary. In the midcervical spine, the distance from the medial border of the foramen transversarium on one side, to the medial border of the same structure contralaterally, is 3 cm. In general, 2 cm of bone should be removed in a transverse direction (Figure 1). Because this leaves only 5 mm from the most lateral extent of bone removal to the medial border of the foramen trans-

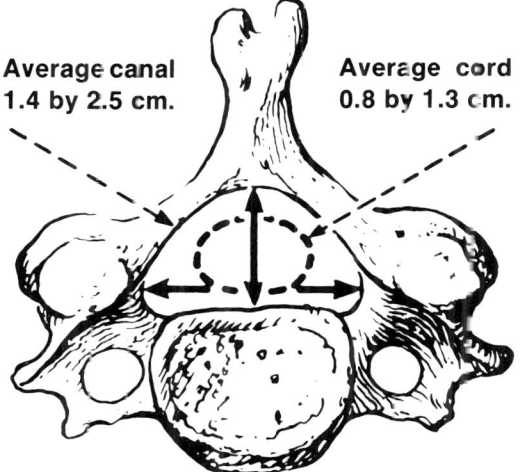

Figure 1. Drawing depicts an axial view of a typical midcervical vertebra. The average transverse diameter of the spinal canal is 2.5 cm. By removing 2 cm of bone in a transverse direction, the spinal cord, which averages 1.3 cm in its transverse diameter, will be well decompressed. Reproduced with permission from Hoff JT, Wilson CB: The pathophysiology of cervical spondylotic radiculopathy and myelopathy. Clin Neurosurg. 1977;24:474-487.

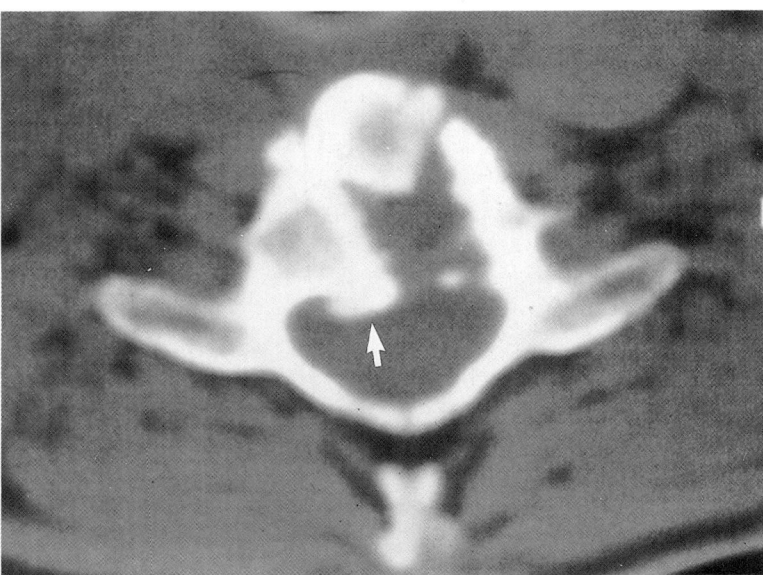

Figure 2. Postoperative CT scan in the axial plane of a patient who underwent anterior cervical decompression and fusion for cervical spondylotic myelopathy. Exposure was obtained from the right side and bone removal was skewed as a result of the surgeon's line of vision, resulting in inadequate osteophyte removal on the right side (arrow).

versarium, the midline must be identified accurately. The midline is usually, but not always, midway between the medial borders of the longus coli muscles; the midline orientation of the longus coli muscles may be distorted by growth of anterior osteophytes. Identification of these same osteophytes on the CT scan also will serve to establish the location of the midline.

The amount of bone drilled in a rostralcaudal direction will be determined by the location of osteophytes in relation to the disk space. The surgeon must be aware that the disk space angles superiorly; by removing bone in a straight anteroposterior direction, more bone will be removed on the superior lip of the vertebra below the disk space and correspondingly less bone will be removed on the inferior lip of the vertebra above the disk space. Thus, it is necessary to direct the bone removal slightly rostrally as the drilling proceeds posteriorly. All cortical bone above and below the disk space should be removed.

The surgeon's line of vision is directed to the contralateral side. Thus, in a right-sided exposure, there is a tendency to remove more bone on the left than on the right. The surgeon must be aware of this and remove adequate amounts of bone on the ipsilateral side. Rotating the operating table toward the surgeon will help expose this "blind" ipsilateral side and avoid asymmetrical bone removal (Figure 2). As the drilling proceeds, further confirmation of bone removal in relation to the midline can be obtained by observing the upward swing of the uncovertebral joints. Bone should be removed to this point but not beyond (Figure 3). As the cortex of the posterior vertebral body and osteophyte are reached, the cutting burr is changed to a diamond burr that will not snag the posterior longitudinal ligament (PLL) or dura. The diamond burr has the disadvantage of removing bone at a much slower rate than the cutting burr; it also produces considerably more heat and should be irrigated continuously.

When the most posteriorly located bone and osteophytes are sufficiently thinned, fine curettes are used to remove the last bits of bone to the edges of the vertebral bodies exposing the PLL. Curettes are preferred to Kerrison[11] rongeurs for this purpose for even

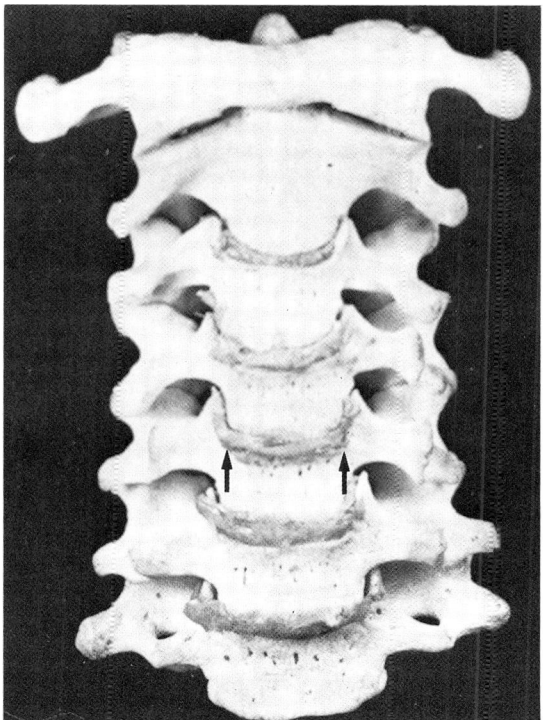

Figure 3. Frontal view of a cervical spine. Arrows depict the most medial border of the uncovertebral joints. Bone should not be removed lateral to this point.

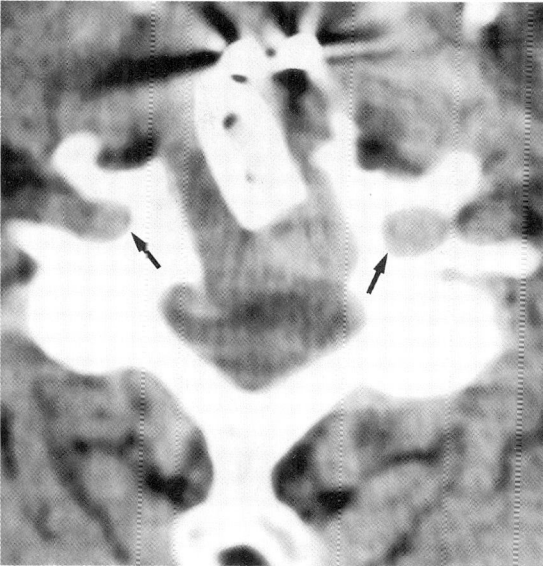

Figure 4. Postoperative CT scan in the axial plane shows wide decompression achieved in a patient with extensive osteophytes. The vertebral artery in the foramen transversarium (arrows) also may be seen to lie anterior to the most posterior portion of the vertebral body and osteophytes. Thus, osteophytes may be removed far laterally without fear of injuring the vertebral artery within the foramen transversarium.

the finest rongeurs take up space within the spinal canal and may injure the spinal cord while there still are osteophytes present. When the intended bone removal is complete, the surgeon should reconnoiter and make certain that adequate decompression has been achieved in all directions. If necessary, additional bone may be removed laterally adjacent to the PLL without fear of injuring the vertebral artery, which now is anterior to this plane (Figure 4). Several authors have stated that osteophyte removal and spinal cord decompression are not necessary[23,41] and fusion of the disk space will result in resorption of ostephytes. There is no valid radiographic evidence that this ever occurs, and it is essential, therefore, that all osteophytes be removed before bone grafting. Although cervical mobility has an adverse effect on the natural history of cervical spondylotic myelopathy,[2] it is unlikely that fusion alone will produce a neurologic result that is superior to decompression followed by infusion. Indeed, a critical reading of series where patients were treated with anterior cervical fusion without an attempt at ostephyte resection reveals that although a high percentage of patients were improved by operation, virtually none were treated for myelopathy and the majority had relief of neck pain or radicular complaints.[23,31]

Although bony compression by osteophytes is responsible for most of the spinal cord compression, spondylosis also results in hypertrophy of the PLL, which in the presence of a narrow spinal canal also can result in compression of the dural tube.[6] Thus, it is important that the PLL be opened and removed to the edge of the bony decompression. The PLL is opened sharply until the shiny white dura mater is exposed. The PLL is a bilayered structure and the most anterior layer may be opened and the posterior layer mistaken for the dura, which may be thought to be adherent to the PLL. However, in previously unoperated patients with spondylosis, the dura is rarely adherent to the PLL. Once all osteophytes are removed, the PLL may be removed safely using fine Kerrison rongeurs. The ligament frequently is vascular, but bleeding is easily controlled using the bipolar cautery at the edges of the ligament.

Bone Grafting

After bony decompression has been achieved, the surgeon must decide whether to use a bone graft. With the extensive amount of bone removal described in previous paragraphs, it is essential that a bone graft be used. If a graft is not placed, disk space collapse with root compression and spinal deformity is likely to occur. With a small amount of bone removal, as may be performed in a patient with herniation of a soft cervical disk, a bone graft may be avoided without any consequence.[19] With time, disk space collapse will occur and spontaneous fusion frequently will take place.

The ideal bone graft "should have structural integrity, be easy to work with, incorporate rapidly, and have a low pseudoarthrosis rate."[3] When a bone graft is employed, the surgeon must decide whether to use bone from the patient's iliac crest or an allograft. Use of allograft avoids the incisional and muscle pain that are inevitable consequences of taking an iliac crest graft. In elderly patients, particularly women, the quality of allograft frequently is better than the patient's own bone. The rate of successful fusion is comparable to that achieved with the patient's own bone, but if one assesses fusion using lateral roentgenograms of the neck, fusion takes longer to occur than is the case with autograft.[40] Transmission of disease such as hepatitis or the human immunodeficiency virus is a theoretical disadvantage of allograft, but the processing of commercially prepared grafts effectively destroys all organisms.

Regardless of the source of the graft, the bone should have at least three cortical surfaces. This assures adequate strength and minimizes the chances of graft collapse. Iliac crest contains three cortical surfaces. Fibular graft contains cortical bone on all its surfaces and resists compression better than iliac crest. Although the authors of one series[3] reported no instances of nonunion with fibula, incorporation of fibular graft may take as long as one to two years and late nonunion and fracturing of a graft that has not been vascularized may occur. In most cases, iliac crest (autogenous or allograft) is a satisfactory graft material. Because of the curve of the iliac crest, graft material from this site frequently is unsatisfactory if three or more vertebral bodies are resected. In this situation, fibula is an ideal material. In most other situations, iliac crest is preferable.

The graft is placed in the area of bone removal so that the cortical surfaces are located anteriorly and laterally. If the graft is too wide to be impacted into place, one lateral cortical surface may be removed using the high-speed air drill. This has the disadvantage of decreasing the strength of the graft and it may be advantageous to widen the area of bone removal of the recipient site to avoid compromising the strength of the graft.

Before the graft is shaped, the Caspar distracting pins[12] are placed in the vertebral bodies above and below the area of bone removal, and the vertebrae are distracted 2-3 mm. The exact amount of distraction achieved may be determined by using the Caspar measuring calipers to measure the space before and after distraction is begun. The Caspar distraction device is powerful and it is easy to overdistract the vertebrae, a maneuver that may produce increased neck pain in the postoperative period.

After distraction is achieved, the measuring calipers are used to determine the rostral-caudal dimensions of the bone graft. The depth of the vertebral bodies adjacent to the graft is measured and the depth of the graft is determined accordingly. A graft 13-14 mm deep will provide sufficient strength and will be well away from the dura in most adult patients even with slight countersinking. It is essential that the contours of the graft exactly match the contours of the recipient site. If too much bone has been removed from one side of the graft, the graft will rotate toward this side as it is impacted into place and the position of the graft will be less than optimal. The graft should be impacted into place with gentle tapping of the impactor using the hammer. As the final position of the graft is reached, one-half of the impactor should overlap the adjacent vertebral body. This will prevent the graft from being pushed against the spinal cord if the graft should suddenly "give" or if impaction is excessively vigorous. The cortical bone of the anterior surface of the graft should be slightly countersunk or even with the cortical bone of the adjacent vertebrae. This will ensure that the stronger cortical bone of the graft resists flexion and axial loading. If the graft is not impacted to a sufficient depth, repetitive flexion and axial loading that occur in the postoperative period despite the use of external orthoses, will cause the graft to collapse and the spine to deform.

Closure and Postoperative Management

After the bone graft is placed, retractors are removed and the wound is inspected for bleeding from soft tissues. A Jackson-Pratt drain is left in the prevertebral space and brought out through a stab wound adjacent to the incision. The platysma muscle is closed with absorbable suture material and a subcuticular suture is placed. The skin is closed with adhesive paper strips. The drain is removed 24 hours after operation.

A Philadelphia collar is worn for 10-12 weeks following operation except when the patient is in bed. Lateral cervical spine x-rays are taken before the patient is discharged from the hospital, two weeks later, and again just before the collar is removed to be certain that the graft is not extruding and the spine is not angulating at the site of bone removal. After the collar is removed, the patient may gradually resume normal activities.

Corpectomy

In patients with extensive osteophyte formation at adjacent levels, corpectomy, or removal of an entire vertebral body, has been proposed as an alternative to osteophyte removal and the placement of two or more bone grafts.[26,40,43-45] This procedure has the advantage of assuring a more complete decompression. There are fewer surfaces at which fusion must take place and the decompression is not compromised by having to leave a thin piece of bone between two adjacent areas of decompression. Moreover, there is no concern that impacting the graft will result in fracturing of the remaining bone between two adjacent levels of decompression. Although the complication rate is reported to be low in some series,[46] the procedure is more extensive than simple osteophytectomy and others[44] have reported a perioperative complication rate of almost 50%.

Adjunctive Instrumentation

The use of anterior cervical plating rarely is necessary as an adjunct to bone grafting in the patient who undergoes removal of osteophytes followed by bone grafting. Instability as a result of bone removal in this situation is unusual and bone graft dislodgement rarely is seen. Anterior cervical plating may be indicated in the patient with preoperative plain-film evidence of subluxation and abnormal movement as a result of the spondylotic process.

In a patient with extensive osteophytes at adjacent disk levels who requires corpectomy, the bone graft is by necessity larger than is the case when multiple adjacent decompressions are performed. With the larger grafts that are inserted for corpectomy, the risk of bone-graft dislodgement is significant. Although this risk may be minimized with "notching" of the vertebrae adjacent to the graft, graft dislodgement may be confidently prevented with the use of an anterior cervical plate and screws.[12]

Complications

Complications resulting from anterior cervical decompression and fusion for spondylotic myelopathy may be divided into three types: (1) injuries to the spinal cord or cervical nerve roots producing new neurologic deficit or exacerbating pre-existing deficit, (2) injuries to the soft tissues or vascular structures of the neck, and (3) mishaps related to the bone graft.

Injuries to the Spinal Cord or Nerve Roots

Incidence

Injuries to the spinal cord or nerve roots after anterior cervical surgery fortunately are unusual. The exact incidence is difficult to ascertain, however. Flynn[21] queried 1,358 neurosurgeons and received replies from just over half. More than 70% of those who replied reported no neurologic complications in a total of 45,457 cases. This figure is not believable and one must wonder whether some of the reporting surgeons had bad memories or were not especially observant. The remaining surgeons reported 311 myelopathic complications in 36,657 patients, an incidence of approximately 0.1%. In another report of a series of patients compiled from a single institution,[6] pre-existing myelopathy worsened in 8.5% of patients. No patient without pre-existing myelopathy developed new neurologic signs. Overall, 3.3% of 450 patients experienced worsening of myelopathy and 1.3% of patients developed additional radicular symptoms. The 3.3% incidence of increased deficit probably is higher than that noted by most neurosurgeons but probably is closer to the real incidence than the figure given by Flynn.[21]

Etiology of Neurologic Deficit

Neurologic complications may be divided into those in which new deficit is apparent immediately after the patient awakens from surgery and those that are not present immediately after surgery but appear in the first 24 hours. Over three-quarters of the myelopathic complications reported by Flynn[21] were the immediate type.

When a patient awakens immediately after operation with new neurologic deficit, neural structures have been injured during the induction of anesthesia, during positioning, or by direct injury to the spinal cord or nerve roots by the surgeon. In a patient with pre-existing myelopathy and a narrow spinal canal, the anesthesiologist must be cautioned to avoid all rapid movements of the neck. Awake intubation has been proposed so that spinal cord function can be monitored in the immediate postintubation period.[47]

Although extension of the neck during the performance of surgery facilitates exposure, this position may cause the hypertrophied ligamentum flavum to buckle inward and compress the spinal cord.[47] In the vast majority of patients who awaken from surgery with increased neurologic deficit, it is likely that the spinal cord or nerve roots have been injured during some aspect of the decompression. Bertalanffy and Eggert[6] reported dural perforation and "jerking of the limbs" in a patient who awoke with markedly increased deficit. Most of the time, however, the surgeon cannot recall producing trauma to the spinal cord.[6,21]

Because the spinal cord already is severely compressed and its function compromised in patients with spondylosis, even small amounts of additional compression may produce spinal cord injury. A crucial part of the operation entails removal of the most posterior portions of bone, osteophyte, disk and the posterior longitudinal ligament. Although some orthopedic surgeons[33] have advocated leaving osteophytes in place to minimize the risk to the spinal cord, this strategy ignores the basic pathogenesis of spondylotic myelopathy and makes little sense. Moreover, the statement that "a significant percentage of those [osteophytes] will resorb postoperative in the presence of a stable interbody fusion"[33] has no basis in fact.

The following "dos and don'ts" may be helpful in minimizing spinal cord trauma: (1) When cortical bone of the posterior vertebral body is visualized, change from a cutting burr to a diamond one to minimize the chances of the burr catching soft tissue or tearing the dura; (2) frequently assess the thickness and location of residual bone and osteophytes using small curettes; (3) never use the drill on osteophytes or bone that is movable; (4) remove loose bone fragments and the last thin shelf of bone with fine curettes; (5) never use rongeurs to remove bone or osteophytes, for even the thinnest-lipped instruments take up space in a narrowed spinal canal where the spinal cord already is compressed; and (6) fragments of bone or osteophytes that are particularly large and adherent to the posterior longitudinal ligament should be removed with the ligament.

The spinal cord also may be injured during placement of the bone graft. Although a graft depth of 13-14 mm in almost all adult patients will provide an adequate margin of safety even with slight countersinking of the graft, the depth of the vertebral body varies and should be measured before placing the bone graft.

Root injury is less common than spinal cord injury; its mechanism probably is direct trauma. For reasons that are not clear, the C5 root is extremely sensitive to trauma. Saunders and others[44] reported a 12.5% incidence of C5 root dysfunction usually occurring two days after corpectomy in patients with spondylotic myelopathy. Fortunately, complete resolution occurred in most patients several months after surgery. We recently have seen one patient who developed C5 root dysfunction after graft collapse. Unless there has been avulsion of the root, most patients recover function over a period of months.

The reasons for the appearance of delayed neurologic deficit generally are more apparent than is the case for immediate deficit. Postoperative epidural hematomas causing neurologic deterioration have been described by U and Wilson[49] and others.[6] In two of the cases reported by U and Wilson, the patient was initially well in the recovery room only to develop the rapid onset of myelopathy. A third patient awoke from anesthesia with severe myelopathy. At re-exploration, each patient had significant extradural hematoma caused by arterial bleeding from the edge of the resected PLL. The authors emphasized that prompt evacuation without delaying to perform diagnostic studies was the most likely reason that none of their patients had a permanent increase in neurologic deficit. Unfortunately, patients in one other reported series had incomplete resolution of their symptoms.[47]

Delayed deficit also has been seen as a result of combined epidural abscess and hematoma.[6] Although the time course of the appearance of neurologic deficit was not given, it is likely that epidural sepsis produces deficit that will be delayed by many days.

Management

In the rare patient known to have had injury to the spinal cord as a result of contusion during the decompressive procedure, re-exploration is not indicated. Such patients should be treated with high doses of methylprednisolone according to a previously published protocol.[10]

In all other patients, including those who awaken with increased deficit and those who are neurologically intact but develop the rapid onset of deficit in the first hours after operation, immediate re-operation is indicated. High doses of corticosteroids should be given intravenously. While waiting for the operating room to be readied, a lateral cervical spine film should be taken to ascertain that operation was performed at the correct level, that angulation of the cervical spine has not occurred, and that the bone graft has not migrated posteriorly against the spinal cord or anteriorly into the soft tissues of the neck.

At re-exploration, the graft should be removed so that the epidural space may be inspected. Any extradural hematoma is removed and bleeding is controlled; the posterior longitudinal ligament is resected to the edges of the bone removal if this has not already been done. A careful search should be made for fragments of osteophyte or soft disk that may not have been removed at the initial operation. The graft is replaced and the wound is closed in routine fashion.

Injuries to Soft Tissue and Vascular Structures of the Neck

Dural Tears and Cerebrospinal Fluid Fistula

Dural tears from injury with the high-speed air drill or curettes may occur during the last stages of bone removal. This complication may be minimized by using the diamond burr rather than the cutting one as the posterior longitudinal ligament is approached, and leaving the posterior longitudinal ligament intact until drilling is concluded. Dural laceration is more likely to occur when drilling is carried out far laterally where the posterior longitudinal ligament is especially thin.

Direct repair of a dural tear generally is not feasible. The hole should be covered with a piece of gelatin foam or muscle. The patient is placed on spinal drainage at the termination of the procedure; the drainage is continued for 4-5 days postoperatively.

Vascular Structures

Injuries to the carotid and vertebral arteries in the neck fortunately are rare. Carotid artery injury most frequently occurs as a result of penetration by the sharp blades of the self-retaining retractor[52] or during the initial soft-tissue dissection in the neck. The latter complication is easily avoided by palpating the carotid artery immediately after the platysma muscle is divided, and placing a hand-held retractor medial to the carotid artery, which then is retracted laterally. Penetration or injury of the carotid artery by the blades of the retractor may be avoided by sufficient removal of the longus coli muscles off the anterior aspect of the vertebral bodies. This will enable the retractor blades to fit beneath the medial borders of the longus coli muscles and make it less likely that the retractor will dislodge and lie against the carotid artery.

Injury to the vertebral artery in the foramen transversarium is unusual but can occur if bone removal is asymmetric and carried too far laterally.[15] In a right-sided approach, the left vertebral artery is the most likely to be injured, for the surgeon's visualization is better on the left, and more bone frequently is removed on the left than on the right. It is difficult to injure the vertebral artery during the soft-tissue dissection because it lies within the bony confines of the foramen transversarium. However, on one occasion, an inexperienced resident at this author's institution injured the vertebral artery by dissecting too far laterally puncturing the vertebral artery between the foramen transversaria of two adjacent vertebral bodies.

Recurrent Laryngeal Nerve

Postoperative voice changes have been reported in 11% of patients undergoing anterior cervical surgery.[29] One must keep in mind, however, that not every patient who awakens with hoarseness has sustained an injury to the recurrent laryngeal nerve. Retraction of the intubated trachea during soft-tissue dissection can cause edema to the vocal cords, resulting in postoperative voice changes.[11,48] This is probably the most common cause of hoarseness and almost always will clear within a few days of surgery. Injury to the recurrent laryngeal nerve can be reliably assumed to have occurred if there is paralysis of a vocal cord on indirect laryngoscopic examination. Cloward[14] reported an incidence of less than 0.5% in a series of 850 anterior cervical operations. In each case, the paralysis was temporary and the patient's voice returned to normal in 3-5 weeks. An incidence of recurrent laryngeal nerve injury of 0.1% to 1% has been reported by others.[6,11,21]

Heeneman[29] has summarized the possible etiologies of recurrent laryngeal nerve injury: (1) division of the nerve during dissection, (2) pinching of the nerves by retractor blades, (3) overstretching of the nerve, (4) postoperative edema of the perineural tissues, (5) nerve included in a ligature, and (6) direct long-standing pressure on the nerve by retractor blades. Injury also may occur as a result of endotracheal intubation,[11] causing compression of the nerve between the thyroid and the cuff of the tube as the branch passes under the mucosa of the larynx.

Bulger and others[11] have emphasized that recurrent laryngeal nerve injury is more likely to occur during a right-sided approach, for the right inferior laryngeal nerve does not recur approximately 1% of the time and is vulnerable to injury as it passes directly into the larynx from the main trunk of the vagus nerve. On the left side, failure of the inferior laryngeal nerve to recur is rare and injury is less likely. Cloward[14] reported that injury always occurred at the sixth to seventh cervical levels in his series of patients with disk lesions. Six of nine injuries occurred in this location in Heeneman's series.[29]

Although recurrent laryngeal nerve injury is unusual and permanent dysfunction is rare, the risk of damage may be minimized by taking into account the following: (1) Recurrent nerve injury is most likely to occur in operations at lower cervical levels; (2) anatomic variation is more common on the right than the left and no structures should be cut until it is absolutely clear that they do not represent aberrant nerves; and (3) sharp retractor blades must remain positioned at all times beneath the longus coli muscles.

Cervical Sympathetic Chain Injury

Injury to the cervical sympathetic chain is an unusual complication manifested by a Horner's Syndrome on the side of the injury. Injury occurs as a result of inadvertent stretching or transection of the sympathetic chain lateral to the longus coli muscles.[25,48] This injury may be avoided by confining dissection to the area medial to the lateral insertion of the longus coli muscles.

Esophageal Injury

Esophageal injury is a rare but potentially lethal complication of the anterior cervical approach. In one large series, there was only one injury in 450 consecutive operations.[6] This occurred during dissection in the upper part of the cervical spine where the hypopharynx tends to be thinner than the more caudally located esophagus. In its location just anterior to the cervical vertebral bodies, the esophagus is vulnerable to injury during the initial soft-tissue dissection if it is mistaken for the strap muscles. It also may be injured by the sharp blades of the self-retaining retractor if these are not securely seated beneath the longus coli muscles. Even when initially placed in their intended location, the blades may dislodge and perforate the esophagus. The position of the retractor blades should, therefore, be inspected from time to time during the decompressive portions of the operation, and repositioned as necessary to avoid esophageal injury. Esophageal perforation by retractor blades also may be minimized by filing the blades to blunt points.[48]

Before closure, the esophagus should be inspected to make certain that occult perforation has not occurred. If it has, a three-layer closure should be performed and the patient should not be allowed to eat or drink for 7-10 days until healing has taken place. Failure to recognize perforation will lead to wound infection and an esophagocutaneous fistula. Esophageal injury in the lower cervical region may result in mediastinitis with high fever and mediastinal widening on chest roentgenograms. Even with treatment with wound drainage, antibiotics, and cervical esophagostomy, this complication has a high mortality.

Graft Complications

In a poll of the members of the Cervical

Spine Research Society, the overall incidence of graft complications from anterior cervical surgery between 1982 and 1986 averaged 1.64%.[25] This figure presumably includes graft collapse, graft displacement, and graft nonunion. This incidence seems particularly low and the figure must remain suspect for only a fraction of the membership reported complications. Indeed, the reported incidence of nonfusion alone in most series is greater than the total incidence of all graft complications reported by the Cervical Spine Research Society members.

Graft Displacement

Graft extrusion is not uncommon in patients who undergo vertebrectomy and who have unstable spines as a result of trauma. It is infrequently seen in patients with spondylosis because their spines usually are stable and the amount of bone removed generally is less than is the case in patients who undergo grafting for traumatic lesions. In a group of patients who underwent corpectomy and the placement of bone grafts for spondylosis, the incidence of graft extrusion was only 2.5%.[44] On the other hand, Aronson and coauthors[1] reported an 8% incidence of graft extrusion requiring reoperation in a series of patients treated for disk herniation and spondylosis.

Graft extrusion may be minimized by distraction of the adjacent vertebral bodies using the Caspar instrumentation. Relaxation of the distraction apparatus after the graft has been hammered into place usually will result in firm impaction of the graft against the adjacent vertebral bodies and will make extrusion unlikely.

Extrusion also may be minimized by slightly countersinking the graft so that the anterior cortical surface of the graft is just below the anterior surface of the adjacent vertebral bodies. The graft must be shaped so that there is excellent contact between the entire rostral and caudal surfaces of the graft and the adjacent vertebral bodies. If the graft is unevenly contoured and there is apposition between the graft and only a small portion of the adjacent vertebra, the graft is more likely to rotate and extrude. Graft extrusion may be further minimized by notching the graft and adjacent vertebral bodies.[23]

Although we ask all patients to wear cervical orthosis postoperatively, the actual amount of restriction of movement provided by such devices is minimal; the collar probably serves more than anything else as a reminder to the patient to avoid excessive neck movement.

Partial graft extrusion usually does not require reoperation unless there is pseudarthrosis, angulation at the grafted interspace, or the position of the graft interferes with swallowing. With time, the portions of the graft anterior to the interspace will resorb in most patients.

Displacement of the graft against the spinal cord is a rare complication that may produce severe neurologic deficit. It may occur from overvigorous hammering during impaction with sudden slip of the graft posteriorly, or as a delayed complication in the days following operation from a graft that did not fit tightly against adjacent vertebrae. Although compression of the spinal cord by a graft that is too large in its anteroposterior dimension is not, strictly speaking, posterior displacement, its occurrence will have the same effect as posterior displacement (Figure 5). Careful measurement of the depth of the graft and recipient site will preclude this disastrous complication.

Graft Collapse

Graft collapse is most likely to occur in elderly patients with osteoporotic bone (Figure 6). If there is any doubt about the integrity of the bone graft, an allograft should be used. Hammering too hard on the graft during impaction also may result in fracture or weakening of the graft that is not immediately apparent.[14] Graft collapse also may be minimized by impacting the graft sufficiently deep so that the anterior cortical bone of the graft is even with or deep to the cortical bone of the adjacent bodies. If the cortical

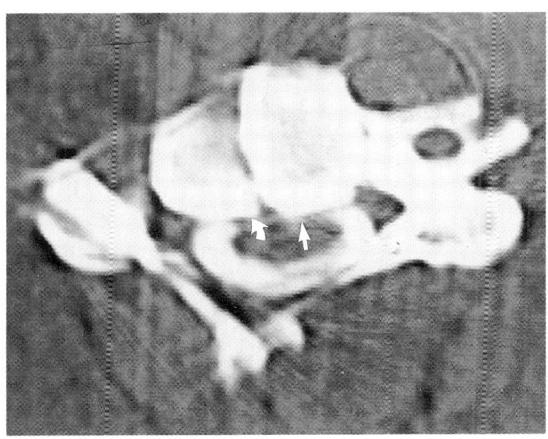

Figure 5. Postmyelogram/CT scan shows spinal cord compression by a graft that was too large (straight arrow). Note also persistent spinal cord compression by retropulsed vertebral body (curved arrow) in this patient who was treated for cervical spine trauma.

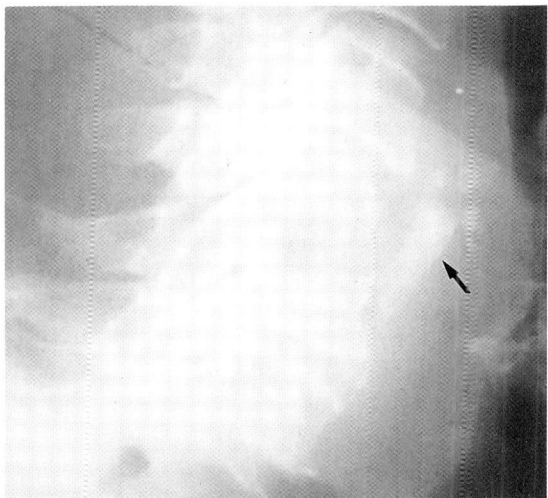

Figure 6. Lateral x-ray of the cervical spine in an elderly woman who underwent anterior cervical decompression and fusion with iliac crest autograft for several spondylotic myelopathy. She suddenly developed bilateral C5 radiculopathy several days after operation. X-ray shows collapse and fragmentation of the graft (arrow). The graft was replaced with an iliac crest allograft, with complete resolution of her radiculopathy 3 months later.

graft and the cortex on the sides of a tricortical iliac crest graft.

Grafts also may collapse as a result of resorption. If the patient remains asymptomatic, as is most often the case, operation is not indicated. Revision is indicated when resorption results in chronic neck pain, progressive spinal deformity, or exacerbation of neurologic deficit.

Graft Nonunion

Graft nonunion or pseudarthrosis may result from insufficient area of contact between the graft ends and recipient site, the interposition of foreign body such as bone wax between graft and adjacent vertebral body, or excessive movement between the graft and vertebral body. The incidence of graft nonunion is more common in patients who have had decompression at multiple levels. A 5% incidence of nonunion for grafts at a single level and 15% for grafts at multiple levels has been reported.[25] There is, however, no relationship betwen the adequacy of fusion and the clinical result.[48] Aronson and coauthors[1] reported an incidence of 4%, but only 0.8% of patients in their series were symptomatic.

Radiographic evidence of nonunion is not uncommon. It may simply be a question of insufficient time from operation to radiographic evaluation. For example, some grafts (all fibular grafts and iliac crest allografts) may take longer to show radiographic evidence of incorporation; evaluation at 12 weeks after surgery will not show fusion. Moreover, plain radiographs cannot show fusion that has occurred over small areas of the graft/vertebral body interface but that may provide quite adequate stability.

Movement between the graft and vertebra on flexion-extension radiographs is a better way to assess pseudarthrosis. Fusion failure commonly produces no symptoms and its existence may be ignored. However, the presence of persistent neck pain, progressive angulation, or subluxation mandate graft revision.

bone of the graft remains anterior to the adjacent vertebrae, collapse is resisted only by the weaker cancellous portions of the bone

Outcome

Results of anterior cervical decompression reported in the literature are difficult to interpret for a variety of reasons: (1) Series often include patients treated for both radiculopathy and myelopathy and, in some cases, neck pain; (2) there is frequently failure to distinguish myelopathy caused by soft disk herniation and bony osteophytes; (3) preoperative neurologic deficit is poorly characterized and outcome is not clearly defined in terms of return to work or residual neurologic deficit; (4) the relationship of outcome to factors such as age, duration of symptoms, the severity of preoperative deficit, or levels treated is not specified; and (5) the duration of followup is too short to obtain a meaningful idea of the efficacy of the procedure.

This author and others[9,45] believe that residual spinal cord compression due to the presence of residual osteophytes is an important cause of persistent neurologic deficit. Despite this, there is no study relating outcome to the adequacy of decompression. In the ensuing section, the relationship of neurologic improvement to the epidemiologic and demographic characteristics of patients with cervical spondylotic myelopathy and the nature of the procedure performed, will be examined in an attempt to delineate those factors that are important in determining outcome.

Type of Procedure

Anterior Cervical Diskectomy and Interbody Fusion

For the purposes of this discussion, anterior cervical diskectomy and interbody fusion refer to decompression confined to the area adjacent to the disk space followed by interbody fusion using bone graft.

In the operation described by Robinson and Smith,[41] neither osteophytes nor the posterior longitudinal ligament were removed. Bohlman[7] reported improvement in 16 of 17 patients treated with the Smith-Robinson technique in which no attempt was made to remove osteophytes. Despite this report, it is likely that long-term outcome has not been satisfactory in patients who have not had osteophyte removal and this author now is quoted as recommending more extensive decompression.[52]

Jomin and coauthors[31] reported the results of anterior decompression in patients who were treated, for the most part, using the technique described by Cloward.[13] Although the exact treatment of osteophytes and the PLL was not specifically stated, Cloward advocated removal of compressive osteophytes. Of patients with myelopathy without radiculopathy, 5% experienced complete recovery, 35% were improved, and 56% were stabilized. Of patients with a combined radiculopathy and myelopathy, the myelopathy was completely relieved in 12%, improved in 60%, and stabilized in 25%. Other authors have reported a rate of improvement ranging from 64% to 82% using Cloward's technique.[5,16,17,27,28,39] Mann and others[36] managed a series of 50 patients utilizing a variation of Cloward's technique. All experienced improvement of at least one neurologic grade.

Galera and Tovi[22] used the Cloward technique, and noted only a 39% improvement rate in their series and a disturbing number of patients who experienced deterioration with long-term follow-up. The implications of a low initial improvement rate and long-term deterioration in this last series is that decompression was inadequate to relieve all spinal cord compression.

Lunsford et al[35] reported that 50% of patients deteriorated or were made worse by anterior operation in which a variety of techniques was utilized.

Anterior Decompression Without Bone Grafting

Anterior cervical decompression without bone grafting has the advantage of shortening operative time and eliminating donor-site complications. In 70% of patients, spontaneous fusion takes place.[26] In the event that the adjacent vertebral bodies do not fuse, movement will be preserved and less stress will be placed on adjacent motion segments. This method may be most appropriate in patients when less extensive bone removal is sufficient to achieve decompression.[9,36] In these instances, angulation and significant movement at the operative site are unusual.[18,54] Bertalanffy and Eggert[4] reported an insignificant mean kyphotic angulation of 4.8° in 450 patients who had anterior diskectomy without fusion.

The use of a graft reduces the incidence of kyphotic deformity, if a large amount of bone removal is necessary because of extensive osteophyte formation. In addition, by preventing collapse of the disk space and preserving the height of the neural foramina, the risk of root compression in the postoperative period is minimized. In one series, 6 of 10 patients who did not have fusion developed neck and arm pain postoperatively.[32] In another series, however, no patient was reported to have postoperative neck pain.[37] Although successful fusion will not result in resorption of osteophytes,[4] if osteophytes are not completely removed, the spinal cord may be less likely to be traumatized by residual osteophytes at the fused motion segment.

The outcome of patients reported in the literature who underwent anterior cervical decompression without fusion probably is comparable to those who are fused, although few series include patients who were treated both with and without fusion. In a prospective series reported by Martins,[37] the percentage of good and excellent results was virtually identical in patients who underwent fusion and those who did not. Kadoya and coauthors[32] found no difference in improvement from myelopathy in patients treated with and without fusion. Nearly identical outcomes in fused and unfused patients were reported in a series treated by Lunsford and others[34] for lateral cervical disk herniations. In a prospective study, Rosenørn and coauthors[42] found a statistically significant increase in excellent results, in patients who did not have fusion compared to those who did. However, when patients with good and excellent results were combined, there was no significant difference between fused and unfused patients.

It is difficult to make sense of this data. When the results of operations in comparable patients are reviewed, the most important factor in determining outcome probably is the adequacy of spinal cord decompression. If decompression can be achieved with only a small amount of bone removal, then decompression without fusion is a reasonable strategy. However, if bone removal is extensive, as may be necessary in patients with spondylosis, fusion is indicated to prevent late kyphotic deformity and instability.

Anterior Decompression Utilizing Corpectomy

The proponents of corpectomy believe that a more radical bone removal will produce a better decompression, and neurologic results superior to that achieved using more conventional techniques of osteophytectomy.

In a series of 72 patients treated by Saunders and coauthors[44] for spondylotic myelopathy, 39 had no signs or myelopathic symptoms postoperatively. Twenty-one of these 39 had severe myelopathy preoperatively. Only 9 patients were considered treatment failures. Similar excellent results were achieved by Seifert and Stolke.[45] Of 19 patients with severe myelopathy, 14 were symptom-free or had only minor residual symptoms. These authors believed that multilevel osteophytectomy frequently results in incomplete decompression of the spinal cord and that incomplete removal of bony compressive lesions is responsible for the high rate of unsatisfactory recovery in many reported series. A number of other authors have reported improvement in 73% to 100% of patients treated with corpectomy for cervical spondylotic myelopathy.[3,8,28,46,53] In a series comparing corpectomy, the Cloward procedure, and the Smith-Robinson operation, good results were achieved with all 3 operations and none was superior to the others when results were analyzed.[30] However, Yonenobu and coauthors[55] found that subtotal spondylectomy produced results that were significantly superior to that achieved by either the Cloward or Smith-Robinson techniques.

Demographic and Epidemiologic Factors

Although there is a general perception that younger patients, those with shorter histories of symptoms, and those with less severe myelopathy are most likely to benefit from operations, the data in the literature supporting this is hard to come by. This is so because in the majority of series reported in the literature, operation was performed for neck pain or radiculopathy. In some series where operation was performed for multiple indications, the results are not classified according to the initial indication for operation. In one such mixed series, a good functional result was significantly more frequent in male patients compared to females (50% versus 38%), in patients less than 40 years old compared to those between the ages of 41 and 59 (63% versus 40%), when symptoms appeared acutely rather than gradually (51% versus 42%), and when the duration of symptoms was less than 6 months as opposed to greater than 1 year (56% versus 38%).[20] Unfortunately, most of the patients had radicular signs and symptoms. Thus, the clinical parameters examined may not be applicable to patients with myelopathy.

Hukuda and coauthors[30] examined similar parameters in a series of 269 patients, all of whom had cervical spondylotic myelopathy. Patients below the age of 50 had better neurologic function both before and after surgery. Thus, the less favorable results in the older patient might be due to more advanced disease and not to their age. Patients who had operations within 1 year of the onset of symptoms fared better compared to those who had symptoms for more than 1 year. This was true regardless of the age of the patient. Bertalanffy and Eggert[5] confirmed the detrimental effect of the following factors on outcome: age greater than 50 years, a duration of symptoms greater than 12 months, and multiple-level involvement.

References

1. Aronson N, Filtzer DL, Bagan M. Anterior cervical fusion by the Smith-Robinson approach. *J Neurosurg.* 1968;29:397-404.
2. Barnes MP, Saunders M. The effect of cervical mobility on the natural history of cervical spondylotic myelopathy. *J Neurol Neurosurg Psychiatry.* 1984;47:17-20.
3. Bernard TN Jr, Whitecloud TS III. Cervical spondylotic myelopathy and myeloradiculopathy: anterior decompression and stabilization with autogenous fibula strut graft. *Clin Orthop.* 1987;221:149-160.
4. Bertalanffy H, Eggert H-R. Anterior discectomy without fusion for treatment of cervical degenerative disc disease. In: Louis R, Weidner A, eds. *Cervical Spine II.* New York, NY: Springer-Verlag; 1988:208-215.
5. Bertalanffy H, Eggert H-R. Clinical long-term results of anterior discectomy without fusion for treatment of cervical radiculopathy and myelopathy: a follow-up of 164 cases. *Acta Neurochir (Wien).* 1988;90:127-135.
6. Bertalanffy H, Eggert H-R. Complications of anterior cervical discectomy without fusion in 450 consecutive patients. *Acta Neurochir (Wien).* 1989;99:41-50.
7. Bohlman HH. Cervical spondylosis with moderate to severe myelopathy: a report of seventeen cases treated by Robinson anterior cervical discectomy and fusion. *Spine.* 1977;2:151-162.
8. Boni M, Cherubino P, Denaro V, et al. Multiple subtotal somatectomy: techniques and evaluation of a series of 39 cases. *Spine.* 1984;9:358-362.
9. Braakman R. Cervical spondylotic myelopathy. *Adv Tech Stand Neurosurg.* 1979;6:137-169.
10. Bracken MB, Shepard MJ, Collins WF, et al. A randomized, controlled trial of methylprednisolone or naloxone in the treatment of acute spinal-cord injury. Results of the Second National Acute Spinal Cord Injury Study. *N Engl J Med.* 1990;322:1405-1411.
11. Bulger RF, Rejowski JE, Beatty RA. Vocal cord paralysis associated with anterior cervical fusion: considerations for prevention and treatment. *J Neurosurg.* 1985;62:557-661.
12. Caspar W, Barbier DD, Klara PM. Anterior cervical fusion and Caspar plate stabilization for cervical trauma. *Neurosurgery.* 1989;25:491-502.
13. Cloward RB. The anterior approach for removal of ruptured cervical disks. *J Neurosurg.* 1958;15:602-614.
14. Cloward RB. Complications of anterior cervical disc operation and their treatment. *Surgery.* 1971;69:175-182.
15. Cosgrove GR, Théron J. Vertebral arteriovenous fistula following anterior cervical spine surgery: report of two cases. *J Neurosurg.* 1987;66:297-299.
16. Crandall PH, Batzdorf U. Cervical spondylotic myelopathy. *J Neurosurg.* 1966;25:57-66.

17. Dereymaeker A, Ghosez J-P, Henkes R. Le traitement chirurgical de la discopathie cervicale: résultats comparés de l'abord postérieur (laminectomie) et de l'abord ventral (fusion corporéale), dans une cinquantaine de cas personnels. *Neurochirurgie.* 1963;9 13-20.
18. de Tribolet N, Zander E. Anterior discectomy without fusion for the treatment of ruptured cervical discs. *J Neurosurg Sci.* 1981;25:217-220.
19. Dunsker SB. Anterior cervical discectomy with and without fusion. *Clin Neurosurg.* 1977;24:516-521.
20. Eriksen EF, Buhl M, Fode K, et al. Treatment of cervical disc disease using Cloward's technique: the prognostic value of clinical preoperative data in 1,106 patients. *Acta Neurochir (Wien).* 1984;70: 181-197.
21. Flynn TB. Neurological complications of anterior cervical interbody fusion. *Spine.* 1982;7:536-539.
22. Galera R, Tovi D. Anterior disc excision with interbody fusion in cervical spondylotic myelopathy and rhizopathy. *J Neurosurg.* 1968;28:305-310.
23. Gore DR. Technique of cervical interbody fusion. *Clin Orthop.* 1984;188:191-195.
24. Gore DR, Sepic SB. Anterior cervical fusion for degenerated or protruded discs: a review of one hundred forty-six patients. *Spine.* 1984;9:667-671.
25. Graham JJ. Complications of cervical spine surgery. In: The Cervical Spine Research Society Editorial Committee, eds. *The Cervical Spine.* 2nd ed. Philadelphia, Pa: JB Lippincott Co; 1989:831-837.
26. Griscli F, Graziani N, Fabrizi AP et al. Anterior discectomy without fusion for treatment of cervical lateral soft disc extrusion: a follow-up of 120 cases. *Neurosurgery.* 1989;24:853-859.
27. Guidetti B, Fortuna A. Long-term results of surgical treatment of myelopathy due to cervical spondylosis. *J Neurosurg.* 1969;30:714-721.
28. Hanai K, Fujiyoshi F, Kamei K. Subtotal vertebrectomy and spinal fusion for cervical spondylotic myelopathy. *Spine.* 1986;11:310-315.
29. Heeneman H. Vocal cord paralysis following approaches to the anterior cervical spine. *Laryngoscope.* 1973;83:17-21.
30. Hukuda S, Mochizuki T, Ogata M, et al. Operations for cervical spondylotic myelopathy: a comparison of the results of anterior and posterior procedures. *J Bone Joint Surg Br.* 1985;67B:609-615.
31. Jomin M, Lesoin F, Lozes G, et al. Herniated cervical discs: analysis of a series of 230 cases. *Acta Neurochir (Wien).* 1986;79:107-113.
32. Kadoya S, Nakamura T, Kwak R. A microsurgical anterior osteophytectomy for cervical spondylotic myelopathy. *Spine.* 1984;9:437-441.
33. Kraus DR, Stauffer ES. Spinal cord injury as a complication of elective anterior cervical fusion. *Clin Orthop.* 1975;112:130-141.
34. Lunsford D, Bissonnette DJ, Janetta PJ, et al Anterior surgery for cervical disc disease, I: treatment of lateral cervical disc herniation in 253 cases *J Neurosurg.* 1980;53:1-11.
35. Lunsford LD, Bissonette DJ, Zorub DS. Anterior surgery for cervical disc disease, II: treatment of cervical spondylotic myelopathy in 32 cases. *J Neurosurg.* 1980;53:12-19.
36. Mann KS, Khosla VK, Gulati DR. Cervical spondylotic myelopathy treated by single-stage multilevel anterior decompression: a prospective study. 1984; 60:81-87.
37. Martins AN. Anterior cervical discectomy with and without interbody bone graft. *J Neurosurg* 1976;44: 290-295.
38. Moussa AH, Nitta M, Symon L. The results of anterior cervical fusion in cervical spondylosis: review of 125 cases. *Acta Neurochir (Wien).* 1983; 68:277-288.
39. Phillips DG. Surgical treatment of myelopathy with cervical spondylosis. *J Neurol Neurosurg Psychiatry.* 1973;36:879-884.
40. Rengachary SS, Redford JB. Partial median corpectomy for cervical spondylotic myelopathy. In: Wilkins R, Rengachary SS, eds. *Neurosurgery Update II.* New York, NY: McGraw-Hill; 1991:356-359.
41. Robinson RA, Smith GW. Anterolateral cervical disc removal and interbody fusion for cervical disc syndrome. *Bull Johns Hopkins Hosp* 1955;96: 223-224. Abstract.
42. Rosenørn J, Hansen EB, Rosenørn MA. Anterior cervical discectomy with and without fusion a prospective study. *J Neurosurg.* 1983;59:252-255
43. Saunders RL. Anterior reconstructive procedures in cervical spondylotic myelopathy. *Clin Neurosurg.* 1991;37:682-721.
44. Saunders RL, Bernini PM, Shirreffs TG Jr, et al. Central corpectomy for cervical spondylotic myelopathy: a consecutive series with long-term follow-up evaluation. *J Neurosurg.* 1991;74:163-170.
45. Seifert V, Stolke D. Multisegmental cervical spondylosis: treatment by spondylectomy, microsurgical decompression, and osteosynthesis. *Neurosurgery.* 1991;29:498-503.
46. Senegas J, Guérin J, Vital JM, et al. Décompression médullaire étendue par voi antérieure dans le traitement des myélopathies par cervicarthrose. *Rev Chir Orthop.* 1985;71:291-300. English abstract
47. Sugar O. Spinal cord malfunction after anterior cervical discectomy. *Surg Neurol.* 1981;15:4-8.
48. Tew JM Jr. Mayfield FH. Complications of surgery of the anterior cervical spine. *Clin Neurosurg.* 1976; 23:424-434.
49. U HS, Wilson CB. Postoperative epidural hematoma as a complication of anterior cervical discectomy: report of three cases. *J Neurosurg.* 1978; 49:288-291.
50. Verbiest H. The management of cervical spondylosis. *Clin Neurosurg.* 1973;20:262-294.
51. Whitecloud TS III. Anterior surgery for cervical spondylotic myelopathy: Smith-Robinson, Cloward and vertebrectomy. *Spine.* 1988;13:861-863.
52. Whitecloud TS III. Cervical spondylosis: the anterior approach. In: Frymoyer JW, ed. *The Adult Spine. Principles and Practice.* New York, NY: Raven Press; 1991;2:1165-1185.
53. Whitecloud TS, LaRocca H. Fibular strut graft in reconstructive surgery of the cervical spine. *Spine.* 1976;1:33-43.
54. Wilson DH, Campbell DD. Anterior cervical diskectomy without bone graft: report of 71 cases. *J Neurosurg.* 1977;47:551-555.
55. Yonenobu K, Fuji T, Ono K, et al. Choice of surgical treatment for multisegmental cervical spondylotic myelopathy. *Spine.* 1985;10:710-716.

CHAPTER 7

Cervical Spondylotic Myelopathy: Posterior Surgical Approaches

Edward C. Benzel, MD

The management of cervical spondylosis is complicated by the inconsistent application of terminology, particularly with regard to the term cervical spondylotic radiculomyelopathy.[36] Cervical spondylotic radiculomyelopathy is a catch-all term that encompasses all neural compressive phenomena related to cervical spondylosis. Management issues are confused by the implication that radiculopathy and myelopathy are intimately interrelated and that they are, thus, treated similarly.

This is probably inappropriate. It may be more rational to consider myelopathy, radiculopathy, and combined symptomatic myelopathy and radiculopathy as three separate entities. The rationale for this terminology is based on the differing clinical manifestations (e.g. myelopathy versus radiculopathy) and surgical approaches (e.g. spinal cord versus nerve root decompression) associated with each. Cervical spondylotic myelopathy (CSM) is usually thought to encompass at least three spinal levels (at least two motion segment diseases);[16,46,48,64] and cervical radiculopathy is most often single-level in origin and multifactorial in nature.

The discussion in this chapter is limited to the treatment of the most disabling and significant aspect of cervical spondylosis, CSM, and does not include radiculopathy, which is discussed in Chapters 8 and 9.

Surgical approaches for CSM include: (1) multiple-level anterior corpectomies with interbody fusion, (2) multiple single-level diskectomies and dural sac decompressions with accompanying multiple single-level interbody fusions, (3) the utilization of either of the prior two with anterior spinal instrumentation techniques, (4) spinal fusion without decompression, (5) cervical laminectomy, (6) cervical laminectomy plus dentate ligament section (DLS), and (7) either of the prior two with an accompanying posterior fusion. Anterior approaches are discussed in Chapter 6.

Rationale for a Posterior Approach to CSM

The fact that CSM exists as a clinical entity has been clearly established. Similarly, posterior surgical approaches to spinal canal decompression have been clearly established as safe and efficacious. [3,6,10,12-15,21,22,33,34,49,51-53]

Although anterior and anterolateral decompression operations have been strongly recommended for the treatment of CSM,[24,25,29,32,40,41,54,62] some have found the ventrally oriented approaches to CSM to be less than satisfactory.[39] Furthermore, significant neurologic and non-neurologic complications associated with anterior surgical approaches to CSM have been reported.[24,29,39,41,54] These may be related to the complexity and degree of difficulty of the operation.

Since anterior operations for CSM usually require spine fusion, one must consider the long-term complications of spinal fusion, such as increased spinal laxity and accelerated degenerative changes immediately above and below the fusion levels.[28] One must also consider an increased chance for neural injury, infection (by virtue of the obligatory increased operation time), and donor site complications.

Conversely, laminectomy is a relatively simple and straightforward operation. The conceptually direct approach to spinal canal decompression and the simplicity and degree of safety offered by laminectomy is very appealing. The complications associated with laminectomy are predictable and preventable,[6,10] and laboratory-based arguments against the utility and safety of laminectomy, such as postlaminectomy diminished spinal cord blood flow, are weak and easily refuted.[1,5]

Both anterior and posterior surgical approaches play a role in CSM managment, however. The advantages and disadvantages of both must be considered in nearly all cases. This chapter emphasizes the importance of a selective approach to CSM management, and a determination of which patients are most likely to benefit from either an anterior or posterior surgical approach. Consideration of spinal geometry is integral to the decision-making process regarding operation selection; appropriate operation selection maximizes the incidence of optimal neurologic outcome while minimizing the incidence of complications.

Patient Selection for Posterior Surgical Approaches: Matching the Operation to the Pathology

Treatment selection for CSM involves both the selection of surgical candidates and the selection of the most appropriate operation. Surgical candidate selection is relatively straightforward. Unfortunately, operation selection is much less so and is, therefore, steeped in controversy.

Significance of the Patient's Symptoms

Primary considerations regarding the selection of surgical candidates include (1) the extent to which the patient's symptoms and physical disability impact upon lifestyle, and (2) confidence that these symptoms and disabilities are secondary to spinal cord compression. Symptoms and degree of disability can be readily quantitated.[2,6,46,67] Their impact on the patient's lifestyle can only be addressed by an honest assessment by the patient. The question must be asked: "Is the chance of alleviation of the negative impact of the patient's symptoms and disability on lifestyle worth the risk of surgery?" In this regard, Ball and Saunders make a compelling case for surgical intervention, even in less severely involved patients.[2]

Certainty of the association of the symptoms and disability with spinal cord compression (as evidenced by imaging studies) may be lacking in some cases. The differential diagnosis of cervical myelopathy includes central nervous system degenerative disorders such as motor neuron disease, complicating the decision-making process. These factors must be considered during surgical candidate selection.

Prophylaxis against sudden catastrophic neurologic deterioration,[23,60] may be indicated in some patients with mild symptomatic disease and significant neural encroachment. The risks of prophylactic surgery must be weighed against the chance of catastrophe associated with untreated cervical stenosis.

Patient Age and Intrinsic Size of the Spinal Canal

A minor consideration in operation selection is patient age. The age of the patient at the time of presentation with symptoms and signs of cervical spinal cord compression may affect the decision-making process by (1) the effect of age on intrinsic spinal stability and (2) the likelihood that CSM is the etiology of the patient's symptoms.

Older patients usually have a greater intrinsic spinal stability, acquired through the aging/spondylotic process. Any operation, such as a laminectomy, which even slightly destabilizes the spine, is less invasive if greater intrinsic stability already exists. On the other hand, the younger the CSM patient, the greater the chance that congenital cervical stenosis is playing a role in the pathologic process.[18,27]

Normal and pathologic sagittal spinal canal diameters have been defined and documented.[26,27,47] These data help the clinician determine what extent congenital stenosis is not associated with dorsally-directed, ventrally-located osteophytes, a laminectomy is expected to offer symptomatic relief and is the operation of choice in most cases.[18] Furthermore, in this younger patient population, there is a greater potential for long-term complications of cervical fusion. Other pathologic processes, such as calcification of the ligamentum flavum, ossification of the posterior longitudinal ligament, and ankylosing spondylitis must also be considered in the differential diagnosis of cervical stenosis.[4,30,35,45,60] (See also Chapters 11 and 12.)

Intrinsic Curvature of the Cervical Spine

Posterior approaches to CSM should be applied to patients in whom a dorsal spinal cord decompressive procedure has a high probability of success. Since a posterior approach to CSM is less complex, faster, and possibly safer than an anterior approach, it may be the most appropriate choice if not otherwise contraindicated. A consideration of spinal geometry is emphasized as an important determinant of the appropriateness of either the anterior or the posterior approach in individual situations.[3]

Patients with an "effective" cervical kyphosis have a high probability of failure associated with a posterior decompressive procedure.[3] An "effective" cervical kyphosis is defined here as a configuration of the cervical spine in which any part of the dorsal aspect of any of the C3-7 vertebral bodies crosses a line drawn in the midsagittal plane (on a lateral cervical spine tomogram, myelogram, or magnetic resonance image) from the dorsocaudal aspect of the vertebral body of C2 to the dorsocaudal aspect of the vertebral body of C7. Conversely, an "effective" cervical lordosis is defined here as a configuration of the cervical spine in which no part of the dorsal aspect of any of the C3-7 vertebral bodies crosses this line.

The definition of this imaginary line is associated with a zone of uncertainty ("gray zone") within which surgeon bias and clinical judgment play a role in the determination of whether lordosis or kyphosis is the predominant spinal configuration in the midsagittal section (Figure 1A). If, in the opinion of the surgeon, there is no gray zone (i.e. only an "effective" kyphosis or an "effective" lordosis is possible), surgical decision-making is simpler. On the other hand, if in the opinion of the surgeon a gray zone exists, the decision-making process is more complex. Patients whose spinal configuration falls in the gray zone, should perhaps be defined as having a "straightened" spine.

One must keep an open mind regarding surgical approaches to the treatment of CSM. Both anterior and posterior approaches are indicated in specific situations. It is suggested that (1) patients with an "effective" kyphosis and with symptoms of CSM be treated with an anterior decompressive operation, and (2) patients with an "effective" lordosis be treated with a posterior decompressive operative approach. Patients with "straightened" spines may be treated either way. Surgeon bias regarding the management approach to the "straightened" spine, as well as its definition, are central to the controversy regarding surgical approach selection.

Surgeon Bias

If one were to draw the imaginary line as described above, and place two points 2 mm

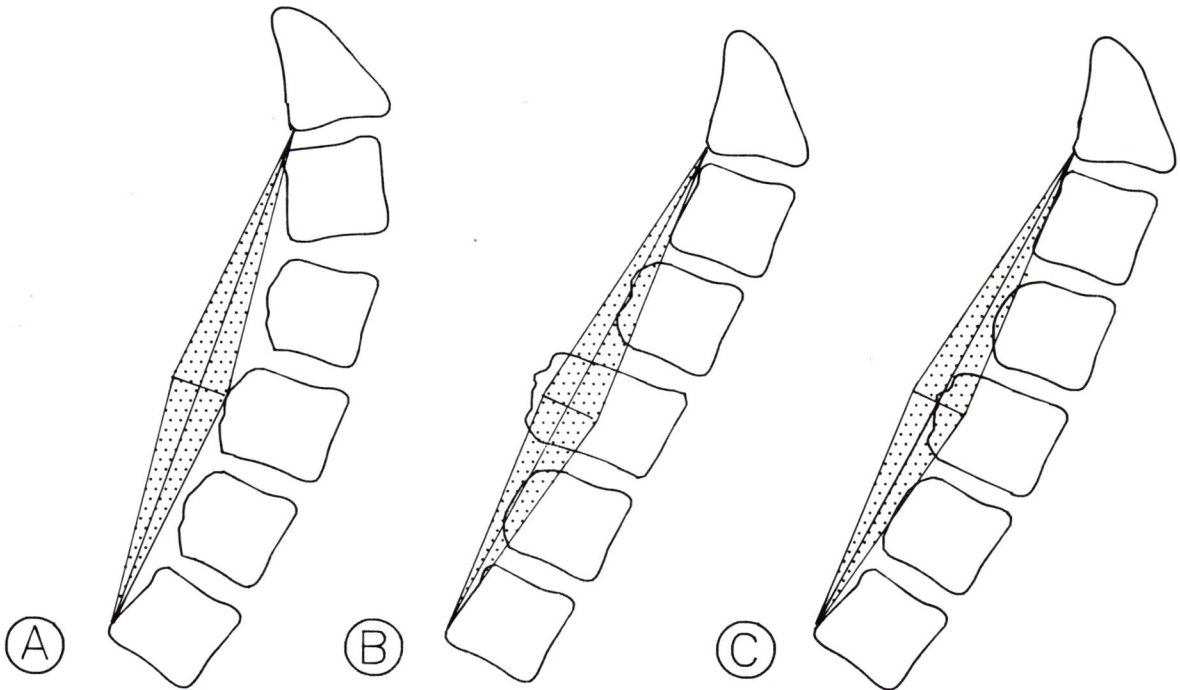

Figure 1. **(A)** Midsagittal section of a cervical spine (as observed by MRI or myelography), which is configured in lordosis ("effective" cervical lordosis). A line has been drawn from the dorsocaudal aspect of the vertebral body of C2 to the dorsocaudal aspect of the vertebral body of C7 (solid line). The "gray zone" is outlined by dotted lines. **(B)** Midsagittal section of a cervical spine, which is configured in kyphosis ("effective" cervical kyphosis). Portions of the vertebral bodies are located dorsal to the "gray zone". **(C)** Midsagittal section of a "straightened" cervical spine. The most dorsal aspect of a cervical vertebral body is located within, but not dorsal to the "gray zone".

on either side of this line at its mid-point, the two points could be connected with each end of the imaginary line, forming an elongated diamond-shaped region (Figure 1A). Within this elongated diamond exists the gray zone—i.e. the width of the diamond is greater than four mm (two mm + two mm). For others, it may be smaller. Patients have an "effective" lordosis (Figure 1A) if no aspect of a vertebral body, disk bulge, or osteophyte between C3 and C7 projects into the gray zone.

Conversely, patients have an "effective" kyphosis (Figure 1B) if some aspect of a vertebral body, disk bulge, or osteophyte between C3 and C7 falls dorsal to the gray zone. Patients have a "straightened" spinal configuration (Figure 1C) if some aspect of a vertebral body, disk bulge, or osteophyte between C3 and C7 falls within, but not dorsal to, the gray zone.

Intrinsic Stability of the Spine

The intrinsic stability of the spine[63] plays a role in operative decision-making. The surgeon may choose an anterior approach (which includes fusion) if the patient's spine is believed to be intrinsically unstable. This approach allows for a decompression and a stabilization procedure to be simultaneously performed. Alternatively, a posterior decompression with an accompanying posterior fusion may be chosen.

Although posterior decompressive operations most certainly diminish intrinsic spinal stability,[65,66] the extent of their effect on stability is often exaggerated. An appropriately performed laminectomy should not significantly diminish intrinsic spinal stability. Raynor et al[50] clearly demonstrated that laminectomy width is related to stability. In series where laminectomy is laterally extended only

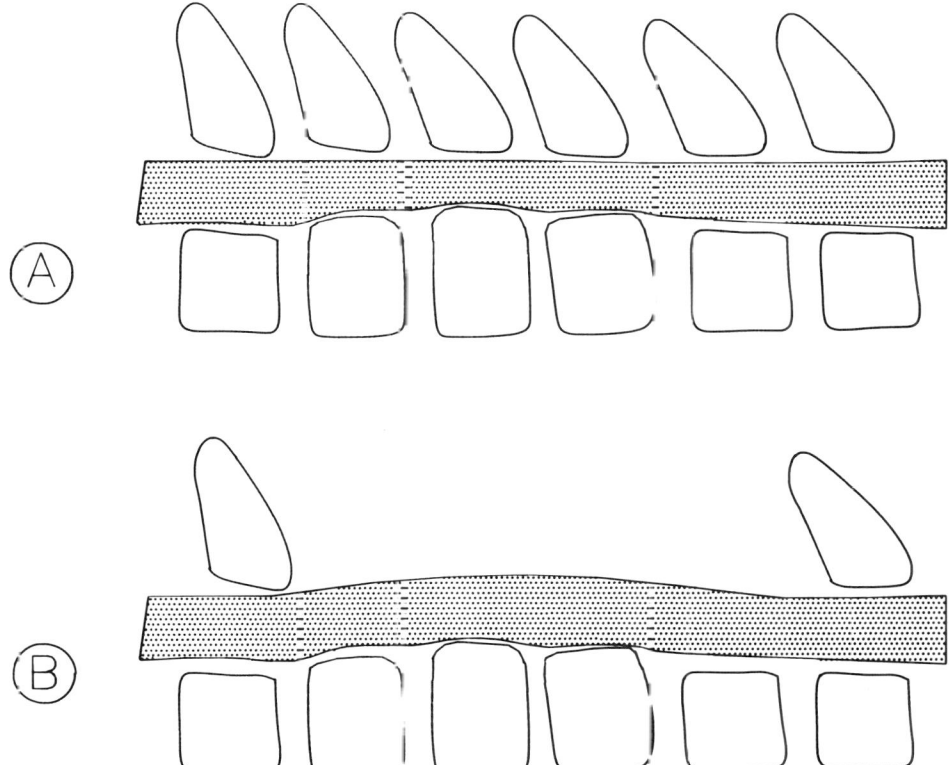

Figure 2. The "sagittal bowstring" effect. The mechanism by which a patient whose spine is kyphotic (**A**) may be worsened neurologically by a dorsal decompressive procedure (**B**) is depicted.

to the most lateral aspect of the dural sac, postoperative instability is rare.[6,10,20,24,31] Therefore, wide laminectomies which are extended past the medial 1/4 to 1/3 of the width of the facet, and foraminotomies which disrupt facet integrity, should be avoided or should perhaps be accompanied by a fusion procedure.

The spondylotic process may be associated with an increase in intrinsic spinal stability. This affords an increased assurance regarding the safety of an appropriately performed laminectomy. This is not always so, particularly in patients with a hyperlordotic configuration.[17]

Hazards Associated with Choosing the Wrong Operative Approach

In general, ventral compressive lesions should be decompressed via a ventral surgical approach, and dorsal lesions decompressed via a dorsal surgical approach. Patients with an "effective" kyphosis have a decreased probability of adequate ventral dural sac decompression following a dorsal decompressive operation (Figure 2). These patients should be approached by an anterior surgical decompression.

In the presence of an "effective" kyphosis, a laminectomy cannot be expected to relieve ventral compression due to a "sagittal bowstring" effect whereby the dural sac and its contents are tethered over ventral osteophytes in a sagittal plane (Figure 2). If an "effective" lordosis is present, a dorsal decompressive operation may be most appropriate (see Figure 1A). If a "straightened" spine is present (recall that the surgeon's bias and clinical judgment play a major role in determining the size of the gray zone), the patient can be treated with either an anterior or posterior decompressive procedure.

A Nonrigid Approach to Operation Selection

An open-minded approach to operation selection for CSM is recommended. The application of both anterior and posterior surgical approaches in a selective manner, maximizes the chance of an optimal outcome.[6,8,10,36,40]

Mechanisms of Spinal Cord Distortion

Three mechanisms of spinal cord distortion play a role in the CSM process: (1) spinal cord compression, (2) tethering of the spinal cord over extrinsic masses in the sagittal plane, and (3) tethering of the spinal cord over extrinsic masses in the coronal plane. Each must be considered and accounted for prior to surgical intervention.

Spinal Cord Compression

Spinal cord compression is most often considered the major cause of neurologic dysfunction in CSM. It causes an annular constriction of the spinal cord which arises from a combination of factors such as ventral osteophyte, dorsolateral facet, and dorsal hypertrophied ligamentum flavum compression.[57] The value of decompression for spinal cord compression has been experimentally documented.[14]

Sagittal Bowstring Effect

An underestimated cause of neurologic dysfunction in CSM is the tethering of the spinal cord over extrinsic masses. In the sagittal plane, this is related to either anterior or posterior structures. Most often, extrinsic masses located anterior to the spinal cord are implicated. The neurologic deficit in a patient with an "effective" cervical kyphosis is, in part, related to tethering in the sagittal plane (sagittal bowstring effect). This explains why some patients may be neurologically worsened by posterior decompression procedures (Figure 2). Bohlman, Morgan and coauthors documented this point clinically in patients with post-traumatic ventral mass lesions.[7,44] This phenomenon has been similarly documented experimentally.[5] The neurologic dysfunction in these cases may be related to spinal cord vascular compromise.[15]

Coronal Bowstring Effect

The spinal cord can occasionally be tethered in the coronal plane as well.[6,33] This coronal plane tethering (coronal bowstring effect) is caused by the tethering of the spinal cord ventrally by a lateral extension of the spinal cord appendages, such as nerve roots or the dentate ligaments (Figure 3A). If coronal bowstringing is present, a laminectomy will often be ineffective in relieving spinal cord distortion (Figure 3B). An anterior decompressive procedure or a laminectomy plus dentate ligament section (DLS) (Figure 3C) is required to relieve the spinal cord distortion.[6]

Choosing a Dorsal Operative Approach

Laminectomy

Laminectomy for CSM has been an accepted treatment of CSM for years.[52,53,55,58,59] It is most clearly indicated in patients who have a compressive myelopathy with an associated "effective" cervical lordosis.[6,10] Due to surgeon bias, the definition of "effective" cervical lordosis will vary from surgeon to surgeon. The "straightened" spine may be treated by either an anterior or posterior decompressive operation. Therefore, the surgical management of those patients whose spinal configuration falls into the gray zone is dictated by surgeon bias.

Laminectomy Plus DLS

The addition of DLS to a laminectomy is safe.[6,49] The efficacy of DLS has been ques-

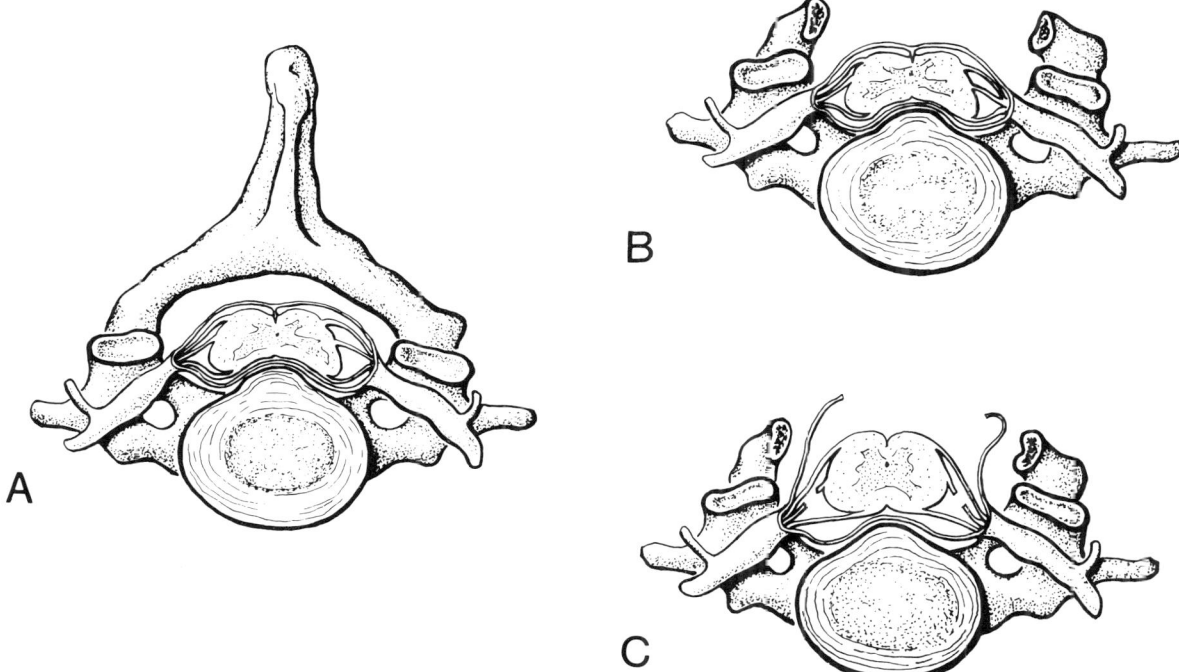

Figure 3. The "coronal bowstring" effect. An axial section through a stenotic region of the cervical spine is depicted. The ventral tethering of the spinal cord by the dentate ligaments is illustrated *(A)*. Note the patent dorsal subarachnoid space. Following a laminectomy, the tethering persists *(B)*. Only following a DLS *(C)* or a ventral decompression operation is the tethering in the coronal plane relieved. (Modified from Benzel et al[6])

tioned, however.[10,42,49] Laminectomy plus DLS is most clearly indicated in patients who are adversely affected by the coronal bowstring effect, as described above (Figure 3), and in whom an "effective" cervical kyphosis does not exist.

Benzel et al assessed the indications for laminectomy and for laminectomy plus DLS in a retrospective study.[6] In this series, laminectomy was observed to be more effective in patients with mild or moderate fixed myelopathic neurologic findings, and a laminectomy plus DLS was observed to offer an advantage in patients with progressive or more severe symptoms. Laminectomy plus DLS produced similar neurologic outcomes as anterior decompressive procedures, particularly in patients with more severe myelopathies.[6] Laminectomy plus DLS is without the associated significant acute risks of ventral bone graft and upper-airway complications,[25,54] and long-term risks of accelerated degenerative changes above and below the fusion.[28]

The similarity of neurologic results may be related to the proposed additional anterior decompression associated with DLS (i.e. relief of the coronal bowstring effect). In selected patients, DLS appears to provide additional ventral spinal cord decompression over that attained with cervical laminectomy alone. This clinical observation has been documented by others.[12,21,22,33] It has also been assessed anatomically and physiologically.[13,51]

In the majority of patients, the potential for response to DLS is difficult or impossible to determine preoperatively. In some patients, magnetic resonance imaging (MRI) or computed tomography myelography (CTM) may be helpful. Since both imaging procedures are performed with the patient in the supine position, the observation of the absence of a patent ventral but presence of a patent dorsal subarachnoid space at the points of maximum compression implies that a laminectomy alone would not be helpful, due to an already patent or decompressed dorsal subarachnoid space. The majority of patients with CSM do not exhibit patent posterior subarachnoid spaces on preoperative imaging studies. The decision regarding the performance of DLS must be made on the basis of other factors, such as neurologic and clinical presentation.

Epstein et al demonstrated that laminectomy with an accompanying ventral osteophyte excision, via a dorsal approach, improves neurologic outcome.[19] This technique offers an effective anterior decompression, as does an anterior decompression and fusion procedure or a laminectomy plus DLS. Although Epstein et al did not observe significant myelopathic or stability-related morbidity in their series, these complications can occur, causing this technique to be a less than desirable choice.

Laminectomy Plus Fusion

The performance of a posterior fusion following a dorsal decompression operation is controversial.[10] A high incidence of instability following laminectomy and/or wide foraminotomy has been reported,[42,56,67] particularly in children.[38,65,66] Others report a negligible incidence.[6,10,20,24,31] If the laminectomy is extended laterally to no farther than the medial 1/4 to 1/3 of the facet joint (only to the lateral aspect of the dural sac), the incidence of postoperative instability is essentially nil (if instability is not present preoperatively). Carol and Ducker emphasized the importance of using a thin-plated 45° angled Kerrison punch while performing foraminotomies, with care taken to avoid disruption of facet integrity.[10]

If preoperative instability exists and the laminectomy is extended farther laterally than 1/4 to 1/3 of the width of the facet joint, or if wide foraminotomies are performed, the chance for instability is greatly increased. Swan neck deformities and even acute loss of stability, which can be catastrophic, may occur. Fusion is indicated in these cases.

The mechanisms by which cervical spondylosis develops and progresses requires movement at the intervertebral joint. Without this movement, the spondylotic process cannot occur or progress. Whether the arrest of the spondylotic process alone is an indication for the performance of a fusion, is most certainly debatable. The short-term and long-term complications of spinal fusion have been alluded to and must be carefully considered in the decision-making process.

Surgical Techniques
Cervical Laminectomy

The prone position is preferred. Complications associated with the sitting position are usually unacceptable, and the advantages minimal. One should use a rongeur, such as a large Leksell, so as to not place any aspect of the instrument underneath the lamina during bone removal. Any encroachment on a maximally compromised spinal canal may result in exacerbation of neurologic deficit.

The author has found it helpful to remove the ligamentum flavum along with the bony elements. This affords an element of safety, makes the ligamentum flavum easier to remove, and allows the removal of the dorsal tissue (bone and ligamentum flavum) in one step rather than two. Following the performance of the laminectomy, the bony defect should be widened to the lateral aspect of the dural sac with a thin-plated Kerrison rongeur. Care must be taken not to extend the laminectomy laterally past the medial 1/4 to 1/3 of the facet joint (Figure 4).

Dentate Ligament Section

The technique of DLS has been described.[6,22] Following laminectomy, a midline dural incision is made. After dural retraction, the arachnoid is incised laterally, allowing the clear visualization of the dentate ligaments. The midline dural incision and the lateral arachnoid incision are associated with an added benefit of the former not overlying the latter. This minimizes the chance for central

Cervical Spondylotic Myelopathy: Posterior Surgical Approaches

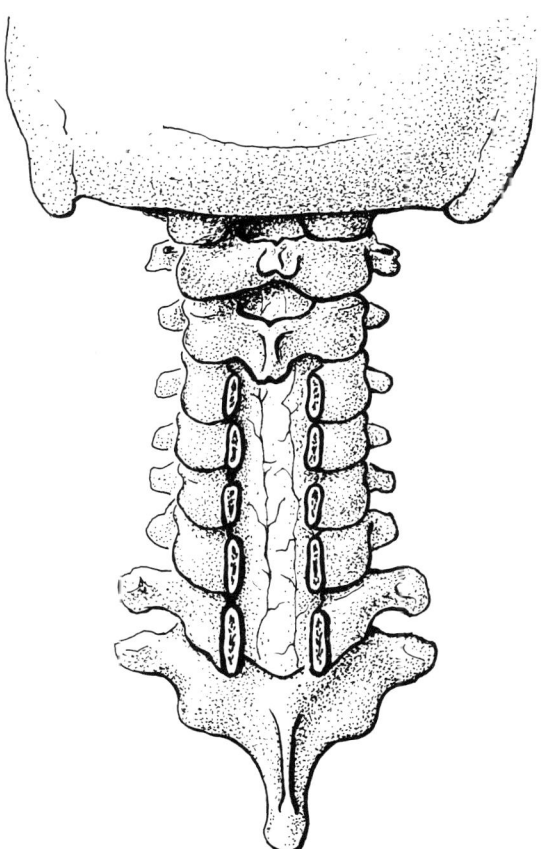

Figure 4. An appropriately performed laminectomy. Note the preservation of the majority of each facet joint.

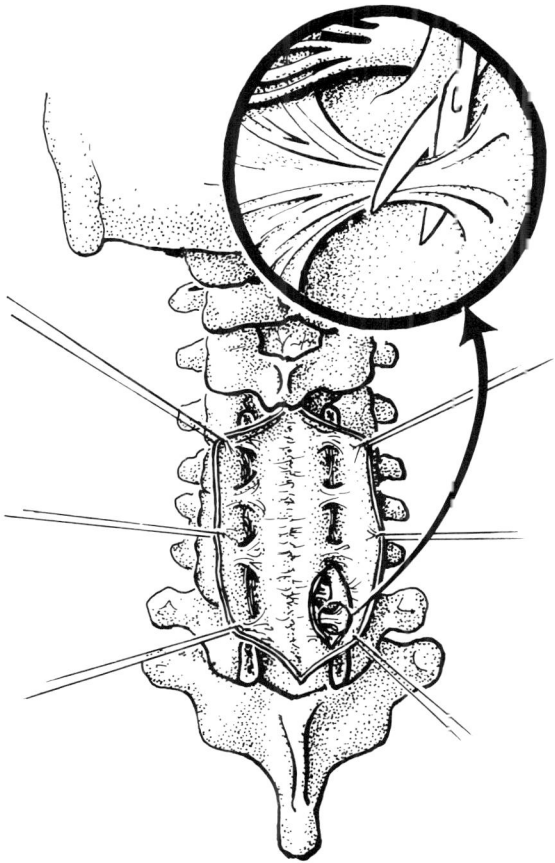

Figure 5. An intradural exposure of the spinal cord and dentate ligaments, one of which is being incised (see insert).

spinal fluid (CSF) leakage. The dentate ligaments are incised, usually with microscissors or Dandy Scissors (Figure 5). Following incision of all accessible dentate ligaments, the dura matter is closed in a water-tight manner.

Leakage of blood into the subarachnoid space must be eliminated or at least minimized and is facilitated by the use of multiple dural retraction sutures. A postoperative febrile course and other symptoms associated with meningeal irritation may ensue if too much blood enters the subarachnoid space. Arachnoid retraction (not spinal cord retraction) also is critical. Two surgeons are necessary for the DLS portion of the case, which should be performed under excellent illumination and possibly with magnification.

Posterior Cervical Fusion

Lateral mass plates or related instrumentation techniques may be used for fixation in combination with bone fusion. The author prefers, due to the limited fusion bed surface area available, to use a split iliac crest graft. The graft is wired at each level to the facet (Figure 6).[9]

Failure of Posterior Decompression Operations

A variety of complications associated with posterior decompression operations have been reported.[11,20,37,43,67] Most are preventable by

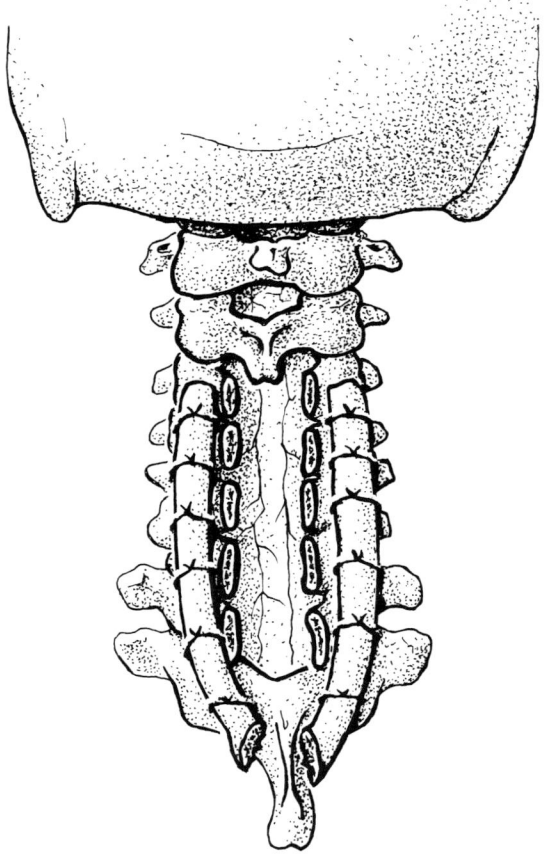

Figure 6. A posterior facet fusion which has been placed following laminectomy. (Modified from Callahan et al[9])

strict attention to detail and operative technique. The avoidance of the sitting position for surgery is emphasized,[11] although some surgeons find this position to be safe and useful. Also important are careful mobilization following operation and the avoidance of hypotension.[37]

The failure of a laminectomy, with or without DLS, to achieve the desired neurologic result or to be associated with an unacceptable complication rate is often predictable. The reasons for these unacceptable results include (1) inappropriate operation selection or the performance of surgery when no operation was indicated, (2) intraoperative spinal cord trauma, (3) inappropriate width of laminectomy, or (4) inappropriate length of laminectomy.

Inappropriate Operation Selection

Inappropriate operation selection as a cause of surgical failure cannot be overemphasized. As discussed above, surgeon bias plays a major role in operation selection. Bias is only relative, however. There are, theoretically, cases where only anterior decompression operations should be considered and, conversely, cases where only posterior decompression operations should be considered. Failure of laminectomy to result in an expected degree of neurologic improvement necessitates a postoperative imaging study. This study should clearly visualize the anterior subarachnoid space using MRI or CT myelopathy. If the dorsal, but not the ventral, subarachnoid space is patent, an anterior dural sac decompression is indicated, either via an anterior decompression and fusion or by the addition of a DLS to the previously performed laminectomy. Care should be taken to avoid surgery in patients who are suspected of having neurodegenerative diseases as the etiology of their myelopathy.

Intraoperative Spinal Cord Trauma

A small incidence of neurologic worsening occurs after posterior procedures.[22] This may be due to intraoperative spinal cord trauma, a preventable cause of an unacceptable operative result. One should avoid both the placement of instruments underneath the lamina and spinal cord retraction.

Inappropriate Width of Laminectomy

A laminectomy that is not wide enough to adequately decompress the spinal canal may result in persistent neurologic dysfunction. Conversely, a laminectomy that is too wide or that is performed in conjunction with a wide foraminotomy may result in spinal instability. A laminectomy, therefore, should be extended laterally to the most lateral aspect of the dural sac—no less and no further. This almost always results in adequate preservation of the stability-preserving effects of the facet joint.[50]

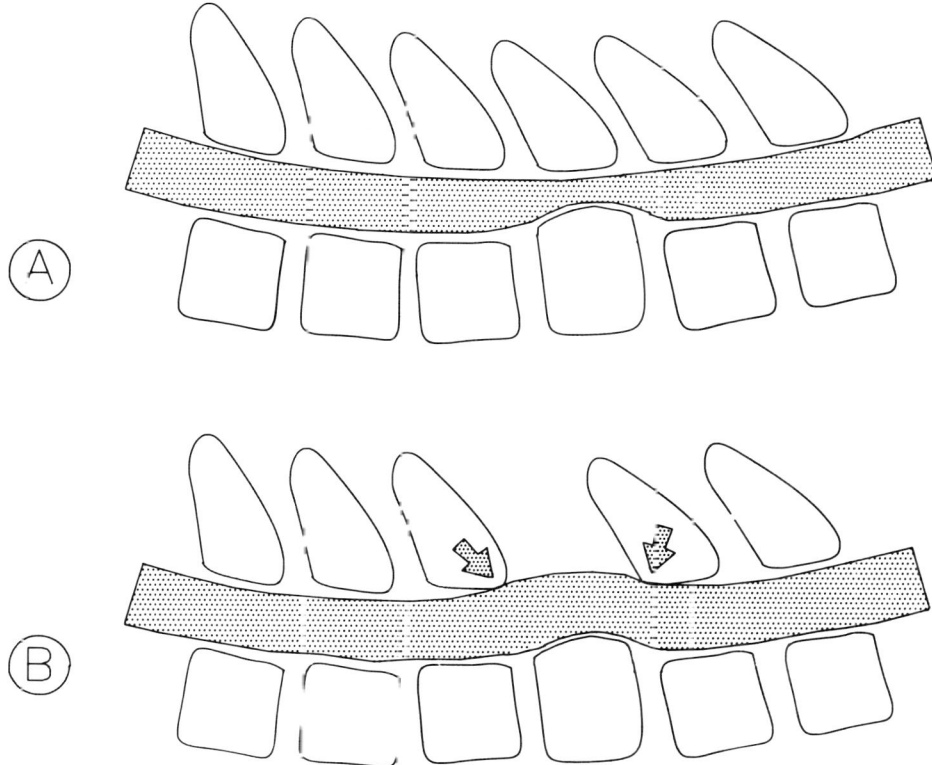

Figure 7. An illustration of the hazards associated with performing a laminectomy which is not long enough to decompress a ventral mass (**A**). A dorsal kinking of the spinal cord, which results from unopposed dorsally directed forces, combined with acute angle deformation of the spinal cord at the margins of the short laminectomy (arrows), may ensue (**B**).

Inappropriate Length of Laminectomy

Similarly, a laminectomy can be too long or too short. If too long, spinal instability or deformity development is encouraged. This is most commonly observed in situations where the first thoracic lamina is removed. The rate of occurrence of postoperative kyphotic deformities may be unacceptable in this patient population. Therefore, unless absolutely necessary, a laminectomy should not be extended inferiorly to include removal of T1.

A laminectomy that is not extended far enough rostrally and caudally to an extrinsic mass located ventral to the spinal cord may result in a worsening of the preoperative neurologic deficit.[20,24] A dorsal kinking of the spinal cord may ensue, which may result from unopposed dorsally directed forces, combined with acute angle deformation of the spinal cord at the margins of the short laminectomy (Figure 7).[10]

Conclusion

Patient selection and operation selection for the surgical management of CSM are key factors that may affect outcome. Posterior approaches for the management of CSM should play an important part in the surgeon's armamentarium. With the appropriate application of posterior approaches to CSM, their true value will be recognized and understood.

References

1. Anderson DK, Nicolosi GR, Means ED, et al. Effects of laminectomy on spinal cord blood flow. *J Neurosurg.* 1978;48:232-238.

2. Ball PA, Saunders RL. The subjective myelopathy. In: Saunders RL, Bernini PM, eds. *Cervical Spondylotic Myelopathy*. Boston, Mass: Blackwell Scientific Publishing. In press.
3. Batzdorf U, Batzdorff A. Analysis of cervical spine curvature in patients with cervical spondylosis. *Neurosurgery*. 1988;22:827-836.
4. Becker DH, Conley FK, Anderson ME. Quadriplegia associated with narrow cervical canal, ligamentous calcification and ankylosing hyperostosis. *Surg Neurol*. 1979;11:17-19.
5. Bennett MH, McCallum JE. Experimental decompression of spinal cord. *Surg Neurol*. 1977;8:63-67.
6. Benzel EC, Lancon J, Kesterson L, et al. Cervical laminectomy and dentate ligament section for cervical spondylotic myelopathy. *J Spinal Disorders*. In press.
7. Bohlman HH. Acute fractures and dislocations of the cervical spine: an analysis of 300 hospitalized patients and review of the literature. *J Bone Joint Surg Am*. 1979;61A:1119-1142.
8. Bose B, Northrup BE, Osterholm JL, et al. Reanalysis of central cervical cord injury management. *Neurosurgery*. 1984;15:367-372.
9. Callahan RA, Johnson RM, Margolis RN, et al. Cervical facet fusion for control of instability following laminectomy. *J Bone Joint Surg Am*. 1977;59A:991-1002.
10. Carol MP, Ducker TB. Cervical spondylitic myelopathies: surgical treatment. *J Spinal Disorders*. 1988;1:59-65.
11. Chadduck WM. Cerebellar hemorrhage complicating cervical laminectomy. *Neurosurgery*. 1981;9:185-189.
12. Crandall PH, Batzdorf U. Cervical spondylotic myelopathy. *J Neurosurg*. 1966;25:57-66.
13. Cusick JF, Ackmann JJ, Larson SJ. Mechanical and physiological effects of dentatotomy. *J Neurosurg*. 1977;46:767-775.
14. Dolan EJ, Tator CH, Endrenyi L. The value of decompression for acute experimental spinal cord compression injury. *J Neurosurg*. 1980;53:749-755.
15. Doppman JL, Girton M. Angiographic study of the effect of laminectomy in the presence of acute anterior epidural masses. *J Neurosurg*. 1976;45:195-202.
16. Epstein BS, Epstein JA, Jones MD. Cervical spinal stenosis. *Radiol Clin North Am*. 1977;15:215-226.
17. Epstein JA, Carras R, Epstein BS, et al. Myelopathy in cervical spondylosis with vertebral subluxation and hyperlordosis. *J Neurosurg*. 1970;32:421-426.
18. Epstein JA, Carras R, Hyman RA, et al. Cervical myelopathy caused by developmental stenosis of the spinal canal. *J Neurosurg*. 1979;51:362-367.
19. Epstein JA, Carras R, Lavine LS, et al. The importance of removing osteophytes as part of the surgical treatment of myeloradiculopathy in cervical spondylosis. *J Neurosurg*. 1969;30:219-226.
20. Epstein N, Epstein JA, Benjamin V, et al. Traumatic myelopathy in patients with cervical spinal stenosis without fracture or dislocation: methods of diagnosis, management, and prognosis. *Spine*. 1980;5:489-496.
21. Fager CA. Reversal of cervical myelopathy by adequate posterior decompression. *Lahey Clin Found Bull*. 1969;18:99-108.
22. Fager CA. Results of adequate posterior decompression in the relief of spondylotic cervical myelopathy. *J Neurosurg*. 1973;38:684-692.
23. Firooznia H, Ahn JH, Rafii M, et al. Sudden quadriplegia after a minor trauma: the role of preexisting spinal stenosis. *Surg Neurol*. 1985;23:165-168.
24. Guidetti B, Fortuna A. Long-term results of surgical treatment of myelopathy due to cervical spondylosis. *J Neurosurg*. 1969;30:714-721.
25. Hanai K, Fujiyoshi F, Kamei K. Subtotal vertebrectomy and spinal fusion for cervical spondylotic myelopathy. *Spine*. 1986;11:310-315.
26. Hinck VC, Hopkins CE, Savara BS. Sagittal diameter of the cervical spinal canal in children. *Radiology*. 1962;79:97-108.
27. Hinck VC, Sachdev NS. Developmental stenosis of the cervical spinal canal. *Brain*. 1966;89:27-36.
28. Hunter LY, Braunstein EM, Bailey RW. Radiographic changes following anterior cervical fusion. *Spine*. 1980;5:399-401.
29. Irvine GB, Strachan WE. The long-term results of localized anterior cervical decompression and fusion in spondylotic myelopathy. *Paraplegia*. 1987;25:18-22.
30. Iwasaki Y, Akino M, Abe H, et al. Calcification of the ligamentum flavum of the cervical spine: report of four cases. *J Neurosurg*. 1983;59:531-534.
31. Jenkins DHR. Extensive cervical laminectomy: long-term results. *Br J Surg*. 1973;60:852-854.
32. Kadoya S, Nakamura T, Kwak R. A microsurgical anterior osteophytectomy for cervical spondylotic myelopathy. *Spine*. 1984;9:437-441.
33. Kahn EA. The role of the dentate ligaments in spinal cord compression and the syndrome of lateral sclerosis. *J Neurosurg*. 1947;4:191-199.
34. Keegan JJ. The cause of dissociated motor loss in the upper extremity with cervical spondylosis: a case report. *J Neurosurg*. 1965;23:528-536.
35. Klara PM, McDonnell DE. Ossification of the posterior longitudinal ligament in caucasians: diagnosis and surgical intervention. *Neurosurgery*. 1986;19:212-217.
36. Lesoin F, Bouasakao N, Clarisse J, et al. Results of surgical treatment of radiculomyelopathy caused by cervical arthrosis based on 1000 operations. *Surg Neurol*. 1985;23:350-355.
37. Levy WJ, Dohn DF, Hardy RW. Central cord syndrome as a delayed postoperative complication of decompressive laminectomy. *Neurosurgery*. 1982;11:491-495.
38. Lonstein JE. Post-laminectomy kyphosis. *Clin Orthop*. 1977;128:93-100.
39. Lunsford LD, Bissonette DJ, Zorub DS. Anterior surgery for cervical disc disease, part II: treatment of cervical spondylotic myelopathy in 32 cases. *J Neurosurg*. 1980;53:12-19.
40. Magnaes B, Hauge T: Surgery for myelopathy in cervical spondylosis: safety measures and preoperative factors related to outcome. *Spine*. 1980;5:211-214.
41. Mann KS, Khosla VK, Gulati DR. Cervical spondylotic myelopathy treated by single-stage multilevel anterior decompression. *J Neurosurg*. 1984;60:81-87.
42. Mayfield FH. Cervical spondylosis: a comparison of the anterior and posterior approaches. *Clin Neurosurg*. 1965;13:181-188.
43. Middleton TH, Al-Mefty O, Harkey LH, et al. Syringomyelia after decompressive laminectomy for cervical spondylosis. *Surg Neurol*. 1987;28:458-462.
44. Morgan TH, Wharton GW, Austin GN. The results of laminectomy in patients with incomplete spinal cord injuries. *Paraplegia*. 1971;9:14-23.
45. Nakajima K, Miyaoka M, Sumie H, et al. Cervical

radiculomyelopathy due to calcification of the ligamenta flava. *Surg Neurol.* 1984;21:479-488.
46. Nurick S. The pathogenesis of the spinal cord disorder associated with cervical spondylosis. *Brain.* 1972;95:87-100.
47. Ogino H, Tada K, Okada K, et al. Canal diameter, anteroposterior compression ratio, and spondylotic myelopathy of the cervical spine. *Spine.* 1983;8:1-15.
48. Payne EE, Spillane JD. The cervical spine: an anatomico-pathological study of 70 specimens (using a special technique) with particular reference to the problem of cervical spondylosis. *Brain.* 1957;30:571-596.
49. Piepgras DG. Posterior decompression for myelopathy due to cervical spondylosis: laminectomy alone versus laminectomy with dentate ligament section. *Clin Neurosurg.* 1977;24:508-515.
50. Raynor RB, Pugh J, Shapiro I. Cervical facetectomy and its effect on spine strength. *J Neurosurg.* 1985;63:278-282.
51. Reid JD. Effects of flexion-extension movements of the head and spine upon the spinal cord and nerve roots. *J Neurol Neurosurg Psychiatry.* 1960;23:214-221.
52. Rogers L. The surgical treatment of cervical spondylotic myelopathy: mobilisation of the complete cervical cord into an enlarged canal. *J Bone Joint Surg Br.* 1961;43B:3-6.
53. Rogers L. The treatment of cervical spondylitic myelopathy by mobilisation of the cervical cord into an enlarged spinal canal. *J Neurosurg.* 1961;18:490-492.
54. Saunders RL, Bernini PM, Shirreffs TG Jr, et al. Central corpectomy for cervical spondylotic myelopathy: a consecutive series with long-term follow-up evaluation. *J Neurosurg.* 1991;74:163-170.
55. Scoville WB. Cervical spondylosis treated by bilateral facetectomy and laminectomy. *J Neurosurg.* 1961;13:423-428.
56. Sim FH, Svien HJ, Bickel WH, et al. Swan-neck deformity following extensive cervical laminectomy: a review of 21 cases. *J Bone Joint Surg Am.* 1974;56A:564-580.
57. Stoltmann HF, Blackwood W. The role of the ligamenta flava in the pathogenesis of myelopathy in cervical spondylosis. *Brain.* 1964;87:45-50.
58. Stoops WL, King RB. Chronic myelopathy associated with cervical spondylosis: its response to laminectomy and foramenotomy. *JAMA.* 1965;192:281-284.
59. Stoops WL, King RB. Neural complications of cervical spondylosis: their response to laminectomy and foramenotomy. *J Neurosurg.* 1962;19:986-999.
60. Stringer WL, Kelly DL Jr, Johnston FR, et al. Hyperextension injury of the cervical spine with esophageal perforation: case report. *J Neurosurg.* 1980;53:541-543.
61. Taylor AR. The mechanism of injury to the spinal cord in the neck without damage to the vertebral column. *J Bone Joint Surg Br.* 1951;33B:543-547.
62. Verbiest H, Paz y Geuse HD. Anterolateral surgery for cervical spondylosis in cases of myelopathy or nerve-root compression. *J Neurosurg.* 1966;25:611-622.
63. White AA III, Johnson RM, Panjabi MM, et al. Biomechanical analysis of clinical stability in the cervical spine. *Clin Orthop.* 1975;109:85-96.
64. Wilkinson HA, LeMay ML, Ferris EJ. Clinical-radiographic correlations in cervical spondylosis. *J Neurosurg.* 1969;30:213-218.
65. Yasuoka S, Peterson HA, Laws ER Jr, et al. Pathogenesis and prophylaxis of postlaminectomy deformity of the spine after multiple level laminectomy: difference between children and adults. *Neurosurgery.* 1981;9:145-151.
66. Yasuoka S, Peterson HA, MacCarty CS. Incidence of spinal column deformity after multilevel laminectomy in children and adults. *J Neurosurg.* 1982;57:441-445.
67. Yonenobu K, Okada K, Fuji T, et al. Causes of neurologic deterioration following surgical treatment of cervical myelopathy. *Spine.* 1985;11:818-823.

CHAPTER 8

Cervical Spondylotic Radiculopathy: Management with Posterior Operation

Ulrich Batzdorf, MD

The first recorded posterior approach in the treatment of brachial neuralgia took place in 1889, when Abbe[1] performed both extra- and intradural nerve root sections in a patient whose radicular pain had already led to an arm amputation, without pain relief. The laminectomy and transdural approach to osteophytes and disks, then known as ventral chondromas, was carried out successfully and was described by Ellsberg[3] in 1931 and by Stookey in 1940.[17] The dura was opened in most instances and dentate ligaments were sectioned to permit rotation of the spinal cord away from the lesions.[17]

While some later authors followed this with refinements of an intradural decompressive approach, better understanding of the pathophysiology of cervical disk and osteophytic disease led to the evolution of a purely extradural decompressive procedure of the nerve root as described by Spurling and Scoville's "keyhole" procedure in 1944.[16] Allen's[2] "window" with extradural dissection was clearly the forerunner of later techniques, although he still opened the dura for decompression in some patients.

Frykholm's[7] comprehensive monograph in 1951 added considerably to our understanding of the problem of cervical nerve root compressive problems and their surgical treatment. Although the basic exposure described by Frykholm, who used a high-speed drill, has remained unchanged to date, he was not quite ready to abandon an intradural approach, and opened the dura over the root sleeve. Scoville's[15] approach became completely extradural and this indeed is the technique generally used today, "unroofing and unwalling" the nerve root sheath at its anterior angulation with a high speed drill.

Advantages and Disadvantages of the Posterior Approach to the Nerve Root

Major advantages and disadvantages are associated with the posterior approach to the nerve root by the foraminotomy technique.

Advantages

1. The compressed segment of the nerve root is under direct vision.[6]
2. The procedure does not involve an intervertebral fusion, which is either deliberately performed or occurs spontaneously with all anterior interbody procedures. It therefore also eliminates the risk of accelerated degeneration at an adjacent interspace, which fusion may entail.
3. The procedure does not carry risk to major vessels, the recurrent laryngeal nerve and the esophagus. While rare complications, these have to be considered in the anterior approach. The spinal cura

is visualized only over its most lateral 3-4 mm, reducing the risk of injury to the spinal cord.

4. The period of postoperative neck immobilization is brief and is determined only by postoperative neck pain. A soft collar usually suffices and seldom needs to be worn for more than a week after surgery. Patients can return to normal activities, including driving, without concern over the status of a fusion.

Disadvantages

1. The osteophytic ridge compressing the nerve root is often not removed by this approach and the root is decompressed by allowing it to move away from the bone spur lying anterior to it. This is not the case when the posterior approach is performed for an acute cervical disk herniation; a fragment of the disk can very often be identified and extracted.
2. Inadvertent removal of too much (more than one-half) of the facet joint may lead to instability, which would require reoperation and fusion.
3. All my patients are advised preoperatively that in rare instances this posterior approach does not relieve the pain or does so incompletely, necessitating a second, anterior operation. These possibly represent patients with extremely large osteophytes that indent the root even when the roof of the neural foramen is no longer present.

Case Selection

Candidates for posterior cervical nerve root decompression procedures are generally:

1. Patients with unilateral nerve root compression syndromes at one or two levels; occasionally, patients with bilateral nerve root compression at one level, in the absence of canal stenosis.
2. Patients with a combined picture of myelopathy and radiculopathy, who have maintained a normal cervical lordosis and who are, by other criteria, candidates for a laminectomy rather than an anterior approach. This would also include patients with multiple levels of spondylotic spinal cord compression and patients with a congenitally narrow spinal canal.
3. Patients who already have undergone an anterior cervical disk and osteophyte removal at the appropriate level and who have gone on to fusion, but who continue to have radicular symptoms and who show imaging evidence of persistent lateral root compression. Multiple root decompression procedures may be performed. In such patients the anterior decompression often was not wide enough, limiting decompression of the more lateral portion of the neural foramen.[12]
4. Patients who, for some other reason such as an open tracheostomy, are not suitable candidates for an anterior approach.

Patients with degenerative subluxation of the vertebral bodies at the level of root involvement, particularly when there is evidence of hypermobility at the interspace, are not good candidates for a posterior root decompression. In these patients interbody fusion will help relieve pressure on the root, while hypermobility could be increased by posterior surgery. Improper selection of patients as well as excessive removal of facets has caused some surgeons to incorrectly abandon facetectomy.[18]

Radiculopathy in association with myelopathy and a kyphotic spondylotic cervical spine deformity is also better treated by an anterior approach as the primary form of therapy. Posterior root decompression may be warranted in a few such patients in whom the anterior approach to the interspace and foramen failed to produce adequate relief of radicular symptoms.

Technique
Anesthesia

Endotracheal intubation should be undertaken with special consideration of the underlying problem of spondylosis. Patients with coexisting myelopathy, due either to spondylotic bars or a congenitally narrow canal, pose a particular risk and should undergo awake fiberoptic intubation. While patients with only spondylotic radiculopathy do not carry the same risk, for most patients with radiculopathy, neck extension is the posture most likely to provoke pain and nerve root compression. Awake fiberoptic intubation with the head and neck in neutral position is therefore also preferred for many of these patients.

Surgical Approach

Patient Position

Some advantages inhere to operating on the cervical spine with the patient in the sitting position. Although the sitting position has been employed by many excellent surgeons,[4,6,14] we believe the disadvantages outweigh the benefits. We prefer to have the patient prone, with the neck in neutral position, the head maintained in a Mayfield head holder. The benefits of easier hemostasis in the sitting position are readily balanced by careful control of bleeding in the prone position. The potential risks of air embolism and the additional time needed to bring the patient to the sitting position further justify operating with the patient prone.

It is important to assess the patient's neck posture preoperatively, and to be aware of a patient's usual posture of comfort, so that a similar posture can be maintained with the patient under anesthesia in the prone position. Both hyperextension and excessive neck flexion must be avoided when positioning a patient. Great care must also be taken in turning the anesthetized patient from the supine to the prone position at the beginning of the procedure. The key to performing the transfer of the patient to and from the operating table safely is to have enough help available to move the patient under full control, slowly and gently, with one person specifically assigned to prevent excessive neck motion. At times we have applied the Philadelphia collar at the conclusion of the procedure as a temporary means of stabilizing the patient's neck during the initial transfer. The head of the operating table is raised slightly, if necessary, to bring the neck into a horizontal plane.

Incision to Expose the Site of Interlaminar Foraminal Decompression

Palpation may help to identify the spinous process at the level of the planned foraminal decompression; a preliminary radiograph may be useful in planning the skin incision. A midline cervical incision through skin and subcutaneous tissue brings the surgeon to the deep cervical fascia. In order to preserve the interspinous ligament the deep fascial layer is incised a few millimeters lateral to the midline on the side of the planned exposure, or on each side of the midline when a bilateral exposure is to be carried out. Sacrificing the interspinous ligament and dissecting out the spinous process adds nothing to the exposure and risks increasing angulation of the spine at the level of the exposure. Meyerding retractors are useful for unilateral exposures; 1-inch-wide blade retractors are available for bilateral exposures. An intraoperative lateral film with a metallic marker on the spinous process is essential unless the characteristic posterior arch of C2 has been exposed, permitting an accurate count. In order to avoid all error it is important to trace the lamina from the marked spinous process to the lamina.

Bone Removal

The local anatomy should be reviewed with aid of a spine model or skeleton if the surgeon is not familiar with this approach (Figures 1A,B). Bone removal is best started in the interlaminar space, in such manner as to identify the lateral margin of the spinal canal, an important landmark, without uncovering the spinal cord itself. The dural sleeve covering the nerve root lies beneath the lamina and between the pedicles of adjacent vertebrae. Anatomic variations occur in

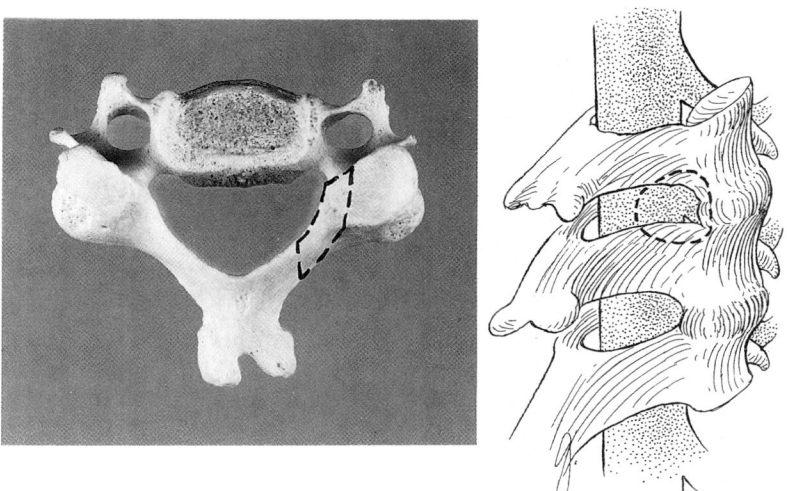

Figure 1A. Outline of laminar drill hole superimposed on axial photograph of a cervical vertebra (left), and superimposed on a drawing of the cervical spine, showing the relationships of the lateral margin of the spinal dura and the root sleeve to the foraminotomy (right).

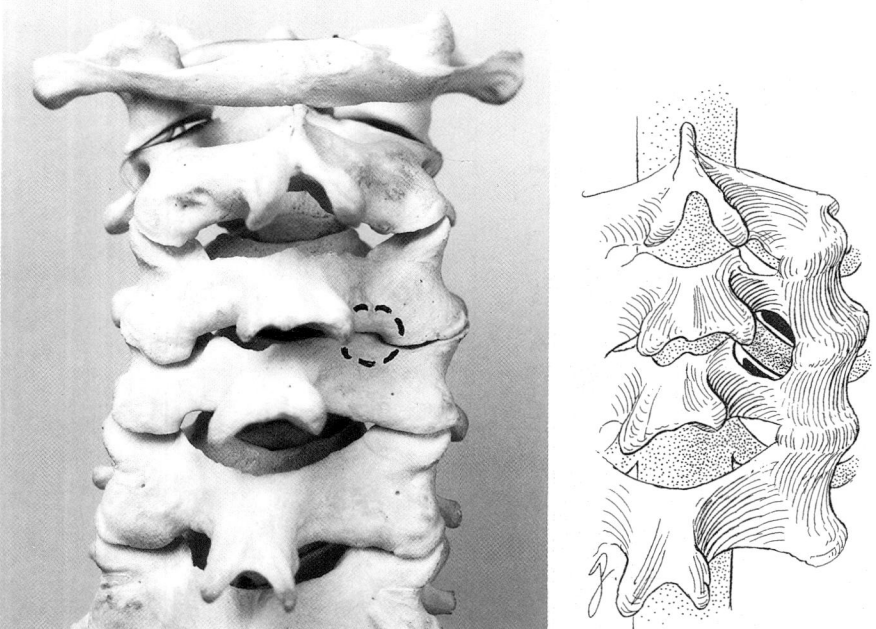

Figure 1B. Outline of initial drill hole into adjacent laminae (left), and close-up of relationship between the lateral margin of the spinal dura, the dural root sleeve, and the walls of the neural foramen, after the decompression has been completed (right). Both the shoulder and axilla of the neural foramen may require drilling. The interspinous ligament, which is preserved, is not shown in this diagram.

Cervical Spondylotic Radiculopathy: Management with Posterior Operation 109

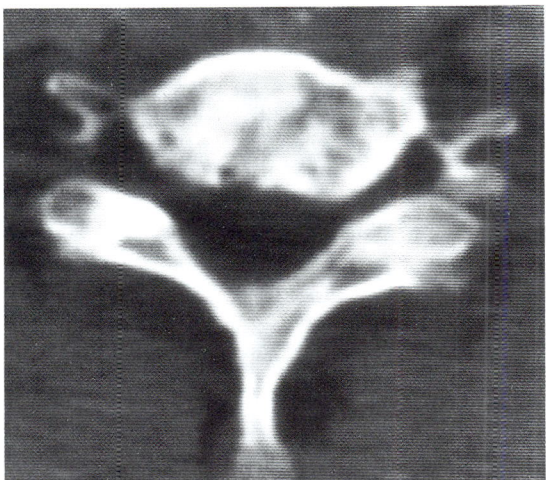

Figure 2. Preoperative (top) and postoperative (bottom) axial computerized tomography (CT) images of the C6 vertebra following bilateral C6-7 foraminotomies, showing the extent of bone removal.

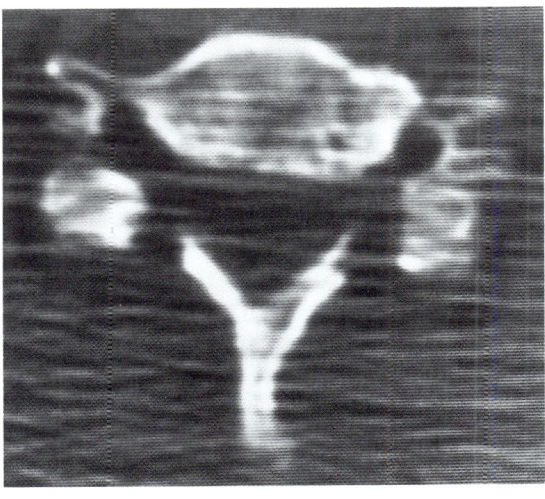

the intimate relationships between the nerve root, its bony surroundings and the disk interspace; these are greater when shingling or telescoping of the laminae alters the relationships of the interlaminar space to the nerve root beneath and when the root itself is displaced by an osteophyte. Generally the undersurface of the lower facet of the interspace is in widest contact with the dorsal surface of the root—e.g. at the C5-6 interspace, the superior facet of C6 has the widest contact with the root.

We prefer to use a limited number of instruments: a high-speed drill, using first a steel burr and changing to a diamond burr once the dura is exposed, has worked well for us. A series of sharp curettes in assorted small sizes and angles are extremely useful. Magnification with either microscope or loupes is essential, both for the preservation of normal structures and for identification of the pathology.

Bone removal for the foraminotomy is generally made with the high-speed drill in the shape of a slanted quadrilateral (parallel to the interlaminar space) or a pear lying on its side (see Figure 2). A steel cutting burr is used initially; as the bone is thinned out, one switches to a diamond burr. As soon as the dural sleeve is first seen, the surgeon can orient himself to the direction that the root takes using a blunt nerve hook, and can proceed to enlarge the opening in order to uncover the root sleeve laterally. It is generally accepted that the medial one-third[4] or even one-half of the facet joint may be sacrificed in order to uncover the root sleeve fully before it turns anteriorly.

This point of forward angulation must be clearly identified, as it represents the lateral margin of bone removal. The very thin layer of bone covering the root can be easily removed with a small curette. The length of root sleeve that can be uncovered before the medial margin of the facet joint is reached is variable, but is usually about 5 mm. A careful study of this was performed by Raynor.[12] He also showed that the root may lie cephalad to the interspace, explaining inadequate root decompression in some patients treated by an anterior transdiskal approach. One can usually expose 8-9 mm of the nerve root beyond the lateral edge of the spinal dura.

We attempt to be as conservative as possible in drilling into the facet joint, and have made it a practice to undercut the facet joint over the root with a small diamond burr rather than sacrificing more full thickness of the joint. We have not encountered any subluxation or facet joint instability after performing a posterior root decompression. Laminectomy or hemilaminectomy in conjunction with posterior root decompression was recommended by Scoville[14,15] to permit removal of the ligamentum flavum, which was regarded a possible source of compression. Today we would perform a laminectomy only if specifically indicated by imaging studies—e.g. focal canal stenosis.

The lateral spinal dura and the root sleeve will be covered by the thinned lateral margin of the ligamentum flavum, and this should be excised. Epidural veins, which may surround the root sleeve, should be coagulated with the bipolar cautery and divided. This maneuver is essential in order to mobilize the root sleeve in search of an osteophyte or disk fragment. While there is general agreement on the need to remove acutely herniated disk fragments pressing on the nerve root, the removal of osteophytes is more controversial. Some authors use a high-speed drill,[5,13] small curettes,[4,5] or even a small osteotome[9] to remove osteophytes; others have found that decompressing the root from the dorsal aspect without any attempt at osteophyte removal suffices.[8,9,15]

Obviously, if a patient has already undergone an anterior osteophyte removal, this issue may not arise; in many instances when the anterior approach has failed to relieve root compression, it is because disk and osteophyte were not removed sufficiently laterally. When nerve roots are decompressed in conjunction with a full laminectomy, great care must be exercised to avoid removing too much of the medial facet. Because of the more extensive ligamentous and muscle disruption that accompanies a full laminectomy, facetectomy should be planned conservatively; ligamentous tissue overlying the root can be removed with small, angled curettes.

The axilla, in particular,[5,14] as well as the shoulder of the root sleeve merit particular attention. A small diamond-tip burr or sharp curette should be used to eliminate any pressure that bone, constituting the rostral and caudal margins of the foramen, might exert against the root sleeve.

When the dural sleeve has been completely uncovered from the posterior approach, a small dissector and nerve hook are used to mobilize the root in its bed, and to be certain that there are no adhesions along the anterior surface of the dural sleeve. Laterally, the root should be free to the point at which it clearly turns anteriorly. We do not open the dural sheath in the manner originally advocated by Frykholm,[7] and we have had excellent symptomatic relief in most patients without taking this additional step. Our concern is that opening the dura eliminates an important barrier to scar tissue that may form postoperatively. The risk that opening the dura may cause injury to small bridging vessels, which supply the nerve root, has also been cited.[14]

Results

While many authors have described favorable results with posterior cervical root decompression for radiculopathy, the reports generally lack the detail one would wish with respect to relief of specific symptoms and findings other than pain. The difficulty in quantitating improvement in any of these parameters further complicates an analysis of postoperative results.

Many surgeons do not distinguish between true osteophytic disease, as seen in spondylosis, and soft-disk herniation, and, from the point of view of surgical technique, treat these conditions in identical manner. Murphey et al[11] summarized their results with more than 600 patients, but these patients all had true disk or annular ruptures. Only the studies by Frykholm[7] and by Henderson et al[8] are helpful in detailed analysis (Table 1); the latter study, detailing exceptionally good results, does include a mixture of "soft"-disk protrusions and osteophytic ridges. The inclusion of these data appears justified, however, since these lesions were treated in identical manner and no effort was made to remove soft disk herniations. while only these studies have been tabulated, the generally more favorable results reported by Henderson et al are

TABLE 1
Outcome of Foraminal Decompression for Cervical Radiculopathy

Series	Number of Patient Procedures	Preoperative Symptoms and Signs			
		Pain	Weakness	Atrophy	Sensory
Frykholm[7]	19[a]	100% (19)	89% (17)	73% (14)	68% (13)
Henderson et al[8]	846[b]	99.4% (841)	68% (576)	Not stated	85% (721)

Series (continued)	Pain				Weakness			Atrophy				Sensory			
	Relief	Improved	Fair	Same or Worse	Relief	Improved	Same	Relief	Improved	Same	Unknown	Relief	Improved	Same	Worse
Frykholm[7] (7)	37% (3)	16% (8)	42% (1)	5% (5)	26% (0)	53% (2)	11% (1)	5% (1)	5% (7)	37% (5)	26% (4)	21% (5)	26% (3)	16% (1)	5%
Henderson et al[8]	95.5% (709)		4.5% (38)		97.7% (564)		2.3% (12)	Not stated				76% 544		24%[c] (177)	

[a]Represents procedures performed for hard disks only
[b]Represents procedures performed for hard disks and soft disks, which are combined, but treated identically
[c]Recalculated from raw data

reflected in the work of other authors as well,[4,15] and are in general agreement with our own experience.

Complications

Spinal instability is a serious potential complication arising from the posterior, facetectomy approach to the root and is due to excessive removal of facets, particularly in patients with pre-existing hypermobility at the particular interspace.[10] This complication has not been seen in patients who underwent a facetectomy as described, removing one-third, or at most, one-half of the facet.[4,15]

Injury to the root may result in new sensory or motor deficit after surgery. A transient increase in radicular pain is not uncommon postoperatively, and presumably is due to retraction and manipulation of the nerve root sheath. Such increased pain usually abates by the third postoperative day. Cerebrospinal fluid leak from the dural sleeve is a potential complication we have not encountered. Reapproximation of the dura with fine suture material is recommended. Injury to the spinal cord could occur from poor control of instruments and from disorientation of the surgeon with respect to the anatomy of the operative field.

The author is aware of one instance of injury to the vertebral artery that occurred when a surgeon reached in front of the root in an attempt to extract what he believed to be a fragment of intervertebral disk. The disk space should not be entered from this posterior approach;[6] if the interspace is not entered, it is extremely unlikely that the vertebral artery will be encountered. Coagulation of the injured vessel or packing the foramen transversarium with muscle may suffice to control hemorrhage, but serious problems may result from vertebral artery occlusion.

Conclusion

Posterior decompression of a cervical nerve root or roots is a relatively simple procedure with generally excellent levels of pain relief and neurologic improvement. Appropriate patient selection and intimate familiarity with the surgical anatomy are important to the success of the procedure.

References

1. Abbe R. A contribution to the surgery of the spine. *The Medical Record*. 1889;35:149-152.
2. Allen KL. Neuropathies caused by bony spurs in the cervical spine with special reference to surgical treatment. *J Neurol Neurosurg Psychiatry*. 1952;15:20-36.
3. Elsberg CA. The extradural ventral chondromas (ecchondroses), their favorite sites, the spinal cord and root symptoms they produce, and their surgical treatment. *Bull Neurol Inst NY*. 1931;1:350-388.
4. Epstein JA, Lavine LS, Aronson HA, et al. Cervical spondylotic radiculopathy: the syndrome of foraminal constriction treated by foramenotomy and the removal of osteophytes. *Clin Orthop*. 1965;40:113-122.
5. Fager CA. Rationale and techniques of posterior approaches to cervical disk lesions and spondylosis. *Surg Clin North Am*. 1976;56:581-592.
6. Fager CA. Management of cervical disc lesions and spondylosis by posterior approaches. *Clin Neurosurg*. 1977;24:488-507.
7. Frykholm R. Cervical nerve root compression resulting from disc degeneration and root-sleeve fibrosis: a clinical investigation. *Acta Chir Scand Suppl*. 1951;160.
8. Henderson CM, Hennessy RG, Shuey HM Jr, et al. Posterior-lateral foraminotomy as an exclusive operative technique for cervical radiculopathy: a review of 846 consecutively operated cases. *Neurosurgery*. 1983;13:504-512.
9. Logue V. Cervical spondylosis. In: Williams D, ed. *Modern Trends in Neurology, Second Series*. London: Butterworth & Co; 1975:259-273.
10. Mayfield FH. Cervical spondylosis: a comparison of the anterior and posterior approaches. *Clin Neurosurg*. 1966;13:181-188.
11. Murphey F, Simmons JCH, Brunson B. Surgical treatment of laterally ruptured cervical disc: review of 648 cases, 1939 to 1972. *J Neurosurg*. 1973;38:679-683.
12. Raynor RB. Anterior or posterior approach to the cervical spine:an anatomical and radiographic evaluation and comparison. *Neurosurgery*. 1983;12:7-13.
13. Raynor RB. Anterior and posterior approaches to the cervical spinal cord, discs, and roots: a comparison of exposures and decompressions. In: The Cervical Spine Research Society, Editorial Committee, ed. *The Cervical Spine, 2nd ed*. Philadelphia, Pa: JB Lippincott Company, 1989:659-669.
14. Scoville WB. Cervical spondylosis treated by bilateral facetectomy and laminectomy. *J Neurosurg*. 1961;18:423-428.
15. Scoville WB, Whitcomb BB. Lateral rupture of cervical intervertebral disks. *Postgrad Med*. 1966;39:174-180.
16. Spurling RG, Scoville WB. Lateral rupture of the cervical intervertebral discs: a common cause of shoulder and arm pain. *Surg, Gynecol & Obst*. 1944;78:350-358.
17. Stookey B. Compression of spinal cord and nerve roots by herniation of the nucleus pulposus in the cervical region. *Arch Surg*. 1940;40:417-432.
18. Verbiest H. The management of cervical spondylosis. *Clin Neurosurg*. 1973;20:262-294.

CHAPTER 9

The Soft Cervical Disk: Natural History and Management

Regis W. Haid, Jr., MD

"Cervical disk disease" is a ubiquitous term that encompasses a multitude of pathologic states. The clinical spectrum of this disorder may range from "diskogenic" neck pain to a myelopathy with quadraparesis. It remains problematic to directly correlate the anatomic degeneration of the cervical disk with the clinical picture and radiographic findings.

Degenerative disease of the cervical spine may present with a variety of clinical signs and symptoms. Nonoperative treatment remains the cornerstone of prudent management in the majority of cases. However, operative treatment is indicated in patients with symptoms and signs of progressive neural compression and/or spinal instability.

This chapter focuses on an isolated entity in the degenerative cascade—the soft cervical disk causing neural compression. Considerable controversy exists regarding the optimal treatment of this condition.

Natural History

To ascertain the true natural history of a lesion so commonly treated with surgery is difficult. The surgeon often intervenes in the treatment before a true determination of natural long-term outcome can be made. The majority of soft disk herniations are posterolateral, producing unilateral radiculopathy. Patients most commonly present with pain and/or neurologic findings in the distribution of a specific cervical nerve root. Radiculopathies tend to improve with time. At least 75% of patients presenting with a unilateral cervical radiculopathy will improve with nonsurgical therapy. Indeed a majority of patients will improve before imaging confirms the presence of a soft disk.[16] Although the sequelae of weakness or dermatomal sensory abnormalities may persist, the pain usually improves. Surgical options are thereby aimed at improving functional status and quality of life. The percentage of patients with soft cervical disks who do not need surgery is unknown.[17]

In one series of young athletes with acute cervical radiculopathy treated without operation, 17 of 20 patients returned to full activity after a mean of 17 weeks. However, neurologic deficits took several months to improve.[28] In a mixed series of patients, cervical radiculopathy rarely progressed to myelopathy, but symptoms persisted in 60% of patients treated nonoperatively.[42] Another study reported outcome after nonoperative treatment. Of the patients in this series, 31% had neck pain and 69% had neck and radicular pain. Of this group, 45% had satisfactory pain resolution.[29]

Rarely, a large midline cervical disk herniation may cause myelopathy and require ur-

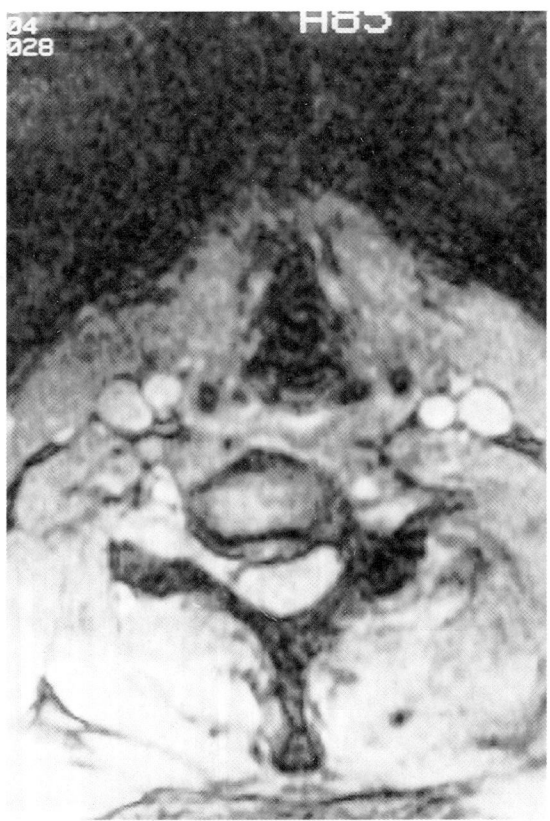

Figure 1. A T-2 weighted axial MRI reveals a broad-based soft disk herniation in a patient who presented with a myeloradiculopathy.

gent decompression (Figure 1). One series of 26 central disk herniations reported a disproportionate incidence at the C3-4 level producing myelopathy, commonly involving the posterior column function of the upper extremities.[36]

Clinical Presentation

Although a soft herniated disk may occasionally produce myelopathy, the most common presentation is a unilateral radiculopathy. However, radicular syndromes may result from a wide variety of pathologic etiologies. The most common causes are posterolateral soft disk herniations and/or spondylotic osteophytes at the neural foramen. Facet joint or ligamentum flavum hypertrophy or congenital canal stenosis may predispose to nerve root compression.[15]

A cervical monoradiculopathy commonly produces medial periscapular pain with radiation into the upper extremity. This brachalgia is commonly associated with specific nerve root signs of weakness, atrophy, decreased deep tendon reflexes, paresthesias or hypesthesias. This clinical sign usually will localize the compression to one level.[46] However, there are anatomic variations that may make the exact level unclear and produce a disparity between the clinical and radiographic findings. Benini evaluated 119 monoradiculopathies resulting from cervical disk herniations. Anatomic variations were explained by anastomoses between adjacent nerve roots, brachial plexus variation, and anastomoses of peripheral nerves in the forearm.[5]

Henderson et al reviewed 846 operative cases of cervical radiculopathy, 98.7% of which occurred at C5-6 or C6-7. He reported a 54% incidence of pain and paresthesia in the normal dermatomal pattern, and 46% in a nondermatomal pattern.[25] One explanation is that sensory dysfunction is dermatomal, whereas pain is myotomal. They further report that specific motor weakness was observed in 68%, deep tendon reflex diminution in 71%, and sensory loss in 85%. Approximately half had periscapular pain, 80% had neck pain, 18% had anterior chest pain, and 10% had headaches.

In this author's experience, medial periscapular pain is almost always present, and isolated neck pain is relatively uncommon. Although the majority of patients have disk herniations at the C5-6 and C6-7 levels, a higher percentage have C3-4 and C4-5 disks than was reported by Henderson et al.[25]

In a retrospective review of 295 patients with cervical radiculopathies, Lunsford et al reported the following distribution of disk herniation: C5-6, 48%; C6-7, 37%; C4-5, 10%; C3-4, 3%, and C7-T1, 2%.[30] It is interesting to note that this incidence corresponds to the degree of movement at each level (i.e. the greater the range of motion of a level, the higher the incidence of pathologic

The Soft Cervical Disk: Natural History and Management

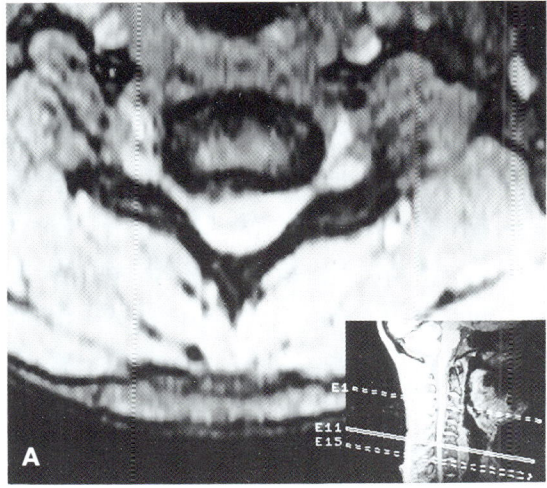

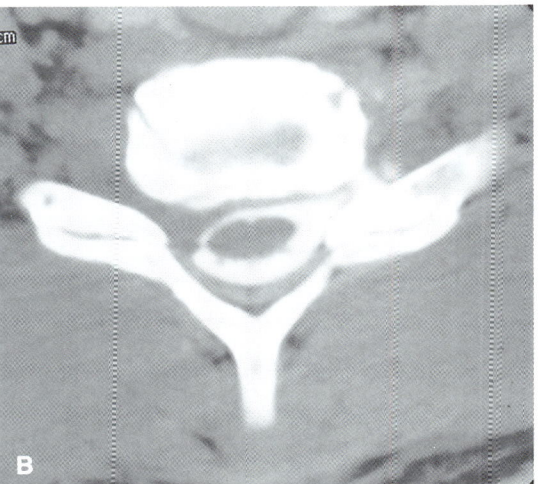

Figure 2. (A) The T2-weighted axial MRI reveals right foraminal narrowing, presumably secondary to mild spondylosis. (B) Because the patient's clinical symptoms seemed disproportionately worse than was indicated by the MRI, a postmyelogram CT (CTM) was obtained. In addition to mild spondylosis, a soft disk herniation could be seen obliterating the right nerve root. In this case, we felt the CTM provided information that was not apparent from examination of the MRI. Either an anterior or posterior approach would be appropriate for this disk herniation.

processes). Lunsford et al observed no difference in the incidence of scapular, neck, arm, or chest pain when patients with hard and soft disks were compared. Similarly, there was no difference in the incidence of unilateral or bilateral presentation. Soft disk herniations more commonly resulted in reflex loss, cervical muscle spasm, restricted motion, a positive Spurling's sign (pain reproduction with cervical spine hyperextension and lateral rotation), and pain or motor deficit in a single dermatomal or myotomal distribution.[31] In the series of Davidson et al, 68% of patients exhibited a positive Spurling's sign.[13] Nerve root tension may frequently be reduced and pain relieved by abducting the shoulder. The patient typically places the forearm on top of the head or rests the hand at the level of the breast pocket in a "Napoleonic" manner. Pain may be increased by sneezing, coughing, straining, or a Valsalva maneuver.

Imaging Evaluation

The goal of imaging of patients with suspected cervical disk herniation is to correlate clinical signs and symptoms with anatomic abnormalities. The most frequently employed imaging modalities are postmyelography computed tomography (CTM) scanning and magnetic resonance imaging (MRI). Several studies correlating preoperative radiographic diagnosis with surgically confirmed cervical disk disease reported a 92% accuracy with water-soluble CTM scanning and 85% to 90% accuracy with MRI. With advances in MRI imaging, the accuracy of this modality should improve and match CTM scanning, which at this time remains the standard against which all other diagnostic modalities are compared. When either myelography or CT are used alone, a lesser degree of accuracy is reported.[3,9,12,33]

On this author's service, MRI is the initial imaging examination after routine plain x-rays are obtained. If the diagnosis is unclear after MRI examination, CTM scanning is performed (Figure 2).

Management

The goals of treatment are to return the

patient to a normal functional level as soon as possible with the least expense and the least risk. There are no prospective, randomized, double-blind studies comparing operative and nonoperative treatment. The choice of treatment depends on the clinician's bias and experience, the patient's age, occupation, and desire for surgical or nonsurgical therapy.

The duration of nonoperative therapy prior to surgery is frequently a difficult decision. Nonoperative treatment should be continued if pain and neurologic deficits are improving. It is commonly accepted that neurologic deterioration is an indication for surgical decompression. Prompt operative intervention also is appropriate in the patient who presents severe neurologic deficit or disabling loss of function.[44]

We advocate earlier surgery for patients with severe deltoid or intrinsic hand muscle weakness, deficits which can be functionally devastating to a patient's vocational or social life. Fortunately, C5 and C8 root lesions are relatively uncommon. The majority of disk herniations involve either the C6 or C7 root, which are less important functionally. A longer duration of nonsurgical therapy may be considered in this latter group.

Nonoperative Treatment

Although no scientific studies have compared operative and nonoperative treatment modalities, most patients should undergo a trial of nonoperative therapy. The mainstay of therapy is immobilization, which can be accomplished by bedrest and/or a soft cervical collar. It is unclear whether continuous or intermittent use of a collar is optimal.[14] Cervical halter or manual traction has also been used but its efficacy is not clear. It is possible that traction is effective because the neck is immobilized and muscle spasm is reduced. However, there is no evidence that axial distraction reduces the degree of disk prolapse.[23] An attempt is made to discontinue the orthotic as soon as possible to prevent muscle atrophy and contracture.

If the patient presents with severe pain, a brief 2—3-day trial of narcotics may be indicated. Severe paraspinous muscle spasm is best treated with benzodiazepines. A 10-14-day course of nonsteroidal anti-inflammatory agents (NSAIDS) should be used unless otherwise contraindicated. Some clinicians prescribe a short course of oral corticosteroids. The continued use of these modalities is dependent on the patient's response.

Boden and Wiesel advocate trigger point injections. There are no true studies to verify the efficacy of this treatment, however. While some patients may respond to this therapy, they are usually not those with a radiculopathy secondary to soft cervical disk herniation.[7]

Although topical corticosteroids and ultrasound may be appropriate for shoulder pain secondary to biceps tendonitis, it has little relevance in the treatment of radiculopathies caused by cervical radiculopathy. Range of motion or muscle strengthening exercises may be useful after the acute symptoms have resolved. However, it is unclear whether a patient's response to exercise has a direct effect on the factors causing the radiculopathy or is related to an overall improved sense of well-being.[8]

Surgical Treatment

What constitutes failure of nonoperative management will vary among surgeons.[44] In general, operative treatment should be considered for those patients with: (1) progressive neurologic deficit, (2) myelopathy, (3) nonprogressive but disabling motor deficit, and (4) failure to respond to nonoperative therapy.

An occasional patient with a large C3-4 disk, severe medial periscapular and posterior shoulder pain, but without motor or sensory dysfunction will respond well to surgery. For the most part, however, removing a soft herniated cervical disk solely for neck pain is not indicated. Most series report a poor response to cervical disketomy in patients whose sole symptom is neck pain.

The approach to a herniated cervical disk in the patient with motor deficit and sensory abnormalities of a radicular nature may be either anterior or posterior. Excellent results are reported with both approaches. The choice of approach is based on several factors—location of the compression, accessibility of the lesion, the patient's age, occupation, and the surgeon's experience. The surgeon should be qualified to treat cervical disk disease by either the anterior or the posterior route. Each approach offers certain advantages.

Posterior Approach

In the 1950s, Scoville and Spurling were among the first to describe the posterior decompressive "keyhole" technique to treat lateral herniated disks and/or osteophytes.[45,46] It has since enjoyed widespread success with low morbidity. The posterior approach has several distinct advantages: (1) there is no threat to soft-tissue structures of the neck such as the major vessels, trachea, esophagus, or the nerves of phonation; (2) the scar is usually hidden by the patient's clothing or hair; (3) if care is taken to preserve the facet complexes, instability is rarely a problem; (4) fusion is rarely needed; and (5) unless pre-existing kyphosis is present, the normal alignment and mobility of the spine is maintained.[18]

The "keyhole" foraminotomy is ideal for laterally placed soft herniated disks. Although some surgeons have reported excellent results with this approach in treating spondylotic osteophytes,[18] osteophytes are more safely and easily removed using the anterior approach. The posterior approach should not be used in patients with pre-existing kyphosis, anterior compression, or hard osteophytes.

Technique

After intubation, the patient is placed in the sitting or prone position with the neck in slight flexion to allow access to the interlaminar space without undue stretch and tightening of the paraspinal muscles. A posterior midline subperiosteal approach or a posterolateral muscle-splitting incision may be chosen. Regardless of the approach, the exposure should allow visualization of the facet-laminar junction. X-ray localization of the correct level is essential, and may be done after the percutaneous placement of a spinal needle or after the incision is made and the posterior elements are exposed. If the correct level is not ascertained after the initial radiograph, it should be repeated with an instrument placed in the facet joint. Depending on the musculature of the patient, the average incision is 3-5 cms in length. A single-bladed self-retaining retractor is used. The remainder of the operation should be done using loupes or the operating microscope. Bone removal may be accomplished with rongeurs, Kerrison punches, a high-speed drill, or a combination of the above; however, the high-speed drill has the advantage of accuracy and safety of bone removal. The initial bone resection is the circular part of the "keyhole" configuration. At the laminar-facet junction, an 8-10 mm bony aperture is created with removal of the inferior aspect of the superior lamina and the superior part of the inferior lamina. The lateral aspect of the "keyhole" is then made by drilling the roof of the foramen, which lies under the medial facet joint complex. The pedicle-to-pedicle exposure of the root can be obtained by judiciously removing the medial facet. No more than 1/3 to 1/2 of the medial facet complex should be removed. Removal of the lateral half of the facet will predispose the patient to instability and should be avoided.

The final unroofing of the nerve root is easily and safely accomplished with angled curettes. The lateral aspect of the ligamentum flavum is removed along with epidural fat. The nerve root should then be clearly visible. It is important that generous bony decompression be finished before root manipulation is attempted. Although some surgeons stop after the bony decompression, it is essential to check for extruded fragments or prolapsed disk compression. All epidural veins are cauterized, and the nerve root is gently mobilized superiorly with a #4 Penfield dissector and freed from the surrounding soft tissues by gentle manipulation. Any extruded fragments may then be removed with blunt nerve hooks.

If there is a large subligamentous prolapse, the annulus may be incised with a #11 blade, cutting away from the neural structures. The root is usually protected with a #4 Penfield dissector in the axilla retracting the root superiorly and medially. The disk often extrudes after a linear incision in the annulus. However, blunt hooks or dissection may "milk" the fragments from a medial to lateral direction. A micropituitary forceps is occasionally used to decompress the most lateral and posterior portion of the interspace. However, this approach precludes removal of any significant amount of material from the disk space. After decompression of the root, hemostasis is obtained with the bipolar cautery and hemostatic agents. The wound is closed in a standard fashion. Postoperative drains are rarely utilized. A soft cervical collar may be worn for comfort if needed.

Results and Complications

Most series report good results in 90% to 95% of patients after posterior operative treatment of cervical radiculopathy. In a series of 846 patients, Henderson et al reported a 96% success rate with a posterolateral foraminotomy without disk removal.[25] Simeone and Dillin cited in 98% of patients "good to excellent" results using this approach with removal of extruded disk fragments as necessary.[44]

The complication rate is uniformly low. The infection rate approaches 1%. New or increased neurologic deficit is unusual. Radiculopathy is said to worsen in 2% to 3% of patients and spinal cord injury occurs in 1 out of 200-300 cases.[18] Other possible complications include operating at the wrong level and recurrence of symptoms. With a "keyhole" foraminotomy technique, late instability does not seem to be a significant problem. Fusion should only be considered in patients with severe kyphosis, pre-existing instability, or excessive facet removal combined with laminectomy.[18,44,50]

Anterior Approach

Difficulty in obtaining access to ventrally placed spinal canal lesions via the posterior route led to the development of the anterior approach to the cervical spine. In 1955, Robinson and Smith described an anterior operation for anterior cervical fusion for disk degeneration. They described a procedure consisting of diskectomy and placement of a horseshoe tricortical iliac crest graft inserted into the interspace. The compressive osteophytes were not removed. They postulated that once arthrodesis and stability was achieved, the offending osteophytes would resorb. They also suggested that widening and fusing the disk space would enlarge the neural foramen and prevent inward buckling of the spinal canal ligaments.[40]

In 1958, Cloward described a technique that emphasized the direct surgical removal of the compressive structures. A cylinder of disk and bone was removed to gain access to the spinal canal. Cloward designed a circular drill with a guard and depth stop that allowed drilling of the disk space and adjacent vertebrae. Drilling is carried out until posterior cortical bone is encountered, then direct decompression is completed with curettes. A dowel of bone was used to maintain the interspace height and produce fusion.[11] The primary difference between the technique of Robinson and Smith and that of Cloward is not the shape of the graft configuration, but rather the direct visualization and removal of compressive osteophytes.[11,40,48]

To prevent injury to the underlying neural structures, meticulous attention is given to the depth of drilling. After decompression, a bone dowel is inserted. The bicortical ends of the dowel should be within the interspace to prevent collapse or extrusion.

Other variations have been proposed for anterior cervical disk decompression. In 1952, Bailey and Badgley performed anterior stabilization utilizing an onlay strut graft for a lytic lesion of C4—C5. This technique was best utilized for neoplasm and trauma.[4] Numerous other techniques have been reported. Biomechanical testing by White and Hirsch concluded that the Robinson and Smith horseshoe graft provided the strongest anterior support.[47]

Robinson and Smith initially advocated removal of the endplates and subchondral bone at the appropriate interspace. Later recommendations advocated *not* removing the subchondral bone. A tricortical iliac crest graft is inserted with the cancellous part directed posteriorly and the cortical segments directed anteriorly and laterally.[40] A modification has been reported in which the graft is reversed 180°. The cancellous portion faces anteriorly and the cortical segment is directed posteriorly. With this technique, the maximum amount of cortical bone is located within the interspace to better withstand axial compressive forces.[6] Whitecloud and others have reported less frequent graft extrusion and collapse and higher fusion rates utilizing this technique.[48]

Some surgeons advocate anterior cervical diskectomy without bone grafting, especially in young patients with a soft herniated disk and no spondylotic changes.[34] Diskectomy without bone grafting precludes the possibility of bone donor site complications and graft extrusion or collapse. Additional theoretical advantages include decreased progression of degenerative changes in the segments above and below the level of the diskectomy, shorter operative times and hospital stays, and a reduced need for a postoperative orthosis.

Disadvantages include interspace collapse with resultant foraminal narrowing or ligamentous buckling, and the potential for an increased incidence of kyphosis or spondylotic changes at the level of the diskectomy, and an increased incidence of late neck pain.[48]

Technique

Although there is variation in the graft configuration and the degree of neural decompression, the operative approach to the anterior cervical spine is fairly standard. The patient is placed supine on the operating table and the neck is slightly extended with a posterior neck roll. The head is *not* turned. The patient may be placed in 2-4 kg of cervical halter traction to distract the disk and aid in positioning the neck in extension. The incision may be made from either the right or left side. Right-handed surgeons generally prefer operating on the right side, and vice versa. The major disadvantage of the right-sided approach is the risk of recurrent laryngeal nerve injury at the C6-7 level and below. However, the thoracic duct may be encountered on the left side at the cervico-thoracic junction. Because it is technically easier to visualize and decompress the side of the spinal canal contralateral to the side of the incision (especially in far lateral foraminal compression) the anatomic site of the compression may determine the side of the incision.

The incision for a one-level soft cervical herniation is transverse, from the midline to the anterior border of the sternocleidomastoid muscle. An incision wider than 2 fingerbreadths is usually not needed if the fascial plane below the platysma is well undermined. The incision may be guided by a preoperative lateral radiograph with a marker. External landmarks are helpful: the hyoid bone is at C3, the thyroid cartilage at C4-5, and the cricoid at C6. The transverse process of C6 is prominent and palpable.[1]

After the incision is made, the platysma is incised in either a transverse or longitudinal direction. To gain wider access with less retraction, the plane below the platysma is widely undermined. Fascial dissection separates the sternocleidomastoid muscle and carotid sheath laterally and the trachea and esophagus medially. The prevertebral fascia is opened with blunt or sharp dissection and the anterior longitudinal ligament is exposed.

A needle 10-12 mm long is placed into the disk space and radiographic verification of the level is obtained. The longus coli muscles are reflected with a 1/4-inch "key elevator" and electrocautery. Caspar self-retaining retractors are placed under the longus coli. For a single level diskectomy, a second set of retractors for the rostral-caudal exposure is usually not needed. Instead of an intervertebral disk space spreader, this author prefers placing the Caspar distraction pins into the vertebral bodies above and below the interspace. This will provide rostral-caudal exposure, excellent unobstructed visualization of the interspace, and allow distraction of the vertebral bodies prior to bone graft placement.

The anterior longitudinal ligament and annulus are incised in a rectangular fashion, and the disk is removed with curettes and pituitary rongeurs. Loupes and a headlight are used to this point after which the operating microscope is utilized. Under the microscope, the posterior aspect of the disk and the posterior longitudinal ligament are removed.

The posterior longitudinal ligament is always opened to inspect the dura and nerve roots and remove any sequestrated fragments. The surgical microscope allows excellent visualization and a thorough decompression.

The posterior longitudinal ligament offers little biochemical support, and disk material may extrude between the ligament and the dural tube. For these reasons, the ligament should be opened to obtain optimal visualization and decompression. It is not necessary to incise the entire ligament, but only the ligament on the side of the herniation. Micro-nerve hooks and micro-curettes are used to verify that adequate foraminal decompression has been accomplished. The disk space is distracted slightly with the Caspar pins, and the height of the interspace is measured. The graft is usually 2-3 mm oversized in height. The average graft height is 8-10 mm. The vertebral body endplates are decorticated, and the graft is gently tapped into place. It should be countersunk 2-3 mm posterior to the anterior cortex. The distraction pins are relaxed, the weight is removed from the halter traction, and the graft is checked to ensure that it is securely impacted (Figure 3). A lateral radiograph is obtained while the soft tissues are closed and a subcuticular closure is performed with self-absorbing suture. Adhesive paper strips are placed to approximate the skin. A rigid collar is placed and worn for 6-12 weeks.

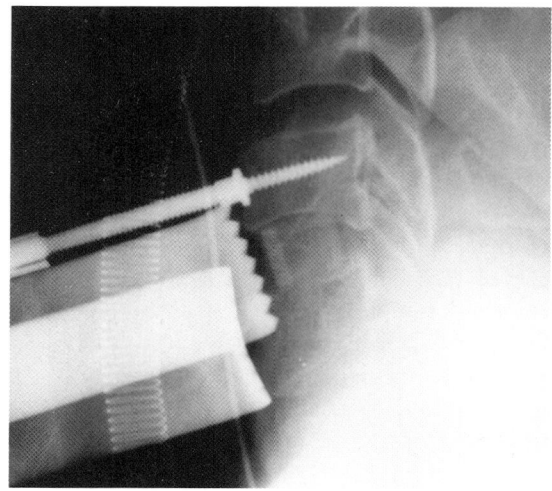

Figure 3. This intraoperative lateral radiograph was taken to confirm graft placement prior to closure. The inferior Caspar distracting pin has been removed. The superior distracting pin has not been unscrewed. The pins allow excellent distraction between the vertebral bodies without obstructing the surgeon's view. The distraction aids in providing a snug graft fit.

The use of allograft bone (human cadaver) eliminates the 14% to 20% morbidity rate of autograft harvesting and provides the same advantages of autograft.[49] Allograft bone eliminates donor site complications, and decreases operative time and hospital stay when compared to autograft fusion. Brown et al reported a 94% fusion rate for anterior cervical grafts employing the Robinson and Smith technique.[10] Utilizing the same technique, Rish reported an 80% allograft fusion rate compared to an 82% autograft fusion rate. There was no clinical difference in outcome.[37] Hanley reported a 92% fusion rate for allograft bone with the same technique. Operative time and hospital stay were decreased by 50%. Good clinical outcomes were obtained in 84%, with no correlation between radiographic pseudoarthrosis and outcome.

Allograft is useful for the majority of anterior cervical fusions. In single-level diskectomy, 92% of patients achieved fusion. Tricortical iliac crest may be placed in a "reverse Smith-Robinson" fashion, i.e. with the cancellous portion directed anteriorly. The quality of allograft bone varies, and iliac crest may collapse. A higher graft collapse rate has been reported with tricortical cancellous bone compared to fibula, which is mostly cortical bone.[22] For this reason, we now use fibular allograft (Figure 4). We have not seen radiographic evidence of collapse, and all patients have been stable in flexion-extension at 3 months. Although radiographic evidence of fusion using fibula is prolonged compared with autograft or allograft iliac crest, this has no apparent effect on outcome. In our series, radiographic evidence of fusion does not occur for 9-15 months (Figure 5). Pseudoarthrosis is not well correlated with clinical outcome, although two patients with nonunion (10% of the patients in our series) underwent reoperation for severe mechanical neck pain.

Results

Whitecloud reviewed the results reported in several series of patients undergoing anterior disk excision and fusion.[49] Utilizing the criteria set out by Odom, et al,[35] out of a total of 1689 patients, 74% had good or excellent results, 17% fair results, and 9% had poor outcomes. However, outcome varied considerably among the series reviewed, and good or excellent results were reported in 51% to 96% of patients. These series include multilevel fusions as well as spondylotic disease cases.[49] In a unilateral single-level radiculopathy secondary to a soft herniated disk, the results should be excellent. Indeed, it is clear that the best results are obtained in patients with a monoradiculopathy of less than 1 year duration. In 88 patients with disk herniation, Aronson reported good or excellent results in 87.[2] There is a great disparity among series with regard to indications, pathology encountered, and the degree of decompression attempted. In comparing the series, it is clear that radicular symptoms responded best to treatment and that patients with "neck pain only" had good results only 25% of the time. In patients with a monoradiculopathy a 90% success rate can be achieved following "disk excision and fusion."[2,49]

There is concern that degenerative processes will accelerate at levels adjacent to those fused. DePalma reported an 81% incidence of degenerative changes at adjacent levels after fusion.[14] However, this group included patients with pre-existing spondylotic disease. The changes were more common at the caudal level than at the rostral level. No clinical sequelae were observed. Other studies have shown no significant acceleration in degenerative changes at adjacent interspaces when compared to a control (nonoperated) group. However, an increased incidence of anterior osteophytes was noted.[20] It remains unclear whether utilizing a graft following diskectomy accelerates the degenerative process compared to diskectomy without grafting.

Clinical results in patients who did not receive grafts is similar to those who did. It is interesting to note that most series report a spontaneous arthrodesis rate of 70% to 98% in cases where a bone graft is not utilized. A variety of techniques has been reported with good clinical results.[1,2,18,34,41,48] Hirsch, et al. noted a good or excellent result in 80% of patients who had removal of only the anterior and middle annulus. The posterior annulus and ligament were left intact.[26] Other series report similar results with fusion rates of 75% to 80% and osteophyte resorption in 40% to 60% of cases.[34,41] In patients who do not "fuse," instability rarely occurs.[1,2,34,39,41,48]

Several other authors, including Robertson,[38] Hankinson and Wilson[21] reported microsurgical removal of the annulus and posterior ligament without bone grafting. Good to excellent results were seen in approximately 80% of patients. Martins advocated radical decompression with a 92% good to excellent outcome. However, in his study, there was no difference between those who

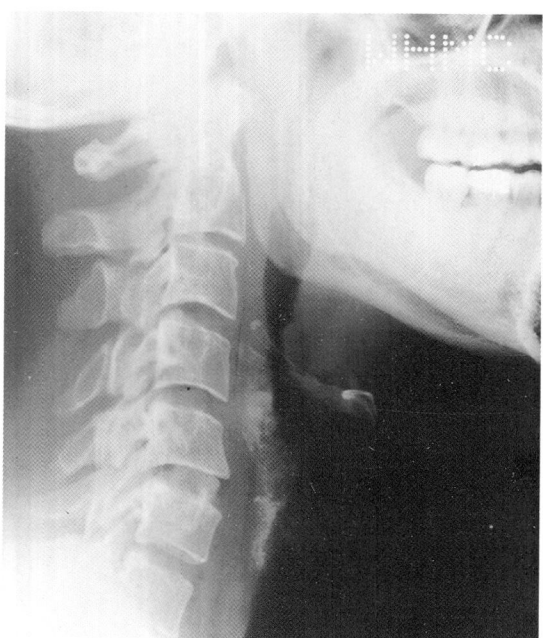
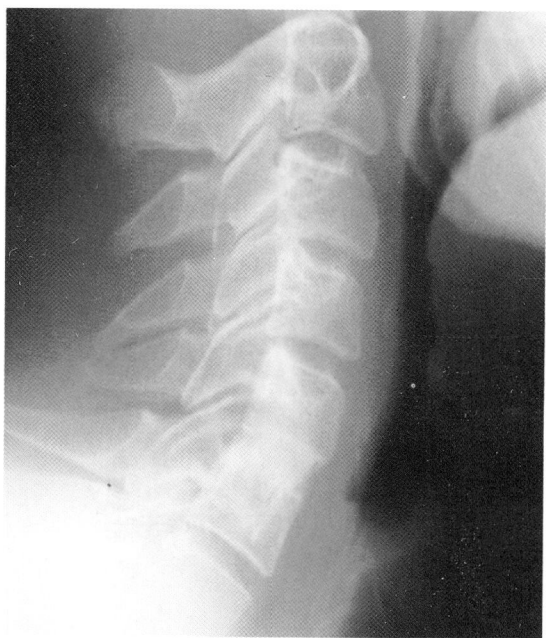

Figure 4. Lateral radiograph of a patient taken 1 week after C5-6 anterior cervical diskectomy with fibular allograft fusion. Note that the graft is oversized 2—3 mm and recessed approximately 2-3 mm. The graft will "settle" prior to arthrodesis. By use of allograft, donor site complications are avoided, cervical lordosis is maintained, and neural foraminal height is maintained.

Figure 5. A lateral radiograph of a 28-year-old male approximately 6 months status—post-C5-6 anterior cervical diskectomy and fibular allograft fusion. Because fibula is mostly cortical bone, collapse is rarely a problem. Although stability in flexion and extension occurs in all patients by 3 months, it may take 9-15 months for radiographic evidence of fusion to appear.

received grafts utilizing the Cloward technique and those who did not receive a graft.[32] In the literature, comparable clinical results have been obtained in patients with bone grafts and those without bone grafts.[1,2,18,21,26,34,38,41,48]

Critics refer to increased postoperative interscapular or neck pain (although temporary), angulation, pseudoarthrosis, or recurrent radiculopathy in patients treated without grafting. However, autograft fusion carries the risk of donor site complications, graft extrusion, prolonged operative time and hospital stay, and possibly a longer duration for orthotic wear.[48]

Complications

Complications may occur at the cervical operative site or at the graft donor site. A review of several series reported a 0.2% morbidity rate at the cervical operative site and a 20% complication rate at the donor site.[49]

Neurologic deterioration is the most feared sequelae. In 1982, Flynn reported a 0.38% incidence of neurologic deterioration. The most common neurologic complication was worsening of the radiculopathy, followed by myelopathy and recurrent laryngeal nerve palsy.[19] The Cervical Spine Research Society reported an incidence of neurologic complications of less than 1% in over 3,800 anterior procedures. Spinal cord injury is reported to occur in less than two per thousand patients. Etiologies of cord injury include epidural hema- include epidural hematoma, instrument mantoma, instrument manipulation within the spinal canal, or bone graft impaction. Approximately 75% of iatrogenic myelopathies occurred immediately postoperatively, with a poor clinical response to immediate reoperation.[48]

Worsening radiculopathy is usually due to root manipulation. It seems the C5 nerve root is the most susceptible to this radiculitis. Some surgeons administer perioperative steroids to decrease the incidence of an inflammatory response.

There are reports of new onset radiculopathy occurring on the contralateral side. This is more common in patients who do not receive interbody grafts. Presumably, settling and foraminal encroachment occur with root compression.[48,49]

Changes in phonation may occur with retraction of the recurrent laryngeal nerve, the superior laryngeal nerve, the vagus nerve, or direct laryngeal pressure. Most of these injuries are transient in nature with a reported 3% incidence of permanent vocal cord paralysis. Excessive retraction or dissection of the longus coli may disrupt the cervical sympathetic chain with a resultant Horner's syndrome. Fortunately Horner's syndrome is usually transient.[24,49]

Injuries to the vascular or visceral structures are reported but are rare. Care must be taken to dissect the medial edges of the longus coli off the anterior aspect of the vertebral bodies, securely placing the edges of the retractor blade beneath the muscle edges.

The incidence of graft extrusion or collapse is higher with cancellous bone, multilevel grafts, or when Cloward dowels are placed at adjoining levels. A kyphotic angulation may occur after graft collapse, but is generally not of clinical significance. Angulation or kyphosis may also develop after diskectomy without fusion. One series reports a 25% incidence of 5° to 15° kyphosis after single-level diskectomy without grafting.[27,45,48,49]

Reported donor site complications range from 14% to 20% and include infection hematoma, hernia, vascular or neurologic injury, and ilium fracture.[49]

Conclusion

A monoradiculopathy secondary to a soft posterolateral disk herniation may respond to a variety of treatment options. Most patients are effectively managed with nonoperative treatment and do not require operation. Although the anterior and posterior operative approaches each have their partisans, both produce excellent clinical success rates, approaching 90% in properly selected patients. The necessity for bone grafting has not been clearly defined. Good results have been obtained without grafts, with various graft configurations, and with allograft or autograft. The treatment of the patient must be individualized to provide the most appropriate treatment. The goal of management is the relief of pain, alleviation of neurologic deficit, and the prevention of long-term sequelae.

References

1. Abitol JJ, Garfin SR. Surgical management of cervical disc disease: anterior cervical fusion. *Semin in Spine Surg.* 1989;1:233-238.
2. Aronson N, Filtzer DL, Bagan M, Anterior cervical fusion by the Smith-Robinson approach. *J Neurosurg.* 1968; 29:397-404.
3. Badami JP, Norman D, Barbaro NM, et al. Metrizamide CT myelography in cervical myelopathy and radiculopathy: correlation with conventional myelopathy and surgical findings. *AJR.* 1985;144:675-680.
4. Bailey R, Badgley C. Stabilization of the cervical spine by anterior fusion. *J Bone Joint Surg Am.* 1960;42A:565-594.
5. Benini A. Clinical features of cervical root compression C5-8 and their variations. *Neural Orthop.* 1987; 4:74-88.
6. Bloom MH, Raney FL Jr. Anterior intervertebral fusion of the cervical spine: a technical note. *J Bone Joint Surg Am.* 1981;63A:842.
7. Boden SD, Wiesel SW. Conservative treatment for cervical disc disease. *Semin in Spine Surg.* 1988;1:229-232.
8. British Association of Physical Medicine. Pain in the neck and arm: a multicenter trial of the effects of physiotherapy. *Br Med J.* 1966;1:253-258.
9. Brown BM, Schwartz RH, Frank E, et al. Preoperative evaluation of cervical radiculopathy and myelopathy by surface-coil MR imaging. *AJR.* 1988;151:1205-1212.
10. Brown MD, Malinin TI, Davis PB. A roentgenographic evaluation of frozen allografts versus autografts in anterior cervical spine fusions. *Clin Orthop.* 1976;119:231-236.

11. Cloward RB. The anterior approach for removal of ruptured cervical discs. *J Neurosurg*. 1958;15:602-617.
12. Daniels DL, Grogan JP, Johansen JG, et al. Cervical radiculopathy: computed tomography and myelography compared. *Radiology*. 1984;151:109-113.
13. Davidson RI, Dunn EJ, Metzmaker JN. The shoulder abduction test in the diagnosis of radicular pain in cervical extradural compressive monoradiculopathies. *Spine*. 1981;6:441-446.
14. DePalma AF, Rothman RH. *The Intervertebral Disc*. Philadelphia, Pa: WB Saunders, 1970.
15. DePalma AF, Subin DK. Study of the cervical syndrome. *Clin Orthop*. 1965;38:135-141.
16. Dillin W, Booth R, Cuckler J, et al. Cervical radiculopathy: review. *Spine*. 1986;11:988-991.
17. Dillin WH, Watkins RG. Cervical myelopathy and cervical radiculopathy. *Semin in Spine Surg*. 1989;1:200-208.
18. Ducker TB. Cervical radiculopathies and myelopathies. In: Frymoyer JW, ed. *The Adult Spine: Principles and Practice*. New York, NY: Raven Press. 1991;2:1187-1205.
19. Flynn TB. Neurologic complications of anterior fusion. *Spine*. 1982;7:536-539.
20. Gore DR, Gardner GM, Sepic SB, et al. Roentgenographic findings following anterior cervical fusion. *Skeletal Radiol*. 1986;15:556-559.
21. Hankinson HL, Wilson CB. Use of the operating microscope in anterior cervical dissections with fusion. *J Neuro Surg*. 1975;43:452-456.
22. Hanley EN, Harvell JC, Shapiro DE, et al. Use of allograft bone in cervical spine surgery. *Semin in Spine Surg*. 1989;1:262-270.
23. Harris PR. Cervical traction: review of the literature and treatment guidelines. *Phys Ther*. 1977;57:910-914.
24. Heeneman H. Vocal cord paralysis following approaches to anterior cervical spine. *Laryngoscope*. 1973;83:17-21.
25. Henderson CM, Hennessy RG, Shuey HM Jr, et al. Posterior-lateral foraminotomy as an exclusive operative technique for cervical radiculopathy: review of 846 consecutively operated cases. *Neurosurgery*. 1983;13:504-512.
26. Hirsch C, Wickbom I, Lidstrom A, et al. Cervical-disc resection: a follow-up of myelographic and surgical procedure. *J Bone Joint Surg. Am*. 1964;46(A):1811-1821.
27. Keblish PA, Keggi KJ. Mechanical problems of the dowel graft in anterior cervical fusion. *J Bone Joint Surg Am*. 1967;49(A):198-199. Abstract.
28. Kumano K, Umeyama T. Cervical disc injuries in athletes. *Arch Orthop Trauma Surg*. 1986;105:223-226.
29. Lees F, Turner WA. Natural history and prognosis of cervical spondylosis. *Br Med J*. 1963;2:1607-1610.
30. Lunsford LD, Bissonette DJ, Jannetta PJ, et al. Anterior surgery for cervical disc disease, 1. Treatment of lateral cervical disk herniation in 253 cases. *J Neurosurg*. 1980;53:1-11.
31. Lunsford LD, Bissonette DJ, Zorub DS. Anterior surgery for cervical disc disease. Treatment of cervical spondylotic myelopathy in 32 cases, 2. *J Neurosurg*. 1980;53:12-19.
32. Martins AN. Anterior cervical discectomy with and without interbody bone graft. *J Neurosurg*. 1976;44:290-295.
33. Modic MT, Masaryk TJ, Mulopulos GP, et al. Cervical radiculopathy: prospective evaluation with surface coil MR imaging, CT with metrizamide, and metrizamide myelography. *Radiology*. 1986;161:753-759.
34. Murphy MG, Gado M. Anterior cervical discectomy without interbody bone graft. *J Neurosurg*. 1972;37:71-74.
35. Odom GL, Finney W, Woodhall B. Cervical disc lesions. *JAMA*. 1958;166:23-28.
36. O'Laoire S, Thomas D. Spinal cord compression due to prolapse of cervical intervertebral disc: treatment of 26 cases by discectomy without interbody bone graft. *J Neurosurg*. 1983;59:847-853.
37. Rish BL, McFadden JT, Penix JO. Anterior cervical fusion using homologous bone grafts: a comparative study. *Surg Neurol*. 1976;5:119-121.
38. Robertson JT. Anterior operations for herniated cervical disc and for myelopathy. *Clin Neurosurg*. 1978;25:245-250.
39. Robertson JT. Anterior removal of cervical disc without fusion. *Clin Neurosurg*. 1973;20:259-261.
40. Robinson RA, Smith GW. Anterolateral cervical disc removal and interbody fusion for cervical disc syndrome. *Bull Johns Hopkins Hosp*. 1955;96:223-224. Abstract.
41. Rosenørn J, Hansen EB, Rosenørn M. Anterior cervical discectomy with and without fusion. *J Neurosurg*. 1983;59:252-255.
42. Rothman RH, Simeone FA. In: *The Spine*. 2nd edition. Philadelphia, Pa: WB Saunders. 1982;477.
43. Scoville WB, Dohrmann GJ, Corkill G. Late results of cervical disc surgery. *J Neurosurg*. 1976;45:203-210.
44. Simeone F, Dillin W. Treatment of cervical disc disease: selection of operative approach. *Contemp Neurosurg*. 1986:1-6.
45. Simmons EH, Bhalla SK, Butt WP. Anterior cervical discectomy and fusion: a clinical and biomechanical study with eight-year follow-up and with a note on discography. *J Bone Joint Surg Br*. 1969;51(B):225-237.
46. Spurling RG. *Lesions of the Cervical Intervertebral Disc*. Springfield, Ill: Thomas; 1956.
47. White A, Hirsch C. An experimental study of the immediate loadbearing capacity of some commonly used iliac bone grafts. *Acta Orthop Scand*. 1971;42:482-490.
48. Whitecloud TS III. Cervical spondylosis; the anterior approach. In: Frymoyer JW, ed. *The Adult Spine: Principals and Practice*. New York, NY: Raven Press. 1991;2:1165-1185.
49. Whitecloud TS III. Complications of anterior cervical fusion. In: *AAOS Instructional Course Lectures*. St. Louis, Mo: Mosby; 1978:27:223-227.
50. Williams RW. Microcervical foraminotomy: a surgical alternative for intractable radicular pain. *Spine*. 1983;8:708-716.

CHAPTER 10

Rheumatoid Arthritis of the Cervical Spine

Michael G. Fehlings, MD, PhD, FRCS(C), Paul R. Cooper, MD, and Thomas J. Errico, MD

Rheumatoid arthritis (RA) is a chronic, idiopathic systemic disorder which, though characterized primarily by inflammatory arthritis of peripheral joints, frequently affects the cervical spine in the following manner[2,12,49]:
At C1-2—
Atlantoaxial subluxation
- anterior (most common)
- posterior (least common)
- lateral

Atlantoaxial impaction
At subaxial—
Subaxial subluxation (especially C2-3, C3-4)
Subluxation below higher fusion
Anterior spondylodiskitis
Intracanalicular rheumatoid granulation
Hyperlordotic deformity
Endplate erosions

Garrod first reported involvement of the cervical spine in chronic RA in 1890.[22] Of 500 patients selected for analysis in this study, 138 (36%) had clinical evidence of cervical spine disease.

Since Garrod's initial work, the pathologic, radiologic and clinical features of rheumatoid disease of the cervical spine have become well recognized. Several large, well-conducted studies reported a prevalence of cervical spine involvement in RA of 50% to 88% (Table 1).[3,13,49,55] The major clinical abnormalities of the cervical spine in RA result from erosive synovitis which leads to pathologic subluxation of the atlantoaxial or subaxial regions, often causing intractable pain and progressive neurologic deficit.[2,19]

Rheumatoid disease of the cervical spine represents a challenge for the spinal surgeon because of the complexity of the spinal deformities and the debilitating nature of this systemic illness. This chapter summarizes current concepts regarding the pathology, pathogenesis, diagnosis, and treatment of rheumatoid cervical spine disease.

Abnormalities of the Cervical Spine in Rheumatoid Arthritis

Pathology

Rheumatoid synovitis of the cervical spine results in ligamentous distension and rupture, articular cartilage destruction, and ultimately abnormalities of bone which include osteoporosis, cyst formation, and erosion.[2,19] These changes lead to a number of well-recognized abnormalities of the atlantoaxial and subaxial regions of the cervical spine as listed previously. The earliest pathologic changes in the cervical spine are noted at the uncovertebral joints[2,19,39,40] and correspond to endplate erosions seen on radiographs.[3,64,67] The pathologic features of the inflammatory synovial

TABLE 1
Prevalence of Cervical Spine Abnormalities and Atlantoaxial Subluxation in Patients with Rheumatoid Arthritis

Authors	Reference No.	Study Design	No. patients	No. with radiologic changes(%)	No. with AAS (%)
Bland et al 1963	3	retrospective	100	88 (88%)	
Conlon et al 1966	13	prospective	335	167 (50%)	84 (25%)
Mathews 1969	40	retrospective	76		19 (25%)
Meikle and Wilkinson 1971	41	retrospective	118		44 (37.3%)
Morizono et al 1987	46	retrospective	100		49 (49%)
Ornilla et al 1972	47	retrospective	100		25 (25%)
Pellici et al 1981	49	prospective	106	74 (70%)	59 (53%)
Rasker and Cosh 1978	51	retrospective	62		26 (42%)
Seze et al 1963	55	retrospective	103	57 (55%)	10 (9.7%)
Summary statistics				386/644 = 59.9%	316/1000 = 31.6%

*Studies with fewer than 50 patients or significant selection bias have been excluded.
AAS = atlantoaxial subluxation.

tissue are similar to those seen in peripheral joints (Figure 1).[33]

Involvement of the cervical spine in RA begins early in the course of the disease and parallels the activity of the disease peripherally.[59,64,66,67,68] In a prospective study of radiologic changes in the cervical spine in early RA, Winfield et al found evidence of cervical involvement within 2 years of diagnosis of RA in the majority of patients.[66]

Abnormalities of Atlantoaxial Region

Atlantoaxial Subluxation

The most common manifestation of rheumatoid involvement of the cervical spine is atlantoaxial subluxation (AAS). The prevalence of AAS in RA has been estimated to be between 9.7%-53% (Table 1).[13,40,41,46,47,49,51,55] By pooling the results of a number of studies, an estimated prevalence of 32% may be calculated (Table 1). In a large surgical series, AAS was seen in 70% of patients with RA who required arthrodesis of the cervical spine.[50] AAS results from erosive synovitis of the atlantoaxial, atlanto-odontoid and atlanto-occipital joints as well as the synovially lined bursae between the odontoid and transverse ligaments.[2,19] AAS may be classified as anterior, posterior, or lateral.[37] Anterior AAS (Figure 2) is the most common single abnormality of the cervical spine in RA and accounts for the majority of all types of AAS.[13,49,57,61]

Atlantoaxial stability depends primarily on the integrity of the transverse, alar, and apical ligaments. An atlantodental interval greater than 3 mm is abnormal in an adult, and anterior subluxation of more than 10-12 mm indicates destruction of the entire ligamentous complex.[20] Most cases of AAS in RA are of this magnitude.[37,46,54]

Posterior AAS is relatively unusual in RA, accounting for only 6.7% of all AAS in one large series.[64] Posterior AAS results from one or a combination of the following abnormalities: incompetence of the anterior arch of the atlas, erosion or fractures of the odontoid, and posterosuperior migration of the atlas.[36] Although posterior AAS has been reported to be a benign abnormality, spinal cord compression from this disorder is well recognized[29,36,62] and may be due to kyphotic "kinking" of the high cervical cord.[36]

Lateral AAS is defined as greater than 2 mm of subluxation of the lateral mass of C1

Rheumatoid Arthritis of the Cervical Spine

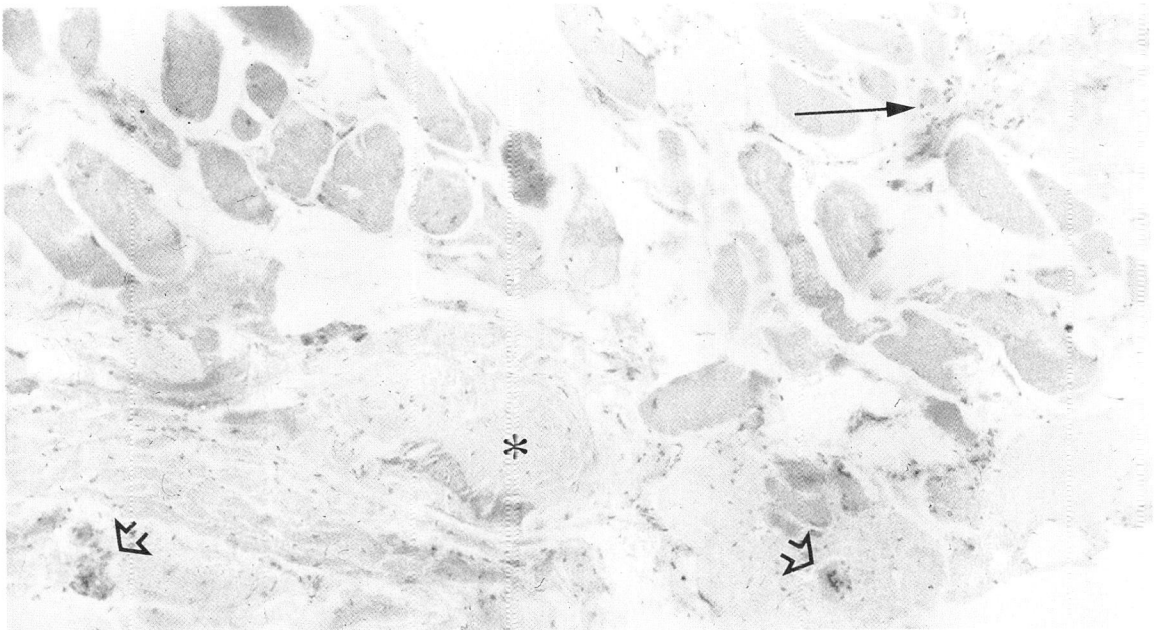

Figure 1. Low-power photomicrograph depicting rheumatoid granulation tissue or "pannus." This section illustrates chronic low-grade inflammatory change with a mononuclear cell infiltrate (arrow), occasional giant cells (arrowheads) and fibrosis (*). This tissue was obtained during posterior decompression of the area of subaxial subluxation depicted in Figure 3 (Hematoxylin-eosin; calibration bar = 400 μm).

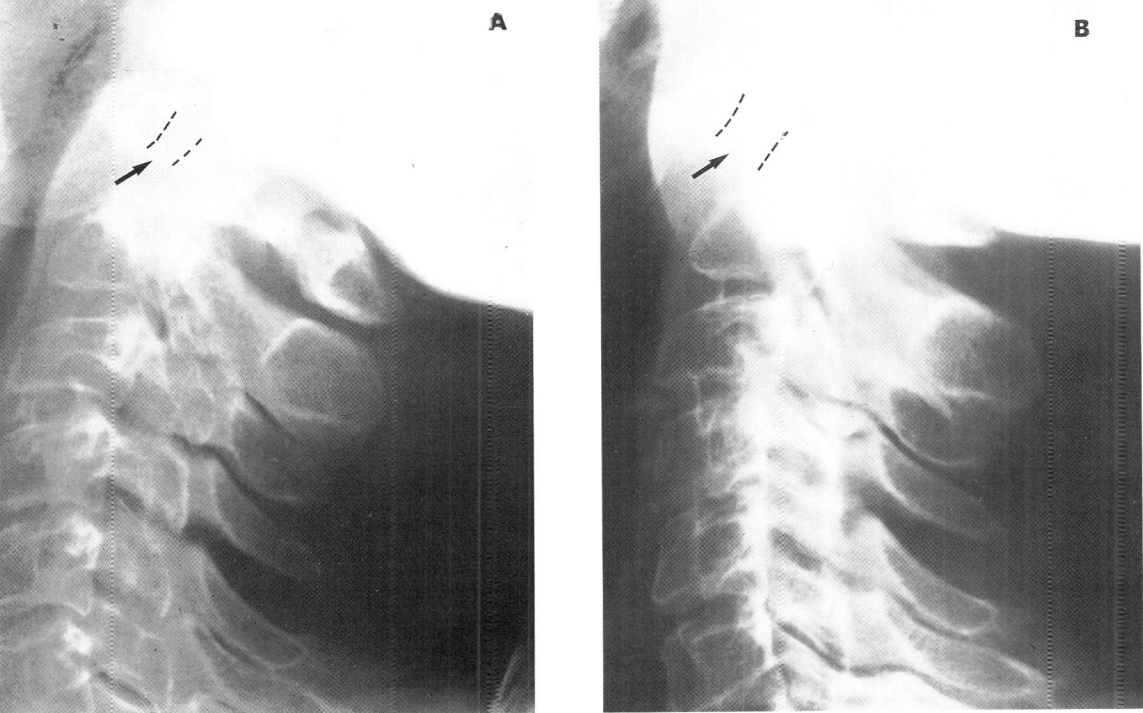

Figure 2. These extension (A) and flexion (B) radiographs of the cervical spine illustrate widening of the atlantodental interval (arrow), indicating anterior atlantoaxial subluxation.

TABLE 2
Radiographic Assessment of Atlantoaxial Region in Rheumatoid Arthritis

Abnormality	Radiographic Criteria
Anterior C1-2 Subluxation	Atlantodental interval (ADI) > 3 mm in adult > 4 mm in child
Lateral C1-2 Subluxation	> 2 mm lateral subluxation of lateral mass of C1 on C2
Atlantoaxial impaction (see Figure 5)	Normal position of odontoid is 1 cm (0.5 cm in child) below anterior edge of foramen magnum
	Chamberlain's Line of Odontoid is: ≥ 6 mm protrusion definitely pathologic.
	McRae's Line: any protrusion of odontoid is abnormal
	McGregor's Line: tip of odontoid should not be > 4.5 mm above line
	Method of Fischgold and Metzger: digastric line (drawn from junction of mastoid to tip of skull on AP view): should be ≥ 1 cm above tip of odontoid
	Method of Ranawat on lateral cervical spine x-ray, line is drawn from anterior to posterior arch of C1; second vertical line is drawn from center of sclerotic ring on C2 body (pedicle) upward along midaxis of C2 to intersect line 1; abnormal if line 2 < 13 mm
	Method of Redlund-Johnell on lateral cervical spine x-ray, line is drawn from the lower endplate of C2 to McGregor's line; this distance should be > 34 mm in men and > 29 mm in women.

on C2.[64] This lesion is probably underreported in RA,[37] and has a clear association with cervical spinal cord compression.[55,64] Weissman et al[64] reported that lateral AAS accounted for 21% of all AAS. Nonreducible head tilt in association with lateral AAS and other deformities has been observed in 10% of patients with RA.[25]

Atlantoaxial Impaction

Atlantoaxial impaction (AAI), also referred to as cranial settling, upward migration of the odontoid, pseudobasilar settling, upward migration of the odontoid, pseudobasilar invagination, and vertical subluxation of the axis[37] occurs secondary to erosive changes in the occipitoatlantal and atlantoaxial joints.[19] AAI accounts for approximately one-fifth of all rheumatoid cervical subluxations[64] and is present in 5% to 32% of patients with RA.[46,49,51]

Methods for assessing AAI are summarized in Table 2 and Figure 3. The method of Ranawat et al[50] avoids the difficulty of defining the hard palate, which may not be seen on a lateral radiograph, and the odontoid, which is often eroded in RA. These are distinct advantages over traditional craniometric techniques, including McGregor's method. The technique of Redlund-Johnell and Pettersson (Table 2) uses the relationship of McGregor's line (Figure 3) to the base of C2 in a manner analogous to the method of Ranawat.[53] Kawaida et al[31] examined the usefulness of the Ranawat and Redlund-Johnell methods in comparison to the McGregor technique. While all three methods were closely correlated, the landmarks for McGregor's line could not be determined in 18% of cases.

Abnormalities of the Subaxial Region

The abnormalities of the subaxial spine in RA are summarized above. They include subaxial subluxation, endplate erosions, subluxation below a higher fusion, anterior spondylo-

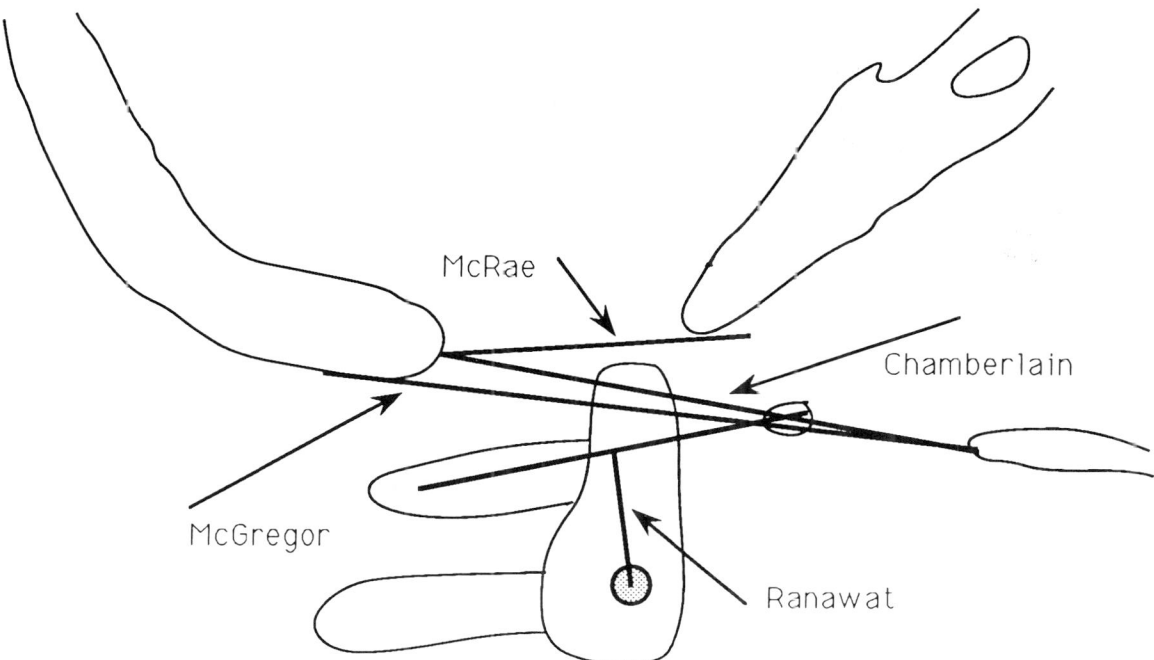

Figure 3. Methods of assessment of basilar invagination on lateral radiograph of the cervical spine are schematically depicted. McRae's line is drawn from the anterior to posterior aspects of the foramen magnum. Any protusion of the odontoid above this line is abnormal. Chamberlain's line connects the posterior aspect of the hard palate to the posterior lip of the foramen magnum. Protrusion of the odontoid by 6mm or more above this line is pathologic. McGregor's line is drawn from the back of the hard palate to the inferior aspect of the most caudal portion of the occiput. Ranawat's line is drawn from the sclerotic ring on the body of C2 which marks the position of the pedicle along the midaxis of the axis and intercepts a line connecting the anterior and posterior arches of C2. A Ranawat measurement of less than 13 mm indicates significant impaction of the odontoid.

diskitis, intracranalalicular rheumatoid granulations, and hyperlordotic deformity.[3,37,52,64]

Subaxial subluxations (Figure 4) are found in 10% to 20% of patients with RA,[41,57] and result from synovitis of the neurocentral joints with secondary erosion of adjacent disk and bone.[2,19] These subluxations most frequently involve the C2-3 and C3-4 segments, typically lack osteophytes, and are often at multiple levels producing a "stepladder" appearance.[3,41]

Subaxial subluxations compromise the cervical spinal cord through compression by bone or pannus (Figure 4), or by the development of pachymeningitis and arachnoiditis.[34,37] Furthermore, the development of subluxation of the subaxial spine in a patient with preexisting AAS is predictive of impending neurologic deterioration.[49] Subaxial subluxations can also develop below a previous fusion. For example, Clark et al[11] reported that 13 of 33 patients (39%) who underwent a C1-2 occipitocervical or high subaxial (rostral to C5) fusion developed radiologic evidence of subluxation. However, in only 5 of these 13 patients was the subluxation greater than 3.5 mm.

Clinical Features and Natural History

Cervical spine involvement in RA begins early in the course of the disease and is progressive. Pellici et al[49] prospectively examined a cohort of 106 patients with RA over a 5-year period. At the beginning of the study, 43% of patients had radiologic evidence of

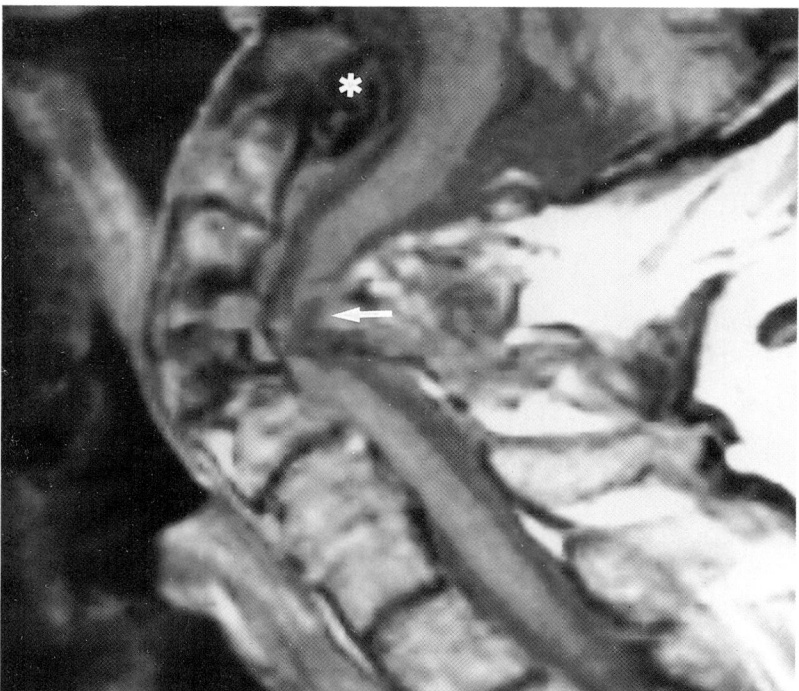

Figure 4A. This T1-weighted MRI study from a patient with rheumatoid disease of the spine illustrates atlantoaxial invagination with compression of the lower medulla and upper cervical cord by pannus (*). In addition, the cervical spinal cord at C3-4 is compressed at this level by a subaxial subluxation and pannus (arrow).

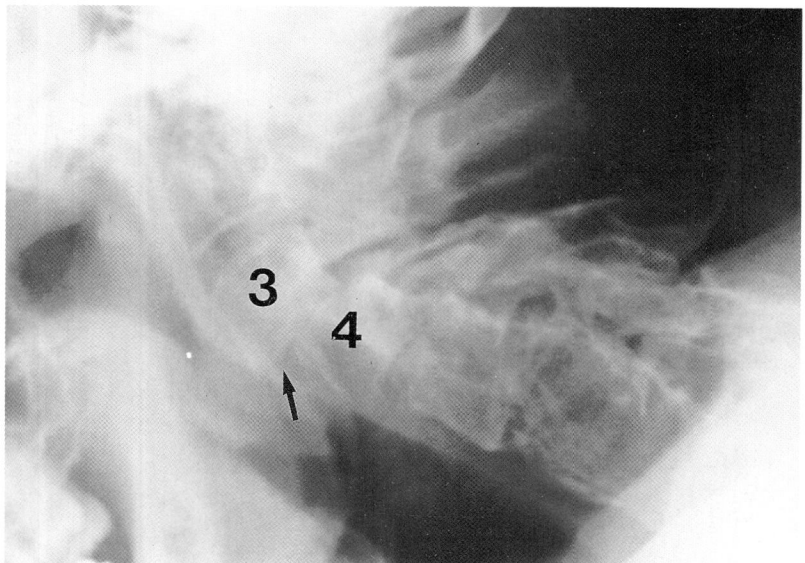

Figure 4B. This radiograph from the same patient whose MRI is seen in Figure 4A illustrates subaxial sublaxation at C3-4, and to a lesser extent at C4-5. Note the spontaneous anterior fusion at C5-6, likely secondary to chronic spondylodiskitis.

rheumatoid involvement of the cervical spine in comparison with 70% of patients 5 years later. Isdale and Conlon also documented radiographic progression of rheumatoid cervical spine disease in a cohort of 171 patients.[28]

The most significant clinical features of rheumatoid cervical spine disease are pain, neurologic dysfunction, and premature death.[37] Neck pain is the commonest clinical manifestation of rheumatoid cervical spine disease, with a prevalence of 40% to 88%.[13,49,56] The pathologic changes in the atlantoaxial region often result in compression of the second cervical nerve root, causing pain which radiates into the neck and occiput. One large prospective series found that 82% of patients had neck pain, which was constant and disabling in 19%.[49] There is a very strong association between AAS and AAI and occipital pain. In a review of 45 patients wit RA and upward migration of the odontoid, all had significant occipital pain.[42]

Neurologic abnormalities occur in 7% to 34% of patients with rheumatoid cervical spine disease.[13,49,56] Neurologic dysfunction is due to direct compression by bone and granulation tissue at the cervicomedullary junction or subaxial regions, by ischemia from compression of the vertebral or anterior spine arteries, or by arteritis of the small perforating vessels of the brain stem and spinal cord.[2,15,26,34,42,44,58] Weissman et al[64] found that AAI was associated with cervical myelopathy in 20% of patients with AAI. In comparison, myelopathy occurred in 7.3% of patients with AAI and other abnormalities of the cervical spine. Similarly, Pellici et al[49] reported that superior migration of the odontoid in patients with pre-existing AAS was a poor prognostic sign. Overall, approximately 36% of patients with documented rheumatoid cervical spine involvement will show progressive neurologic dysfunction.[49]

Patients with cervical spine involvement by RA are at risk for premature death,[17] although the role that subluxations play is still uncertain.[28] An autopsy study of 104 patients with RA revealed 11 with AAS and compression of the cervicomedullary junction.[44] Seven of these 11 patients died suddenly, presumably from fatal medullary compression. Although reports suggest that subluxations of the cervical spine do not adversely affect survival,[28] patients with RA have a significantly shorter life expectancy than the general population. Pellici et al[49] found that patients with cervical spine involvement by RA had a 17% 5-year mortality rate in comparison with 7% for age-matched controls. Although death could not be attributed directly to AAS in this study, subluxations worsened in 80% of patients and neurologic dysfunction progressed in 36% of cases with documented cervical involvement over the course of this 5-year prospective study.

Clinical evaluation of the rheumatoid patient involves a careful evaluation of the systemic features of the disease. The classification of the functional capacity of patients with RA may be objectively defined using the American Rheumatism Association scale (Table 3).[60] In most series, the majority of patients undergoing surgery of the cervical spine fall into functional class III or IV,[45,50] which emphasizes the fact that these patients are often severely crippled by arthritic changes. The systemic factors which correlate with the severity of cervical spine involvement by RA are (1) male sex; (2) seropositivity; (3) the presence of rheumatoid subcutaneous nodules; (4) the presence of erosive and mutilating articular disease; and (5) therapy with corticosteroids.[3,13,64]

There is an excellent correlation between the severity of the peripheral manifestations of RA and the changes seen in the cervical spine.[66,67] Pellici et al,[49] on the basis of a careful prospective analysis of a cohort of patients with RA, proposed a classification of rheumatoid disease of the cervical spine using objective clinical and radiologic criteria (Table 4). The use of this scale in selecting patients for surgery will be discussed subsequently.

Radiology

Plain radiographs of the cervical spine with flexion-extension views are essential in

TABLE 3
American Rheumatism Association Classification of Functional Capacity

Class	Definition
I	Complete ability to carry on all usual duties without handicaps
II	Adequate for normal activities, despite handicap or discomfort or limited motion at one or more joints
III	Limited to little or none of duties of usual occupation or self-care
IV	Incapacitated, largely or wholly, bedridden or confined to wheelchair; little or no self-care

*Classification of Steinbrocker et al[60]

the initial evaluation of a patient with known or suspected involvement of the cervical spine by RA (Fgure 2).[3,64] Bland et al defined 10 radiographic criteria for the diagnosis of rheumatoid cervical spine disease.[3] They are:

- Atlantoaxial subluxation of 2.5 mm or more
- Multiple subluxations of C2-3, C3-4, C4-5, C5-6
- Narrow disk spaces with little or no osteophytosis
  a) Pathognomonic of RA at C2-3 and C3-4
  b) Probable RA at C4-5 and C5-6
- Erosions of vertebrae, especially vertebral plates
- Odontoid small, pointed and eroded with loss of cortex
- Basilar impression ("platybasia")
- Apophyseal joint erosion; blurred facets
- Generalized osteoporosis in cervical spine
- Wide space (5 mm or more) between posterior arch of atlas and the spinous process of the atlas (in flexion)
- Osteosclerosis, secondary, of atlantoaxial occipital complex.

Although these authors defined the presence of AAS on the basis of an atlantodental interval exceeding 2.5 mm, most investigators use 3mm as the upper limit of normal.[20,50,64] The criteria for evaluation of the atlantoaxial region on plain radiographs are

TABLE 4
Clinical and Radiographic Classification of Rheumatoid Cervical Spine Disease

Grade	Pain	Neural Involvement	Radiographic Involvement
0	None	None	None
I	Intermittent, relieved by non-narcotic analgesics	Hyperreflexia, dysesthesias	2.5 mm < AAS < 5 mm; 15% < SAS < 25%; SM: 6-12 mm
II	Intermittent, requiring collar and narcotics for relief	Mild weakness, posterior column deficit	5 mm ≤ AAS < 8 mm; 25% ≤ SAS ≤ 33%; SM: 0-5 mm
III	Constant and disabling	Severe weakness resulting in significant functional disability	AAS ≥ 8 mm; SAS ≥ 33% SM: C2 pedicles above C1 line

*From Pellici et al[49]

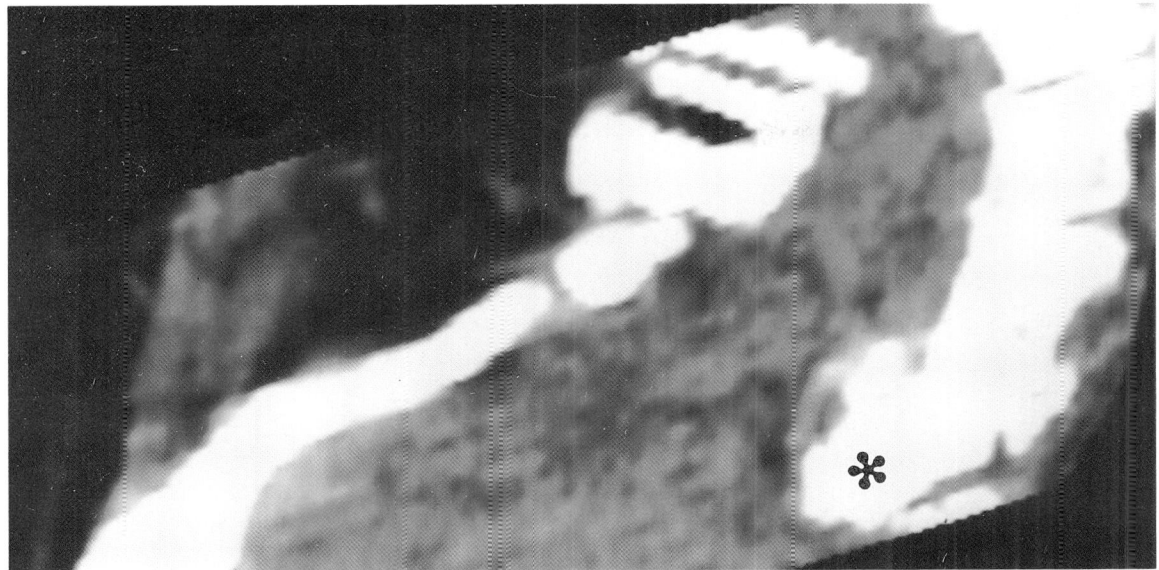

Figure 5. Sagittal reconstruction of a computed tomographic study of the upper cervical spine. The upward migration of the odontoid (*) into the foramen magnum is readily appreciated.

summarized in Table 2 and Figure 5. On the basis of a detailed evaluation of plain radiographs, Weissman et al[64] defined risk factors which predispose to symptomatic compression of the cervical spinal cord: (1) anterior AAS exceeding 9 mm, (2) the presence of AAI, and (3) lateral AAS.

Computed tomography (CT) is valuable in assessing the extent of erosive changes, defining the severity of spinal cord compression, and revealing with precision axial and sagittal relationships (Figure 5).[6] While CT has largely superseded conventional tomography, the latter study may occasionally be of value in delineating sagittal relationships.[26] Although the addition of intrathecal contrast enhances the ability of CT to define areas of cord compression, magnetic resonance imaging (MRI) has reduced the necessity for this invasive procedure.

The cervicomedullary junction and the cervical spinal cord can be imaged with precision using MRI (Figure 4A).[7,10,52] Bundschuh and Modic found that a cervicomedullary angle of less than 135° (normal = 135°-175°) correlated with clinical evidence of neural dysfunction.[10] Compression of the spinal cord documented by MRI correlates closely with clinical evidence of myelopathy.[7] Dynamic MRI images of the craniovertebral junction in flexion and extension may provide further diagnostic information.[18]

Management

Conservative Management and Indications for Surgery

Treatment in the early stages of rheumatoid cervical disease commonly consists of a firm collar that affords some protection against sudden trauma and provides relief of occipital pain due to atlantoaxial instability.[7,49] The principal indications for surgery are pain which is refractory to conservative measures and neurologic dysfunction.[37,49] The presence of a subluxation alone does not mandate surgical intervention, since radiologic involvement of the cervical spine is common, and in a large proportion of patients does not lead to neurologic disability.[28,37,49]

Pellici et al[49] found that only 10% of patients with radiographic signs of cervical RA developed neurologic dysfunction or pain mandating surgery. These authors proposed a clinical classification of rheumatoid disease of the cervical spine (Table 4) and listed the following indications for surgery: (1) intractable pain associated with any neurologic deterioration; (2) progression to Grade II neurologic dysfunction when caused by superimposition of subaxial subluxation or superior migration on pre-existing AAS; and (3) progression to Grade II neurologic dysfunction.

Other authors have advocated a more aggressive surgical approach to the treatment of patients with cervical spine RA. Papadopoulos et al[48] suggested that in patients less than 65 years of age and with a good functional classification (Table 3), prophylactic atlantoaxial arthrodesis should be considered if the AAS exceeded 6 mm. The role of cervical arthrodesis in otherwise asymptomatic patients with AAS remains to be established.

Operative Approaches and Preoperative Planning

Patients with rheumatoid cervical spine disease severe enough to warrant surgical treatment present difficult preoperative, intraoperative, and postoperative challenges. These patients are often physically debilitated, have difficult airways for endotracheal intubation often compounded by cervical instability, are susceptible to infection, and may have poor wound healing.[37] Each of these factors needs to be considered in operative planning.

Preoperative skeletal traction may be necessary to reduce subluxation and alleviate compression of the spinal cord.[42] If rigid internal fixation is not achieved at the time of surgery, postoperative immobilization in a halo orthosis is recommended. Some authors recommend the routine use of a halo device postoperatively to augment internal fixation.[1,30,48]

Surgical management of rheumatoid cervical spine disease may be conveniently divided into a consideration of lesions of the atlantoaxial and subaxial regions. The goals of treatment are to ensure decompression of neural structures and to stabilize areas that are abnormally mobile.

Operative Management of the Atlantoaxial Region

Fusion Techniques

Posterior arthrodesis is the most common surgical method to deal with rheumatoid disease of the atlantoaxial region. Most authors recommend an atlantoaxial fusion for isolated AAS and inclusion of the occiput in the fusion in the presence of AAI.[1,24,26,50,54] Conaty and Mongan[12] recommended the use of C1-2 fusion for reducible AAS and occipitocervical fusion for nonreducible AAS.

Since compression of the cervicomedullary junction by periodontoid pannus is decreased in many cases after posterior arthrodesis, it is recommended that a fusion be performed as an initial procedure in most cases of symptomatic AAI.[35,69] Larsson et al[35] performed MRI examinations on rheumatoid patients with AAI before and 6 months following occipitocervical fusion. The amount of residual periodontoid pannus decreased significantly in all nine patients studied, and only three patients had residual compression of the cervicomedullary junction. Transoral decompression should thus be reserved for cervicomedullary compression which does not resolve after posterior stabilization.

Posterior Atlantoaxial Arthrodesis

The rheumatoid patient presents several challenges which complicate C1-2 fusion procedures. The posterior arch of C1 may be thin and eroded, making wiring or instrumentation difficult.[21,48] The presence of epidural granulation tissue or significant AAS may impede the safe passage of sublaminar wires. Furthermore, the poor quality of bone and impaired tissue healing in patients with RA result in a significant rate of pseudoarthrosis.[8,11,21,48]

A number of techniques have been used to achieve a posterior atlantoaxial fusion in

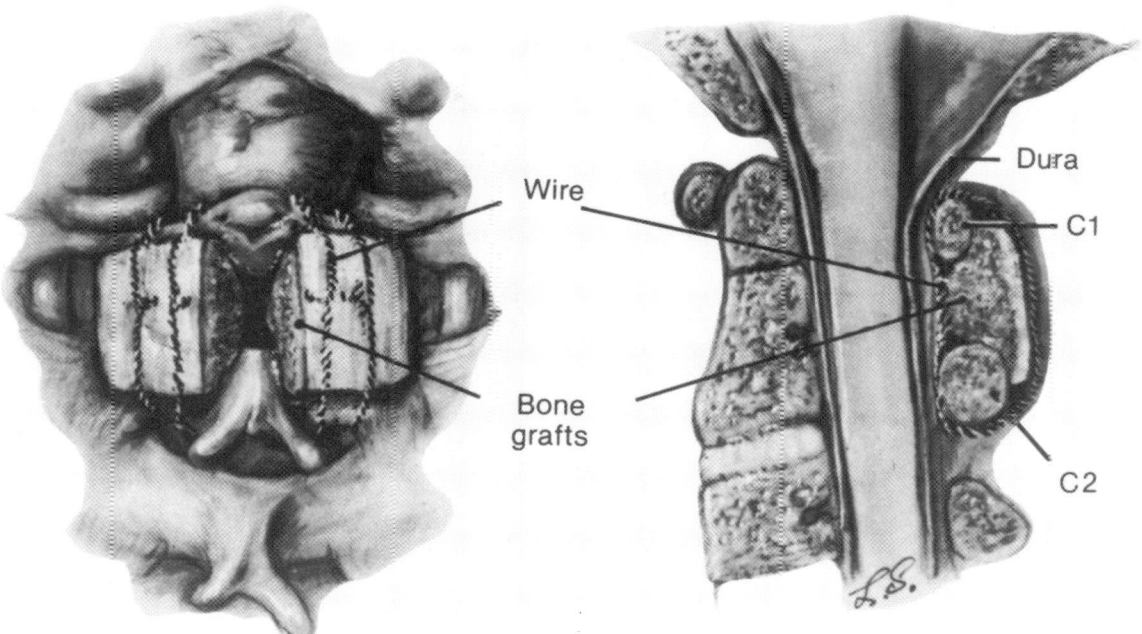

Figure 6. The technique for performing a Brooks fusion of C1-2 is illustrated. Tricortical iliac crest blocks are wedged between the posterior arch of C1 and the lamina of C2 as shown. These grafts are held in position by bilateral sublaminar wires between C1 and C2. (From Griswold et al[23] with permission of the publisher.)

patients with RA. Fielding et al[21] advocated the use of a modified Gallie H-graft from the iliac crest, contoured to fit over the posterior arches of C1 and C2. A doubled, U-shaped 18- or 20-gauge wire is passed under the arch of C1 from inferior to superior. The loop of the wire goes over the bone block and the spinous process of C2. The ends of the wire are then tightened around the graft between C1 and C2. However, these authors indicated that in patients with RA the presence of extensive, erosive bone disease or AAI would mandate occipitocervical fusion. Papadopoulos et al described a modification of the Gallie-type fusion, using a contoured tricortical iliac crest shaped to fit between the posterior arch of C1 and the lamina of C2.[48] Despite the use of postoperative halo immobilization, these authors reported a 25% incidence of pseudarthrosis.

In the Brooks type of fusion[3,23] (Figure 6) doubled, twisted 24-gauge wires are passed under the arch of C1 and then under the lamina of C2. Rectangular iliac crest grafts are beveled to fit in the space between the arch of C2 and each hemilamina of C2. The wires are then tightened to secure the graft in position. This construct has biomechanical advantages over the Gallie-type fusion,[23] but necessitates the use of sublaminar wires under the arch of C2.

To avoid the use of sublaminar wires, several instrumentation techniques have been used. Mitsui or Halifax interlaminar clamps (Figure 7) have been advocated as an alternative to conventional Gallie or Brooks fusion techniques.[16,27,45] Cybulski et al[16] recommended the use of supplemental methylmethacrylate, whereas Holness and Huestis[27] suggested including an additional level in the fusion (Figure 7) when using interlaminar clamps for atlantoaxial instability. Alternatively, bilateral interarticular screw fixation of C1-2, by the technique of Magerl, has been used to achieve rigid atlantoaxial arthrodesis with good results.[65]

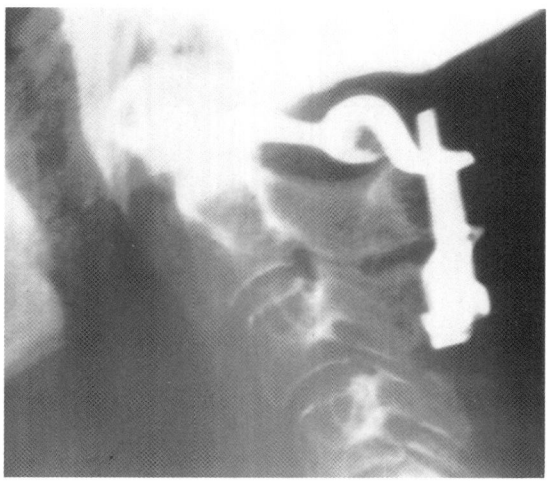

Figure 7. This lateral radiograph of the upper cervical spine from a rheumatoid patient with anterior atlantoaxial subluxation illustrates a C1-3 arthrodesis using Halifax clamps. With this technique, we recommend that C3 be incorporated into the fusion to provide greater biomechanical stability.

Posterior Occipitocervical Fusion

Occipitocervical fusion is recommended if AAS is accompanied by AAI, extensive erosive changes at C1-2, subaxial subluxation. It has also been recommended following decompression of the craniovertebral junction.[1,5,11,14,15,21,42,50] It is also appropriate in patients whose spinal canals are narrowed by pannus or irreducible subluxations which make sublaminar wire passage dangerous. Several techniques have been advocated. As illustrated in Figure 8, we favor a modification of the techniques of Itoh et al[30] and Mackenzie et al,[38] who use Luque rectangles and interspinous wiring to perform craniocervical stabilization.

Our technique uses a U-shaped pediatric Cotrel-Dubousset rod which is secured to the cranium by suboccipital wires and to the cervical spine by spinous process wires. This method provides rigid fixation, obviating the need for routine halo immobilization and avoids the use of sublaminar wires. Other authors have recommended using wire mesh or plates and methylmethacrylate to supplement bony fusion.[5,9,11,42] It is our belief that methylmethacrylate does not add to stability of posterior constructs and should be avoided except in those patients with malignant disease and limited life-span. Grob et al and Weidner combine transarticular screw fixation of C1-2 with occipitocervical plating[24,63] to achieve rigid fixation.

Decompressive Procedures

Most patients with atlantoaxial instability and neural compression should be treated initially with traction and posterior fusion. Menezes et al[42] reviewed a large series of patients with "cranial settling" secondary to RA. Of 45 patients, 36 had good reduction of AAI with halo traction and were treated with occipitocervical fusion, which was occasionally combined with C1 decompression. The remaining patients in this series were considered for transoral anterior decompression.

As discussed above, when the major compression of the cervicomedullary region is caused by periodontoid pannus, posterior fusion alone will often alleviate the compression.[33,69] Thus, transoral decompression should be reserved for patients with irreducible AAI or those patients with persistent cervicomedullary compression after a posterior fusion. The techniques of transoral decompression have been reported extensively elsewhere.[5,14,15,42,43]

Operative Management of the Subaxial Region

Subaxial involvement of the cervical spine in RA includes anterior subaxial subluxation, subluxation below higher fusion masses, anterior spondylodiskitis with spinal cord compression, compression from epidural rheumatoid granulations, and apparent subaxial hyperlordosis which responds to halo traction and immobilization.[37] The primary indication for surgery with subaxial disease is the development of neurologic impairment.[49] Santavirta et al suggested posterior decompression combined with posterior and posterolateral fusion for patients with progressive myelopathy.[54] Anterior decompression and

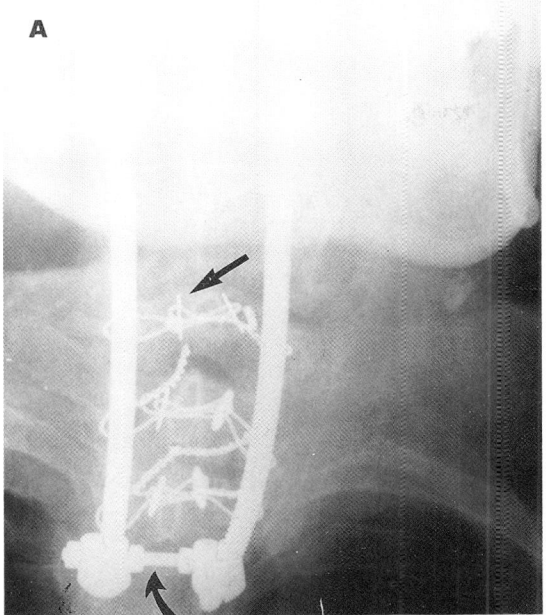 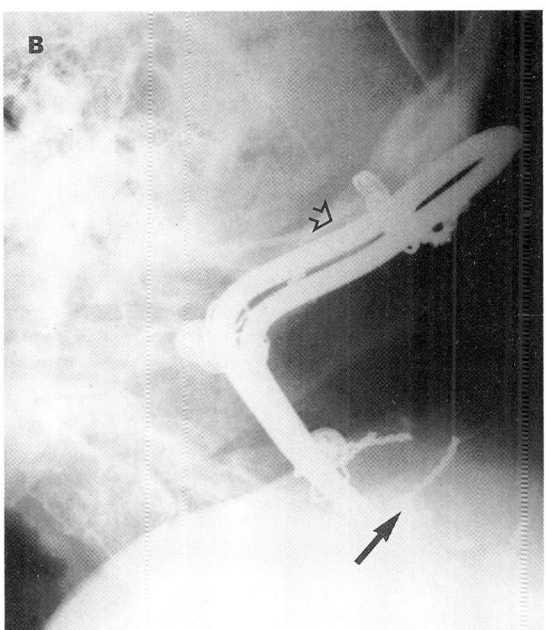

Figure 8. Anteroposterior **(A)** and lateral **(B)** radiographs of the cervical spine from the patient depicted in Figures 4 and 5 illustrate an occipitocervical fusion from occiput to T1. The technique uses a 5 mm pediatric Cotrel-Dubosset rod (open arrowhead) which is bent to form a "U". Fixation to the occiput is obtained by wires passed under burrholes. Fixation to the cervical spine is obtained segmentally by interspinous wiring (straight arrow) and obviates the need for sublaminar wiring. A device for transverse traction (DTT) is incorporated into the construct to provide greater biomechanical stability (curved arrow). It is recommended that the occiput be incorporated into the fusion in cases of atlantoaxial invagination (cf Figures 4A, 5). It is important to fuse to a stable motion segment at least one level below a region of subaxial subluxation (cf Figure 4B).

fusion may be occasionally indicated. Resorption and collapse of the graft have been reported in a high proportion of patients due to the brittle nature of the bone.[50,69]

Conclusion

The cervical spine is involved in approximately 60% of patients with RA. Erosive synovitis can lead to pathologic subluxation of the atlantoaxial and subaxial regions, producing pain and compression of neural structures. The primary indications for surgery are intractable pain and progressive neurologic dysfunction. The role of prophylactic atlantoaxial arthrodesis in asymptomatic patients with AAS is controversial. The majority of patients with symptomatic atlantoaxial instability may be managed by posterior arthrocesis. Transoral decompression should be reserved for patients with irreducible C1-2 subluxation and those who have persistent compression after posterior fusion. The majority of patients with symptomatic subaxial subluxation should be treated with posterior decompression and fusion, although anterior procedures may play a role in carefully selected patients.

References

1. Awerbuch MS, Henderson DRF, Milazzo SC, et al. Longterm follow-up of posterior cervical fusion for atlantoaxial subluxation in rheumatoid arthritis. *J Rheumatol.* 1981;8:423-432.
2. Ball J, Sharp J. Rheumatoid arthritis of the cervical spine. In: Hill AGS, ed. *Modern Trends in Rheumatology.* New York, NY: Appleton-Century-Crofts; 1971;2:117-138.

3. Bland JH, Davis PH, London MG, et al. Rheumatoid arthritis of cervical spine. *Arch Intern Med.* 1963;112:892-898.
4. Brattström H, Elner Å, Granholm L. Transoral surgery for myelopathy caused by rheumatoid arthritis of the cervical spine. *Ann Rheum Dis.* 1973;32:578-581.
5. Brattström H, Granholm L. Atlantoaxial fusion in rheumatoid arthritis: a new method of fixation with wire and bone cement. *Acta Orthop Scand.* 1976;47:619-682.
6. Braunstein EM, Weissman BN, Seltzer SE, et al. Computed tomography and conventional radiographs of the craniocervical region in rheumatoid arthritis: a comparison. *Arthritis Rheum.* 1984;27:26-31.
7. Breedveld FC, Algra PR, Vielvoye CJ, et al. Magnetic resonance imaging in the evaluation of patients with rheumatoid arthritis and subluxations of the cervical spine. *Arthritis Rheum.* 1987;30:624-629.
8. Brooks AL, Jenkins EB. Atlanto-axial arthrodesis by the wedge compression method. *J Bone Joint Surg Am.* 1978;60A:279-284.
9. Bryan WJ, Inglis AE, Sculco TP, et al. Methylmethacrylate stabilization for enhancement of posterior cervical arthrodesis in rheumatoid arthritis. *J Bone Joint Surg Am.* 1982;64A:1045-1050.
10. Bundschuh CV, Modic MT. Rheumatoid arthritis of the cervical spine. *Orthop Trans.* 1987;11:7. Abstract.
11. Clark CR, Goetz DD, Menezes AH. Arthrodesis of the cervical spine in rheumatoid arthritis. *J Bone Joint Surg Am.* 1989;71A:381-392.
12. Conaty JP, Mongan ES. Cervical fusion in rheumatoid arthritis. *J Bone Joint Surg Am.* 1981;63A:1218-1227.
13. Conlon PW, Isdale IC, Rose BS. Rheumatoid arthritis of the cervical spine: an analysis of 333 cases. *Ann Rheum Dis.* 1966;25:120-126.
14. Crockard HA, Calder I, Ransford AO. One-stage transoral decompression and posterior fixation in rheumatoid atlantoaxial subluxation. *J Bone Joint Surg Br.* 1990;72B:682-685.
15. Crockard HA, Pozo JL, Ransford AO, et al. Transoral decompression and posterior fusion for rheumatoid atlantoaxial subluxation. *J Bone Joint Surg Br.* 1986;68B:350-356.
16. Cybulski GR, Stone JL, Crowell RM, et al. Use of Halifax interlaminar clamps for posterior C1-2 arthrodesis. *Neurosurgery.* 1988;22:429-431.
17. Davis FW Jr, Markley HE. Rheumatoid arthritis with death from medullary compression. *Ann Intern Med.* 1951;35:451-454.
18. Dvorak J, Grob D, Baumgartner H, et al. Functional evaluation of the spinal cord by magnetic resonance imaging in patients with rheumatoid arthritis and instability of upper cervical spine. *Spine.* 1989;14:1057-1064.
19. Eulderink F, Meijers KAE. Pathology of the cervical spine in rheumatoid arthritis: a controlled study of 44 spines. *J Pathol.* 1976;120:91-108.
20. Fielding JW, Cochran GVB, Lawsing JF III, et al. Tears of the transverse ligament of the atlas: a clinical and biomechanical study. *J Bone Joint Surg Am.* 1974;56A:1683-1691.
21. Fielding JW, Hawkins RJ, Ratzan SA. Spine fusion for atlantoaxial instability. *J Bone Joint Surg Am.* 1976;58A:400-407.
22. Garrod AE. *A Treatise on Rheumatism and Rheumatoid Arthritis.* London: C Griffin; 1890.
23. Griswold DM, Albright JA, Schiffman E, et al. Atlanto-axial fusion for instability. *J Bone Joint Surg Am.* 1978;60A:285-292.
24. Grob D, Dvorak J, Panjabi M, et al. Posterior occipitocervical fusion: a preliminary report of a new technique. *Spine.* 1991;16(suppl 3):S17-S24.
25. Halla JT, Fallahi S, Hardin JG. Nonreducible rotational head tilt and lateral mass collapse: a prospective study of frequency, radiographic findings, and clinical features in patients with rheumatoid arthritis. *Arthritis Rheum.* 1982;25:1316-1324.
26. Hildebrandt G, Agnoli AL, Zierski J. Atlanto-axial dislocation in rheumatoid arthritis: diagnostic and therapeutic aspects. *Acta Neurochir (Wien).* 1987;84:110-117.
27. Holness RO, Huestis WS. Halifax interlaminar clamps. *Neurosurgery.* 1988;23:127-128. Letter.
28. Isdale IC, Conlon PW. Atlanto-axial subluxation: a six-year follow-up report. *Ann Rheum Dis.* 1971;30:387-389.
29. Isdale IC, Corrigan AB. Backward luxation of the atlas: two cases of an uncommon condition. *Ann Rheum Dis.* 1970;29:6-9.
30. Itoh T, Tsuji H, Katoh Y, et al. Occipito-cervical fusion reinforced by Luque's segmental spinal instrumentation for rheumatoid diseases. *Spine.* 1988;13:1234-1238.
31. Kawaida H, Sakou T, Morizono Y. Vertical settling in rheumatoid arthritis: diagnostic value of the Ranawat and Redlund-Johnell methods. *Clin Orthop.* 1989;239:128-135.
32. Kawaida H, Sakou T, Morizono Y, et al. Magnetic resonance imaging of upper cervical disorders in rheumatoid arthritis. *Spine.* 1989;14:1144-1148.
33. Konttinen Y, Santavirta S, Bergroth V, et al. Inflammatory involvement of cervical spine ligaments in rheumatoid arthritis. *Acta Orthop Scand.* 1986;57:587. Abstract.
34. Kudo H, Iwano K, Yoshizawa H. Cervical cord compression due to extradural granulation tissue in rheumatoid arthritis: a review of five cases. *J Bone Joint Surg Br.* 1984;66B:426-430.
35. Larsson E-M, Holtås S, Zygmunt S. Pre- and postoperative MR imaging of the craniocervical junction in rheumatoid arthritis. *AJR.* 1989;152:561-566.
36. Lipson SJ. Cervical myelopathy and posterior atlanto-axial subluxation in patients with rheumatoid arthritis. *J Bone Joint Surg Am.* 1985;67A:593-597.
37. Lipson SJ. Rheumatoid arthritis in the cervical spine. *Clin Orthop.* 1989;239:121-127.
38. MacKenzie AI, Uttley D, Marsh HT, et al. Craniocervical stabilization using Luque-Hartshill rectangles. *Neurosurgery.* 1990;26:32-36.
39. Martel W. Pathogenesis of cervical discovertebral destruction in rheumatoid arthritis. *Arthritis Rheum.* 1977;20:1217-1225.
40. Mathews JA. Atlanto-axial subluxation in rheumatoid arthritis. *Ann Rheum Dis.* 1969;28:260-266.
41. Meikle JAK, Wilkinson M. Rheumatoid involvement of the cervical spine: radiologic assessment. *Ann Rheum Dis.* 1971;30:154-161.
42. Menezes AH, VanGilder JC. Transoral-transpharyngeal approach to the anterior craniocervical junction: ten-year experience with 72 patients. *J Neurosurg.* 1988;69:895-903.
43. Menezes AH, VanGilder JC, Clark CR, et al. Odon-

toid upward migration in rheumatoid arthritis: an analysis of 45 patients with "cranial settling." *J Neurosurg.* 1985;63:500-509.
44. Mikulowski P, Wollheim FA, Rotmil P, et al. Sudden death in rheumatoid arthritis with atlanto-axial dislocation. *Acta Med Scand.* 1975;198:445-451.
45. Mitsui H. A new operation for atlanto-axial arthrodesis. *J Bone Joint Surg Br.* 1984;66B:422-425.
46. Morizono Y, Sakou T, Kawaida H. Upper cervical involvement in rheumatoid arthritis. *Spine.* 1987;12:721-725.
47. Ornilla E, Ansell BM, Swannell AJ. Cervical spine involvement in patients with chronic arthritis undergoing orthopaedic surgery. *Ann Rheum Dis.* 1972;31:364-368.
48. Papadopoulos SM, Dickman CA, Sonntag VKH. Atlantoaxial stabilization in rheumatoid arthritis. *J Neurosurg.* 1991;74:1-7.
49. Pellici PM, Ranawat CS, Tsairis P, et al. A prospective study of the progression of rheumatoid arthritis of the cervical spine. *J Bone Joint Surg Am.* 1981;63A:342-350.
50. Ranawat CS, O'Leary P, Pellicci P, et al. Cervical spine fusion in rheumatoid arthritis. *J Bone Joint Surg Am.* 1979;61A:1003-1010.
51. Rasker JJ, Cosh JA. A radiological study of cervical spine and hand in patients with rheumatoid arthritis of 15 years' duration: an assessment of the effects of corticosteroid treatment. *Ann Rheum Dis.* 1978;37:529-535.
52. Redlund-Johnell I. Subaxial caudal dislocation of the cervical spine in rheumatoid arthritis. *Neuroradiology.* 1984;26:407-410.
53. Redlund-Johnell I, Pettersson H. Radiographic measurements of the cranio-vertebral region: designed for evaluation of abnormalities in rheumatoid arthritis. *Acta Radiol.* 1984;25:23-28.
54. Santavirta S, Slätis P, Kankaapää U, et al. Treatment of the cervical spine in rheumatoid arthritis. *J Bone Joint Surg Am.* 1988;70A:658-667.
55. Sèze S de, Djian A, Debeyre N. Luxations atloïdo-axoidiennes au cours de la polyarthrite rheumatoïde. *Rev Rhum Mal Osteoartic.* 1963;30:560-565.
56. Sharp J, Purser DW. Spontaneous atlanto-axial dislocation in ankylosing spondylitis and rheumatoid arthritis. *Ann Rheum Dis.* 1961;20:47-77.
57. Sharp J, Purser DW, Lawrence JS. Rheumatoid arthritis of the cervical spine in the adult. *Ann Rheum Dis.* 1958;17:303-313.
58. Smith HP, Challa VR. Alexander E Jr. Odontoid compression of the brain stem in a patient with rheumatoid arthritis. *J Neurosurg.* 1980;53:841-845.
59. Smith PH, Benn RT, Sharp J. Natural history of rheumatoid cervical luxations. *Ann Rheum Dis.* 1972;31:431-439.
60. Steinbrocker O, Traeger CH, Batterman RC. Therapeutic criteria in rheumatoid arthritis. *JAMA.* 1949;140:659-662.
61. Stevens JC, Cartlidge NEF, Saunders M, et al. Atlanto-axial subluxation and cervical myelopathy in rheumatoic arthritis. *Q J Med.* 1971;40:391-408.
62. Teigland J, Magnaes B. Rheumatoid backward dislocation of the atlas with compression of the spinal cord. *Scand J Rheumatol.* 1980;9:253-256.
63. Weidner A. Fusionen bei rheumatischer subluxation des kraniozervikalen übergangs. *Neurochirurgia (Stuttg).* 1990;33:50-53.
64. Weissman BNW, Aliabadi P, Weinfeld MS, et al. Prognostic features of atlantoaxial subluxation in rheumatoid arthritis patients. *Radiology.* 1982;144:745-751.
65. Wertheim SB, Bohlman HH. Occipitocervical fusion. *J Bone Joint Surg Am.* 1987;69A:833-836.
66. Winfield J, Cooke D, Brook AS, et al. A prospective study of the radiological changes in the cervical spine in early rheumatoid arthritis. *Ann Rheum Dis.* 1981;40:109-114.
67. Winfield J, Young A, Williams P, et al. Prospective study of the radiological changes in hands, feet, and cervical spine in adult rheumatoid disease. *Ann Rheum Dis.* 1983;42:613-618.
68. Wolfe BK, O'Keefe D, Mitchell DM, et al. Rheumatoid arthritis of the cervical spine: early and progressive radiographic features. *Radiology.* 1987;165:145-148.
69. Zygmunt SC, Ljunggren B, Alund M, et al. Realignment and surgical fixation of atlanto-axial and subaxial dislocations in rheumatoid arthritis (RA) patients. *Acta Neurochir Suppl (Wien).* 1988;43:79-84.

CHAPTER 11

Ankylosing Spondylitis

Deborah A. Blades, MD, and Russell W. Hardy, MD

Definition and Epidemiology

Ankylosing spondylitis (AS), generally thought to represent the prototype of the spondyloarthropathies, was described during the years 1884-1898 by the neurologists Strumpel, Marie, and Bechterew. Bechterew is credited with describing the characteristic thoracic kyphosis which ultimately makes it impossible for the patient to look ahead or to lie flat in bed. The disease occurs predominantly in in men. The relative incidence for men versus women has ranged from 10:1 to 3:1.[7] In women, a prevalence rate of 0.3% to 0.6% has been reported.[12]

The disease shows a very strong association with HLA-B-27; however, the recognition of HLA-B-27 in a particular patient must be interpreted with caution. A 7% frequency of HLA-B-27 in normal individuals has been noted. Despite the determination of HLA-B-27 positively in 90% of patients with clinical AS, less than 2% of HLA-B-27 positive individuals will ultimately develop AS.[2] Therefore, as a marker for the disease in as yet asymptomatic patients, it is essentially useless.

The prevalence of AS roughly corresponds with the prevalence of B-27 in the population. Thus, African blacks do not have B-27 and AS is virtually absent among them. American blacks, because of racial heterogeneity, do possess B-27, but less commonly (2% to 4%) than whites (8%),[14] and the prevalence of AS in American blacks may be about one-third of that in whites although no formal epidemiologic studies have been performed. Although B-27 negative AS is far less common than B-27 positive AS, in blacks B-27 negative AS forms a much greater proportion of AS patients.

Etiologic Factors

A host response, albeit genetically determined, to an environmental factor(s) seems to be the most likely basis for the pathogenesis of AS and other related spondyloarthropathies. Environmental factors such as infectious agents have long been suspected of triggering the disease. Bacteria—Shigella, Yersinia, Salmonella, Chlamydia, and certain members of the *Enterobacteriaceae* species—have been thought to initiate the disease process.[13,15,20-24] Investigators have proposed that Gram-negative bacteria such as Klebsiella possess antigens that resemble B-27. The inflammatory component of the disease with secondary tissue damage is caused by anti-Klebsiella antibodies binding to B-27 positive cells, causing a reactive arthritis.[8] AS according to this proposal, would be the end stage of repeated episodes of Klebsiella-reactive arthritis.

Geczy et al showed that antibodies raised

in animals against certain strains of Klebsiella react very specifically with cells from about 80% of B-27 positive patients, but not with B-27 positive cells from normal individuals.[11] These investigators suggested that the absorption of a Klebsiella-derived factor onto B-27 may be an important element in the pathogenesis of AS, since it may specifically modify B-27 or a B-27 associated receptor.

Due to the inability of many other investigators to independently confirm the findings of the above mechanism, the role of Klebsiella-triggered AS is still quite controversial. Other factors, specifically gut derived, may be involved in triggering AS since there is a high frequency of subclinical ileitis diagnosed by ileocolonoscopy and bowel histology, particularly in AS patients with peripheral joint disease. There appears to be elevation of serum IgA in AS patients, and there is an association of AS with inflammatory bowel diseases such as ulcerative colitis, Crohn's disease, and Whipple's disease.[17]

Clinical Manifestations

The presenting symptoms and signs of AS are specific and well-defined. They include low back pain and stiffness, a limited range of motion in extension, flexion, and lateral planes, progressive limitation of chest expansion, and advanced sacroiliitis.

Interestingly, other clinical entities are often seen in association with AS. These include acute anterior uveitis, cardiac conduction disturbances, inflammatory bowel disease, aortic insufficiency, psoriasis, pulmonary fibrosis, amyloidosis, Reiter's syndrome, and peripheral arthropathy.[2]

Laboratory data that support the diagnosis include an elevated sedimentation rate and positive HLA B-27. On clinical examination, a positive Mennell's sign (pain in the sacroiliac—SI) joint on hyperextension of the thigh) is often seen. Rheumatoid factor and antinuclear antibody are negative and complement levels are not decreased. Positive straight leg raising, sciatic pain, and limitation of spinal movement characteristically seen in lumbar disk disease are absent in AS.

Diagnostic Criteria

The diagnostic criteria for AS were first proposed in 1961 at the Rome symposium on Population Studies in Relation to Chronic Rheumatic Diseases. The Rome Symposium required the presence of four of the five clinical criteria or a sixth criterion, that of radiographic sacroiliitis in addition to one of the clinical criteria, to make the diagnosis.

The diagnosis of AS is dependent on radiographs, but the interpretation of SI joints according to the Atlas of Standard Radiographs was highly unsatisfactory. A new grading system of radiographic abnormalities of the SI joints was devised. Grade 0 was considered normal; grade 1 suspicious; grade 2 consisted of small, localized areas showing erosions or sclerosis without alteration in joint width; grade 3 was consistent with more advanced sacroiliitis with one or more erosions, evidence of sclerosis, widening, narrowing, or partial ankylosis; grade 4 was consistent with total ankylosis.

Based upon this new grading system, the Rome criteria were revised, and a committee of experts developed the New York criteria for use in population studies. The entity of asymptomatic radiographic sacroiliitis was recognized by the new criteria and the term "probable AS" was recommended for the presence of grade 3 or 4 bilateral sacroiliitis without any clinical criteria.

Further evaluation of the New York criteria was performed by Moll and Wright in conjunction with a family study.[18] They determined that both the Rome and the New York criteria were not ideal for population surveys because a sizable proportion of individuals with radiographic sacroiliitis do not satisfy the clinical criteria needed for the diagnosis of AS. Van der Linden et al[25] recommended that the New York criteria be revised based on their family study of probands with AS, thus making the revised criteria more sensitive and equally specific. (Table 1)

TABLE 1
Criteria for Ankylosing Spondylitis

ROME, 1961

Critical criteria
1. Low back pain and stiffness for more than 3 months, not relieved by rest
2. Pain and stiffness in the thoracic region
3. Limited motion in the lumbar spine
4. Limited chest expansion
5. History or evidence of iritis or its sequelae

Radiologic criterion
6. Roentgenogram showing bilateral sacroiliac changes characteristic of ankylosing spondylitis (this would exclude bilateral osteoarthritis of the sacroiliac joints)

Definite AS
1. Grade 3-4 bilateral sacroiliitis with at least one clinical criterion
2. At least 4 clinical criteria

NEW YORK, 1966

Clinical Criteria
1. Limitation of motion of the lumbar spine in all 3 planes: anterior flexion, lateral flexion, and extension
2. Pain at the dorsolumbar junction or in the lumbr spine
3. Limitation of chest expansion to 2.5 cm or less measured at the level of the 4th intercostal space

Grading of radiographs
Normal 0; suspicious 1; minimal sacroliitis 2; moderate sacroliitis 3, ankylosis 4

Definite AS
1. Grade 3-4 bilateral sacroiliitis with at least 1 clinical criterion
2. Grade 3-4 unilateral or grade 2 bilateral sacroiliitis with clinical criterion 1 or with both clinical criteria 2 and 3

Probable AS
Grade 3-4 bilateral sacroiliitis with no clinical criteria

MODIFIED NEW YORK CRITERIA, 1984

1. Low back pain at least three months' duration improved by exercise and not relieved by rest
2. Limitation of motion of the lumbar spine in sagittal and frontal planes
3. Chest expansion decreased relative to normal values for age and sex
4. Bilateral sacroiliitis grade 2-4
5. Unilateral sacroiliitis grade 3-4

Definite AS if unilateral grade 3 or 4, or bilateral grade 2-4 sacroiliitis and at least one of the three clinical criteria

Reference 14.

Radiographic Features

The classic radiographic features of AS include bilateral symmetric SI joint involvement progressing from erosion to bony ankylosis. The early radiographic findings of grade 1 or 2 sacroiliitis and lateral syndesmophyte may not be well visualized on plain radiographs. Computed tomography (CT) is particularly useful for demonstrating the early changes in sacroiliitis. The technique is ideally suited to studying the curved, oblique SI joints in a transaxial plane, minimizing inter-

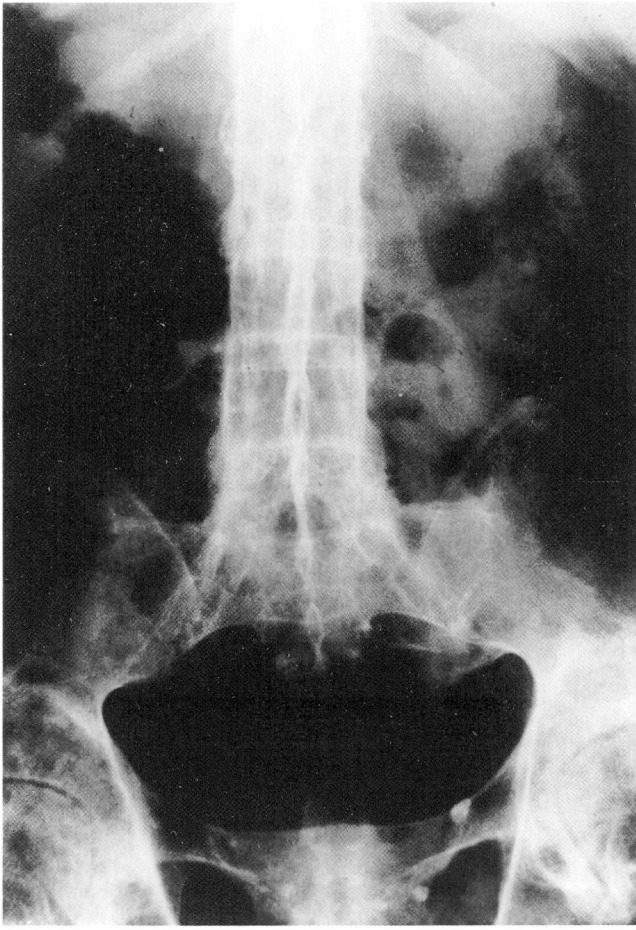

Figure 1. Squaring of lumbar vertebral bodies with evidence of lateral bridging bony syndesmophyte formation. (Courtesy of Dr. Geoffrey Wilbur, Department of Orthopedic Surgery, Case Western Reserve University. Reprinted with permission.)

ference from the overlying soft tissues and bony structures.[9]

As the disease progresses, its radiographic features become increasingly more complex and vary from individual to individual. The disease process called enthesopathy is at the root of the bone and soft-tissue changes.[1,4] The enthesis, or the point of contact between ligament and bone, is the site of a nongranulomatous inflammation resulting in gradual destruction of the ligament, followed by bony replacement. This typically occurs throughout the pelvis, at the hips, greater trochanters, heels, and spine. The outer fibers of the annulus are typically affected first, leading to the typical lateral bridging bony syndesmophyte formation and squaring of the vertebral body (Figure 1).

Ankylosis and ossification at the level of the facet is followed by endochrondral ossification of the disk. The synovitis that is usual to rheumatoid arthritis is commonly seen in the peripheral joints of AS patients. Its development during the first 10 years of the illness is usually indicative of eventual spinal involvement. The C1-2 unit is usually not ankylosed, but may actually become hypermobile with subluxation similar to that seen in rheumatoid arthritis.

The differential diagnosis of patients suspected of having AS includes such entities as Forestier's disease and diffuse idiopathic skeletal hyperostosis (DISH). Although these disorders demonstrate an exuberant bony overgrowth anterior and lateral to the disks, as does AS, they spare the facet and SI joints and occur in men characteristically over the age of 50. The spondylitis of psoriasis and Reiter's syndrome may closely resemble that of AS, but it is characteristically milder and less uniform.

Natural History

The natural history of ankylosing spondylitis is fairly benign for most patients. A large percentage of patients remains undiagnosed, despite radiographic findings, possibly because of the tendency for pain to resolve as the SI joint ossifies. For those who are diagnosed, the onset of peripheral arthritis is slow and occurs early. Its course is characterized by exacerbations and remissions. The disease in females is milder and frequently does not affect the spine. The spinal deformity typically progresses slowly. The majority of patients remain quite functional despite considerable spinal involvement, and most never require surgical treatment.

Nonsteroidal anti-inflammatory agents such as indomethacin appear to be the most effective medical therapy, although it does not affect the progressive nature of the disease. Physical therapy, bracing, and extension exercises are helpful for many patients. Deaths in these patients are largely attributable to falls with spinal fracture, respiratory insufficiency, renal disease, and aortic insufficiency. Patients who had been treated in the past with spinal radiation have had moderately decreased spinal morbidity, but greatly increased mortality from hematologic malignancies.[19]

Spinal Complications of AS

The radiographically recognized spinal complications of AS commonly include acute fracture, pseudoarthrosis, and the cauda equina syndrome.

Acute fractures are usually seen in late-stage AS when the spines are completely fused. Seventy-five percent of the spinal fractures occur in the cervical region. The mechanism is usually that of hyperextension and the neurologic deficit is usually severe.[3,6] The site of the fracture is usually at the level of the intervertebral disk or across the vertebral body. The neurologic sequelae are usually more severe with the latter than the former fracture site.

The clinical picture in AS patients with fractures is often complicated by the development of spinal epidural hematomas.[5] Delays in diagnosis of fractures contribute heavily to the increased morbidity and mortality in this population. Radiographic detection of fractures is often made difficult because of osteoporosis, anatomic distortion, and absence of fracture displacement. In cases of apparently mild trauma, the presence of a fracture may not be suspected and diagnostic studies would not be performed. Radionuclide studies have been helpful in evaluating AS patients since an increase in uptake is noted in the region of the fracture.

As with fractures of the spine, pseudoarthroses occur in late-stage disease following extensive spinal fusion. Radiographically, pseudoarthroses appear as irregular destruction of adjacent endplates with an associated reactive sclerosis. The disk appears to represent the center point of the process and it often appears more lucent than its adjacent counterparts. The posterior elements are often fractured as well. Fang et al described a series of 35 AS patients with 49 pseudoarthroses; 37 lesions occurred as a result of nonunion of fractures through an ankylosed disk and 3 lesions occurred through the vertebral bodies and extended into the posterior elements.[10] Histopathologic examination supported the hypothesis that a pseudoarthrosis was of traumatic etiology and nonunion occurred as a direct result of mechanical stress and continued motion at the fracture site.[10]

Other, less frequently seen complications include atlantoaxial subluxation, upward migration of the axis and ossification of the posterior longitudinal ligament.

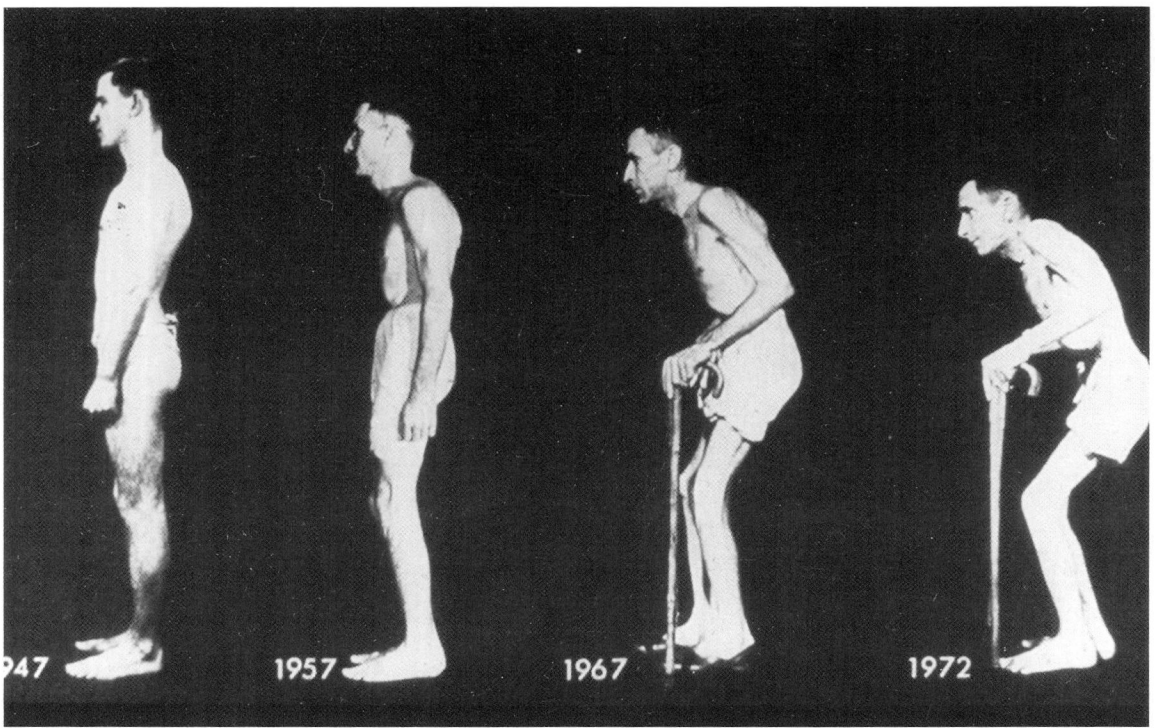

*Figure 2. Progressive deformity over the span of 25 years in an AS patient. (*American Journal of Medicine. *Vol. 60; Feb. 1976. Reprinted with permission.)*

Surgical Correction of Flexion Deformity

AS is an arthritic process that progressively ravages the spine. Treatment depends on the stage of the disease process (Figure 2). The earliest stage, represented by the beginning of inflammatory changes, requires the administration of anti-inflammatory agents. The second stage, representing not only the presence of inflammation but the beginning of flexion deformity without evidence of bony fusion of articular facets and longitudinal ligaments, has been controlled with postural exercises, braces, hyperextension frames, and casts. The final stage, characterized by fixed flexion deformity, can be corrected only with spinal osteotomy (Figures 3, 4).

Smith-Petersen, Larson, and Aufranc are credited with the first-described spinal osteotomy. In 1945, they reported the results of six cases of lumbar spine osteotomies. Successful cases have been described since that time using certain variations.[16]

The severe kyphotic deformities make it impossible for the patient to see ahead, lie flat in bed, and to have adequate and effective chest expansion during repiration. Few contraindications for correction of flexion deformity have been cited. These include the existence of fixed flexion deformity of one or both hips and the presence of aortic calcifications, which can be detected radiographically. Flexion deformity of the hips is a particular contraindication. If correction of the hip deformity is not undertaken first, correction of the spinal deformity in the presence of ankylosed hips will allow the patient to see ahead when standing but would cause the patient considerable disability while sitting.

Spinal instrumentation for fixation after fracture and osteotomy have been used with inceasing success. For cervical instability, Luque rods can be wired to spinous pro-

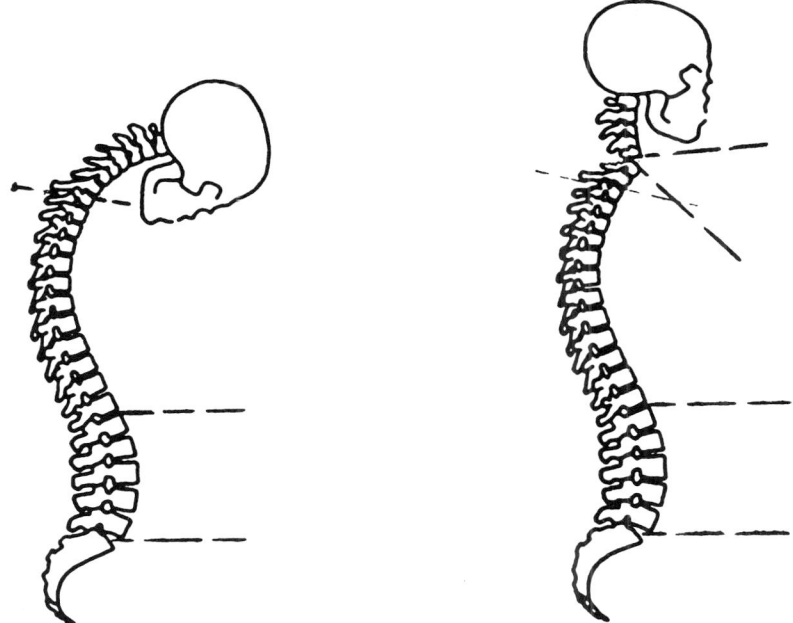

Figure 3. Kyphosis of low lumbar origin followed by osteotomy at the upper lumbar column, allowing for tilting of the upper vertebral segment. (Herbert JJ. Vertebral osteotomy for kyphosis, especially in Marie-Strumpell arthritis. J Bone Joint Surg. 1959;41-A:291. Reprinted with permission.)

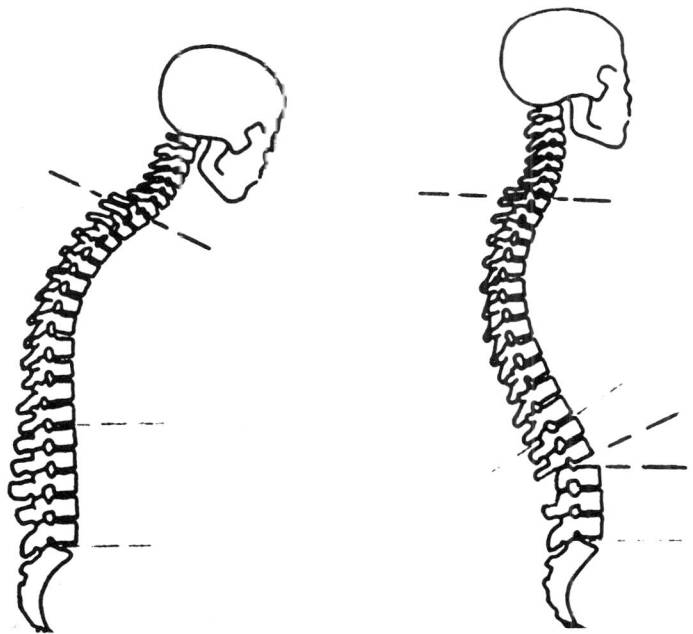

Figure 4. Kyphosis of cervical spine followed by osteotomy at lower cervical column with re-establishment of cervical lordosis. (Herbert JJ. Vertebral osteotomy for kyphosis, especially in Marie-Strumpell arthritis. J Bone Joint Surg. 1959;41-A:291. Reprinted with permission.)

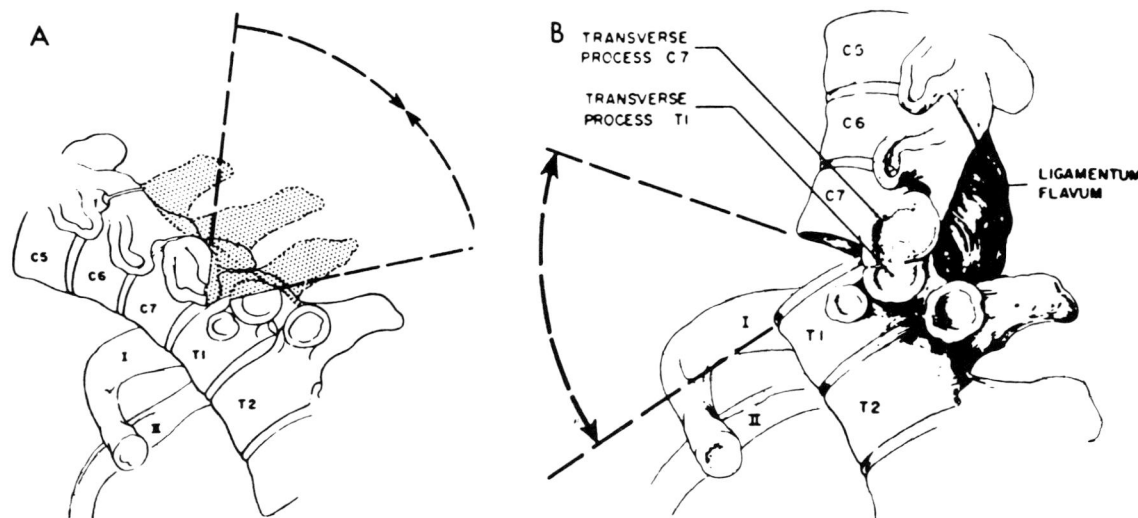

Figures 5A, B. *The plan for osteotomy at C7-T1 with opening of a 64° angle at the level of the disk space for fixed flexion deformity. (Urist M. Osteotomy of the cervical spine: Report of a case of ankylosing rheumatoid spondylitis.* J Bone Joint Surg. *1958;40-A:833. Reprinted with permission.)*

cesses, providing internal fixation if external halo stabilization is not adequate.

Osteotomy of the cervical spine is rarely employed since the risk of death, injury to the brachial plexus, and failure to alter the deformity is considerable. The procedure essentially is an adaptation of that performed by Smith-Petersen, Larson, and Aufranc on the lumbar spine (Figures 5A & B). The feasibility of the procedure was determined after studying fractures of the cervical spine in AS patients. Treatment of those fractures often resulted in correction of the flexion deformity.[3]

Conclusion

Ankylosing spondylitis is a progressive disorder with a pathogenesis that remains unclear; however, its effects are protean and debilitating. For the majority of patients, symptomatic treatment is all that is required. It is of utmost importance, that patients be informed of the risks of even the most minor traumatic event. A high index of suspicion of every injury is essential and radiographic recognition of fractures is of extreme importance since, if undetected, spinal instability is accompanied by a high morbidity and mortality. When fixed flexion deformity is associated with considerable disability, it can be successfully treated surgically in certain circumstances with osteotomy.

References

1. Ball J. The enthesopathy of ankylosing spondylitis. *Br J Rheumatol.* 1983;22(suppl 2):25-28.
2. Bennett G. Ankylosing spondylitis. *Clin Neurosurg.* 1989;37:622-635.
3. Bergmann EW. Fractures of the ankylosed spine. *J Bone Joint Surg Am.* 1949;31A:669-671.
4. Bluestone R. *Ankylosing Spondylitis, Arthritis and Allied Conditions: A Textbook of Rhematology.* In: McCarty DJ, ed. Philadelphia, Pa: Lea & Febiger; 1985:819-840.
5. Bohlman HH. Acute fractures and dislocations of the cervical spine. *J Bone Joint Surg Am.* 1979; 61A:1119-1142.
6. Broom MJ, Raycroft JF. Complications of fractures of the cervical spine in ankylosing spondylitis. *Spine.* 1988;13:763-766.
7. Carter ET, McKenna CH, Brian DD, et al. Epidemiology of ankylosing spondylitis in Rochester, Minnesota, 1935-1973. *Arthritis Rheum.* 1979;22: 365-370.
8. Ebringer A. The relationship between Klebsiella infection and ankylosing spondylitis. *Baillieres Clin Rheumatol.* 1989;3:321-338.
9. Fam AG, Rubenstein JD, Chin-Sang H, et al. Computed tomography in the diagnosis of early ankylosing spondylitis. *Arthritis Rheum.* 1985;28:930-937.
10. Fang D, Leong JCY, Ho EKW, et al. Spinal pseudoarthrosis in ankylosing spondylitis. *J Bone Joint Surg Br.* 1988;70-B:443-447.

11. Geczy AF, Van Leeuwen A, Van Rood JJ, et al. Blind confirmation in Leiden of Geczy factor on the cells of Dutch patients with ankylosing spondylitis. *Hum Immunol.* 1986;17:239-245.
12. Gran JT, Husby G, Hordvik M. Prevalence of ankylosing spondylitis in males and females in a young middle-aged population of Tromso, northern Norway. *Ann Rheum Dis.* 1985;44:359-367.
13. Khan MA, Abdul-Karim A. Interaction between HLA antigens and bacteria. *Rev Mex Rheumat.* 1989;4(suppl 1):14-16.
14. Khan MA, Van der Linden SM. Ankylosing spondylitis and other spondyloarthropathies. *Rheum Dis Clin North Am.* 1990;16:551-579.
15. Leirisalo M, Repo H. Reactive arthritis. In: Calin A, ed. *Spondyloarthropathies*. Orlando, Fla: Grune & Stratton; 1984:383-401.
16. McMaster PE. Osteotomy of the spine for fixed flexion deformity. *J Bone Joint Surg Am.* 1952; 44A:1207-1216.
17. Mielants H, Veys EM. The gut in the spondyloarthropathies. *J Rheumatol.* 1990;17:7-10. Editorial.
18. Moll JMH, Wright V. New York clinical criteria for ankylosing spondylitis. *Ann Rheum Dis.* 1973;32: 354-363.
19. Radford EP, Doll R, Smith PG. Mortality among patients with ankylosing spondylitis not given x-ray therapy. *N Engl J Med.* 1977;297:572-576.
20. Saag MS, Bennett JC. The infectious etiology of chronic rheumatic disease. *Semin Arthritis Rheum.* 1987;17:1-23.
21. Taylor-Robinson D, Thomas BJ, Dixey J, et al. Evidence that Chlamydia trachomatis causes seronegative arthritis in women. *Ann Rheum Dis.* 1988;47 295-299.
22. Toivanen A, Granfors K, Lahesmaa-Rantala R, et al. Pathogenesis of Yersinia-triggered reactive arthritis: immunological, microbiological and clinical aspects. *Immunol Rev.* 1985;86:47-70.
23. Toivanen A, Lahesmaa-Rantala R, Stahlberg TH, et al. Do bacterial antigens persist in reactive arthritis? *Clin Exp Rheumatol.* 1987;5(suppl 1):25-27.
24. Toivanen A, Lahesmaa-Rantala R, Vuento R, et al. Association of persisting IgA response with Yersinia-triggered reactive arthritis: a study of 104 patients. *Ann Rheum Dis.* 1987;46:898-901.
25. Van der Linden S, Valkenburg HA, Cats A Evaluation of diagnostic criteria for ankylosing spondylitis: a proposal for modification of the New York criteria. *Arthritis Rheum.* 1984;27:361-368

CHAPTER 12

Ossification of the Posterior Longitudinal Ligament

Noel Perin, MD

Ossification of the posterior longitudinal ligament (OPLL) as a cause of spinal cord compression was first reported by Key in 1838 in the Guy's Hospital report.[10A] Tsukimoto, in 1960, first described this condition as a pathologic entity with autopsy findings.[31A] Soon after Tsukimoto's report the number of reported cases of OPLL increased rapidly in Japan. This disorder is more common among Asians than Caucasians.[13] In 1974 the Ministry of Public Health in Japan appointed a study group to evaluate the frequency, etiology, and salient clinical and radiologic features of OPLL, and to formulate proper guidelines for treatment (Investigation Committee Report on OPLL).[27A]

Incidence and Epidemiology

OPLL is common in East Asia, especially in Japan. A comprehensive epidemiologic study in Japan showed the incidence of radiographically defined OPLL to be 2.4%.[27] Its prevalence was 23.01% among relatives of patients with OPLL.[27] Another study showed the incidence of OPLL among family members of second-order kinship to the patient to be about 30%, much higher than the general population.[32] In another study, OPLL was noted in 1.7% of all cervical roentgenograms performed on outpatients in Japan, Korea, and Hong Kong, as opposed to a 0.2% incidence at the Mayo Clinic and 0.6% in Hawaii.[8]

OPLL manifests most frequently in the sixth decade of life and shows a male-to-female ratio of about 2:1. The mean age of Japanese patients was 56 years, whereas European patients were older (more than 60 years). In the Japanese population the pathohistologic incidence of OPLL was reported to be 20% in those over the age of 60 years (1974 investigation committee).[27A]

Diffuse idiopathic skeletal hyperostosis (DISH) occurs in middle-aged and elderly patients. In the United States, 50% of patients with DISH demonstrate associated OPLL; thus, OPLL is considered one of the partial phenotypes of DISH. Other studies indicated a dominant inheritance with variable penetrance.[15]

OPLL frequently is seen in well-built, pyknic individuals. The association with glucose intolerance,[32] and the incidence of diabetes mellitus in patients with OPLL, is reported to be 12.4%.[32] It has been postulated that the relationship between the ossifying tendency of the ligament and glucose metabolism may partially be explained by the higher incidence of OPLL among people eating large quantities of rice.[32]

HLA antigen studies demonstrate that antigens BW 40 and SA 5 were more commonly associated with OPLL than one would expect by chance.[32] The frequency of OPLL in adults with familial hypophosphatemic rickets and hypoparathyroidism suggests the presence of abnormal calcium metabolism. Calcium-

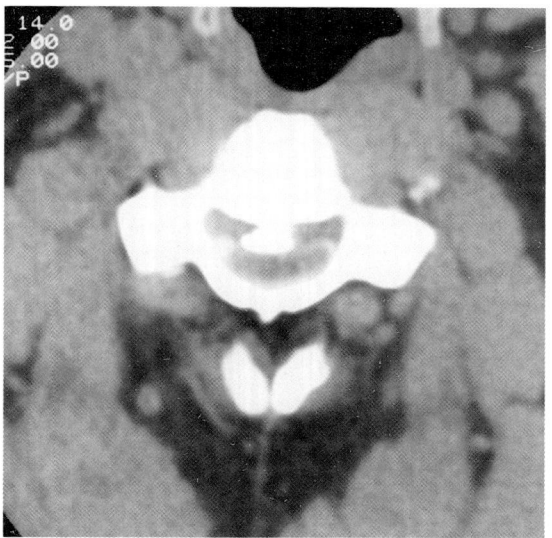

Figure 1. Transaxial postmyelogram CT image showing a hook type of segmental OPLL.

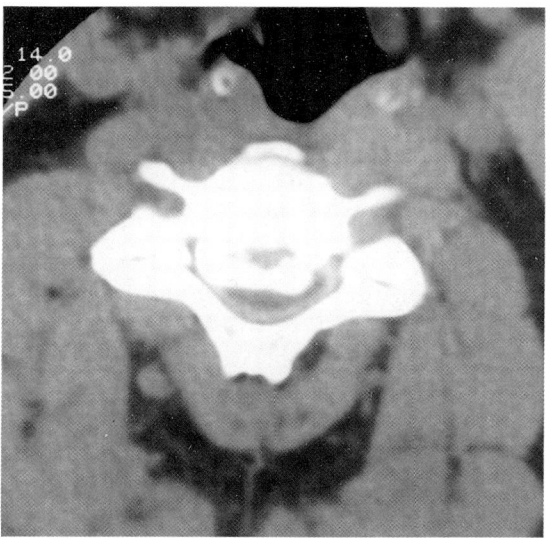

Figure 2. Transaxial postmyelogram CT scan showing extensive OPLL of the continuous type with significant cord compression.

uptake tests revealed a tendency toward low enteral calcium absorption in OPLL and other spinal ligament ossifying syndromes.[32]

Imaging Studies

OPLL usually develops in the cervical spine,[6] and is difficult to detect using plain lateral cervical spine films, even when there is extensive calcification of the ligament.[4] However, lateral tomograms will clearly demonstrate ossification. Postmyelographic high-resolution computed tomography (CT) is extremely useful in evaluating the site, size and height of the ossified mass, the sagittal diameter of the canal,[36] and the degree of cord and/or root compression (Figures 1 and 2).

OPLL is classified as one of four types: (1) continuous, (2) segmental, (3) mixed, and (4) other (Figure 3). The 1975 pilot study[33] of the epidemiology of OPLL reported

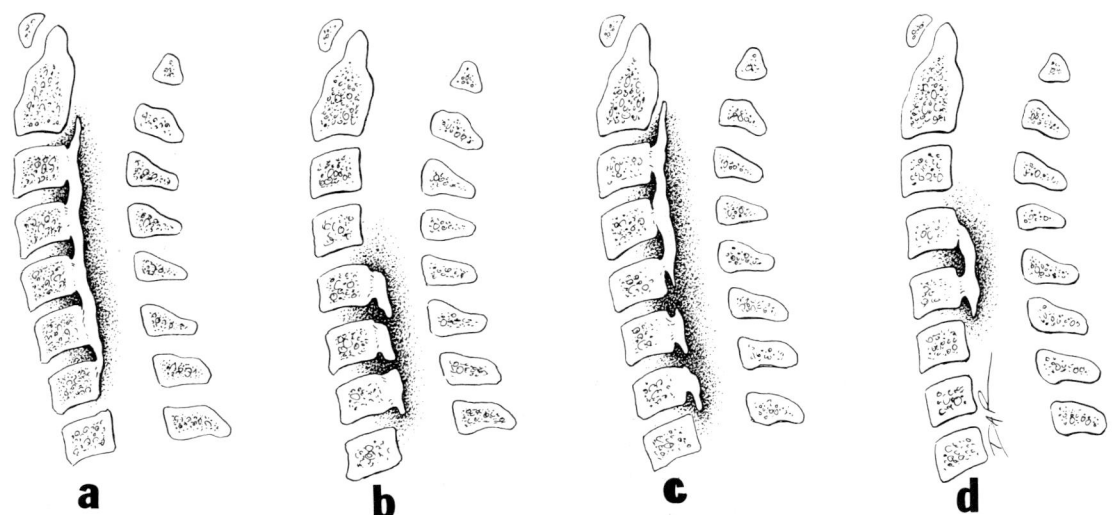

Figure 3. Classification of the types of OPLL: (A) continuous, (B) segmental, (C) mixed, and (D) other.

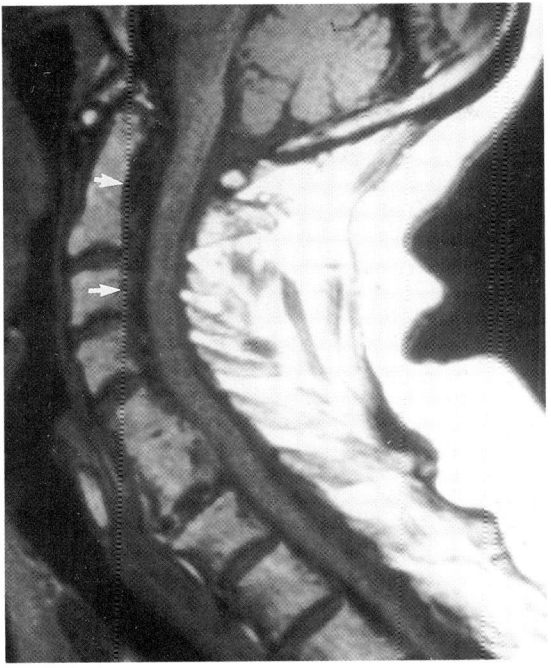

Figure 4. Saggital T1-weighted MR spinal image, showing area of hypointensity anterior to the cord from C2-5; representing continuous type of OPLL (previous surgery at C5-6).

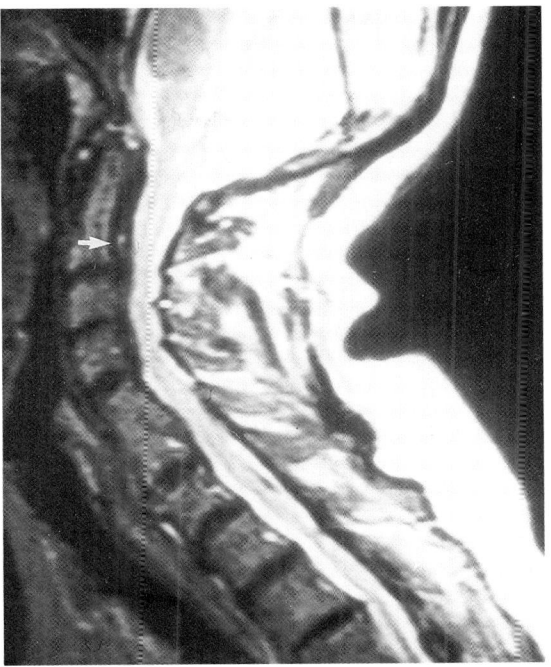

Figure 5. Saggital T2-weighted image showing the same area of hypointensity anterior to the spinal cord.

a 39% incidence for the segmental type, 27.3% for the continuous type, 29.2% for the mixed, and 7.5% for other types.[27A] OPLL is most frequently noted at the C5, C4, C6 levels in that order; the average number of vertebral bodies involved was 3.1. Spinal canal narrowing (measured as the ratio of the thickness of the ossified mass to the anteroposterior diameter of the canal on lateral x-rays) was most severe in the continuous and mixed types.

Magnetic resonance imaging (MRI) in OPLL,[34] using different pulse sequences, shows the ossification as a thick area of hypointensity; a band of intermediate or high signal intensity within the areas of hypointensity is thought to represent marrow (Figures 4-6). The segmental type of OPLL appears as a thin area of hypointensity and is more closely associated with disk degeneration. Magnetic resonance imaging cannot distinguish ossification from hypertrophy of the ligament.[34]

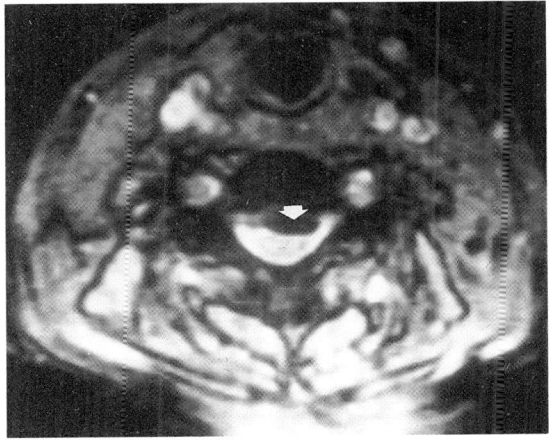

Figure 6. Transaxial gradient-echo image (T2) showing OPLL as an area of hypointensity (arrow).

Pathology and Pathophysiology

The posterior longitudinal ligament extends from the basi-occiput to the sacrum and is composed of stout bundles of randomly arranged thick collagen fibers and narrow bundles of streamlined fine collagen fibers. The posterior longitudinal ligament is connected by fibrous tissue to the vertebral bodies. In the midline this attachment is noted throughout, but more laterally it only attaches to the upper and lower margins of the vertebral bodies.[7]

Proliferation of cartilaginous tissue occurs first at points of fibrous tissue attachment to the vertebral bodies where stresses due to cervical spine motion converge maximally. Proliferation and then calcification of cartilaginous tissue occurs, followed by ossification, suggesting an enchondral mechanism of ossification in OPLL. The ossified mass consists mainly of lamellar bone with some irregular woven bone surrounding the fibrocartilage.[7]

Yamamura[33] reported that connective tissue proliferation as well as mucoid degeneration occurred first within the posterior longitudinal ligament before enchrondral ossification. Others have suggested that the pathophysiology was similar to heterotopic calcification in response to mechanical stresses. Cartilaginous cells proliferate first in the periosteum of the vertebral bodies and then in the annulus, posterior longitudinal ligament, and the dura (in that order). Mature lamellar bone eventually forms. In one study, the mean annual increase in OPLL size was 4.07 mm in a rostral-caudal dimension and 0.67 mm in the anterior-posterior dimension.[25]

Although the segmental type of OPLL does not progress to the continuous type,[27] the underlying mechanisms are essentially the same. The continuous type frequently occurs in the upper cervical spine and the segmental type occurs in the lower cervical spine where there is increased mobility.

Ossification of the Dura

Two types or ossification patterns occur. In the first, an ossified dura is separate from the ossified ligament; in the second, continuous ossification of ligament and dura is present. The mechanism of ossification of the dura is unknown. While dural ossification is usually not thick enough to cause spinal cord compression, dural ossification may protect the spinal cord from incidental trauma.[7]

Pathologic Changes in the Spinal Cord

Spongy degeneration of the anterior and lateral columns has been reported.[33] Anterior horn cells may be affected more than the white matter tracts due to the greater sensitivity of the gray matter to hypoxia. Circulatory disturbances caused by the compression of the anterior spinal artery and venous drainage may be responsible for these changes.

Clinical Presentation

Onset of symptomatology is insiduous except in patients who present after spinal trauma. Symptoms usually include a steadily progressive myeloradiculopathy, weakness and clumsiness of the upper extremities with numbness or paresthesias, difficulty with walking, leg weakness, and neck pain. Lower extremity numbness, paresthesias, urinary incontinence, upper extremity pain, and impotence are noted less often. The mean duration of the interval between the initial occurrence of symptoms and diagnosis is 12.5 months (range 0-36 months).[6]

At presentation, the most common signs include limitation of neck movement, sensory loss and weakness with increased tone, and a Hoffman's Sign in the upper extremities. Lower extremity weakness with signs of myelopathy is also noted. Unlike patients with cervical spondylosis, those with OPLL do not initially present with radiculopathy.[36] Overall in 70% of patients, the initial presentation was myelopathy.[4]

Some suggest that in any patient with paraplegia or tetraplegia of unknown cause, silent OPLL should always be suspected. The differential diagnosis of OPLL should always include: (1) structural spinal disorder, (2) tumor of the spine or spinal cord, (3) vascular insufficiency or malformation, (4) myelitis/multiple sclerosis, or (5) motor neuron disease and other inherited or degenerative myelopathies.

Treatment

Both operative and nonoperative management have been proposed for patients presenting with symptoms related to OPLL. Nonoperative treatment consists of bed rest with or without a neck brace. Although continuing cervical traction has been proposed as a method of management and may result in temporary relief of signs and symptoms, this modality is obviously impractical over the long term.

These measures may eliminate or decrease the dynamic factors of repeated impacts and friction of the ossified mass against the spinal cord. Because almost 70% of patients initially respond favorably to nonoperative treatment,[32] conservative measures should be tried at the outset in all patients.

Indications for Surgery

Surgery is recommended for patients with (1) progressive neurologic deficit refractory to conservative treatment, (2) incomplete recovery of quadriparesis following trauma, or (3) complete neurologic recovery after trauma, with persistent neck pain or as prophylaxis against further cord injury.

Operative results in OPLL are influenced by: (1) the patient's age—patients over 60 years of age sustain lesser degrees of improvement than younger patients; (2) preoperative duration of symptoms (especially myelopathy)—if present for over two years, myelopathy generally does not improve following treatment; (3) extensive canal compromise—patients with greater than 60% canal compromise do not recover significant neurologic function; and (4) type of operation—inadequate or inappropriate operative treatment may prevent optimal recovery.[8,28]

Surgical Treatment

Considerable controversy surrounds the optimal operative approach for the treatment of patients with OPLL. Wide laminectomy has been frequently used, especially in the continuous type of OPLL. As proposed by Miyazaki,[16] this involves a wide laminectomy, 1—1.5 segments above and below the mylographic abnormality. Laminectomy may extend to four or even six segments. Extensive wide laminectomy may produce spinal deformity and instability several years after surgery with ensuing neurologic deficits.

After the spinous processes are removed with a rongeur, an air drill is used to thin the bone to a cortical shell in both gutters to the medial aspect of the facet joints, and across the laminae at the rostral and caudal extent of the planned laminectomy. The two halves of the lamina are then freed by cutting the ligamentum all around and lifting the shell of bone off the spinal cord.[16] This method prevents both sudden decompression and swelling of the spinal cord and strangulation against the edges of the lamina. To prevent spinal cord hypoxia, Miyazaki[16] recommended that the systolic blood pressure be maintained above 100mm Hg systolic intraoperatively and for 24 hours postoperatively. When the anterior dura is calcified and adheres to the ossified ligament, the dura is opened posteriorly and the dentate ligaments are divided to allow the cord to move posteriorly.

More recently Hirabayashi,[8] Nakano,[17] and others performed a so-called open-door expansive laminoplasty, which theoretically prevents the loss of structural integrity produced by laminectomy. Although the technique can be a disadvantage because of an inability to decompress the root on the hinged side (Figure 7), it may be as effective as laminectomy for the relief of long-tract signs. In one study the results of laminectomy and open-door laminoplasty were similar.[17] Although no instability was noted in either group, recovery from symptoms was quicker with laminoplasty.

Anterior decompression in OPLL is the

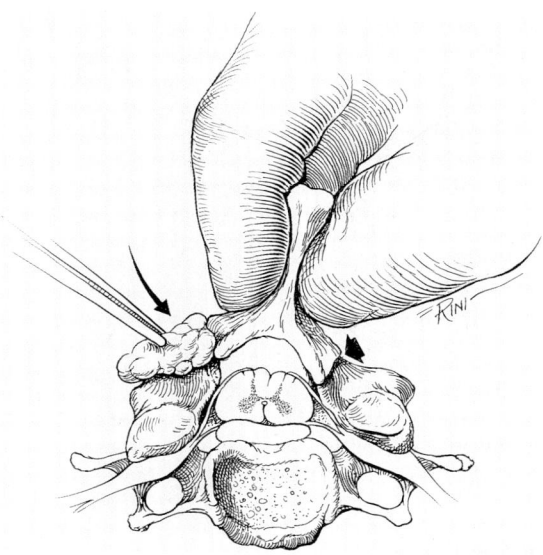

Figure 7. Schematic representation of the open-door expansive laminoplasty. Free fatty tissue over the open-door laminoplasty (long arrow), hinge on the opposite lamina adjacent to the facet joint (short arrow).

calcification involves the dura without a plane between the ossified ligament and dura, the whole mass is removed en bloc and the dura is closed with a patch graft. Autogenous fibula or a fibular allograft may be used for fusion.[1]

Selection of anterior versus posterior decompression depends on the type of OPLL. In the continuous type involving more than three vertebral segments, laminectomy or open-door laminoplasty is appropriate.[31] In the segmental and other types of OPLL involving three levels or less, anterior decompression may be more appropriate, especially for patients under 60 years of age. In the mixed type, however, a two-stage combined posterior decompression followed by anterior decompression three to six weeks later may be performed when indicated. Posterior decompression followed by an anterior procedure is considered safer than an anterior procedure followed by a posterior approach.[8]

method that most directly deals with the anterior pathology. Anterior decompression is usually performed in segmental and other types when four or fewer vertebral segments are involved. Anterior operation consisting of fusion without decompression has been utilized to decrease movement and minimize spinal cord trauma. A second method involves freeing the ossified ligament from its attachment to bone, especially when there is dural involvement, without removing the freed calcified mass but performing interbody bony fusion.[5] The most extensive of these procedures consists of anterior decompression, removal of the ossified segments, and bone graft fusion.[6]

In the anterior operation, a longitudinal groove 1.2-1.5 cm wide (side to side) is made anteriorly in the vertebral body; however, on the posterior aspect of the body, bone removal extends further laterally to decompress the roots on either side. Normal dura is exposed above and below the ossified mass initially, and subsequently the dissection is carried down into the calcified areas. When

Postoperative Progression of OPLL

Postoperative progression does not depend on the type of operative procedure but rather on the type of OPLL. Postoperative progression was noted in two-thirds of patients after laminectomy, three-fourths of patients progress after anterior fusion, and two-thirds after combined posterior-anterior operations.[5] Interestingly progression of OPLL after surgery is noted more frequently than the 16% rate noted among nonoperated cases.

The progression rate in the segmental type is much lower than in the continuous or mixed types. Patterns of progression consist of rostral or caudal thickening. Upward or downward elongation, noted about 6 months after laminectomy, ceased by 4½ years. Progression from the mixed to the continuous type terminated when the ossification between the short spaces was complete. Six months after laminectomy, observed thickening was of two types, postdiskal and postvertebral. Although postoperative progression of OPLL was noted in a number of cases, no clinical deterioration occurred that required a second operation.⁸

Summary

OPLL is a degenerative disorder common in East Asia, especially in Japan, and occurs less frequently in Caucasian populations. Operative management depends on the surgeon's preference, the type of OPLL, and the extent of involvement. A greater understanding of the pathophysiologic progression of OPLL, including rapid and slow-growth phases during its evolution, will be essential in the future to better manage this condition.

References

1. Abe H, Tsuru M, Ito T, et al. Anterior decompression for ossification of the posterior longitudinal ligament of the cervical spine. *J Neurosurg.* 1981; 55:108-116.
2. Bakay L, Cares HL, Smith RJ. Ossification in the region of the posterior longitudinal ligament as a cause of cervical myelopathy. *J Neurol Neurosurg Psychiatry.* 1970;33:263-268.
3. Correa AV, Beasley BAL. Ossification of the posterior longitudinal ligament. *N Y State J Med.* 1980; 80:1972-1974.
4. Dietmann JL, Dirheimer Y, Babin E, et al. Ossification of the posterior longitudinal ligament (Japanese disease): a radiological study in 12 cases. *J Neuroradiol.* 1985;12:212-222.
5. Hanai K, Inouye Y, Kawai K, et al. Anterior decompression for myelopathy resulting from ossification of the posterior longitudinal ligament. *J Bone Joint Surg Br.* 1982;64B:561-564.
6. Harsh GR IV, Sypert GW, Weinstein PR, et al. Cervical spine stenosis secondary to ossification of the posterior longitudinal ligament. *J Neurosurg.* 1987;67:349-357.
7. Hashizume Y. Pathological studies on the ossification of the posterior longitudinal ligament (OPLL). *Acta Pathol Jpn.* 1980;30:255-273.
8. Hirabayashi K, Miyakawa J, Satomi K, et al. Operative results and postoperative progression of ossification among patients with ossification of the posterior longitudinal ligament. *Spine.* 1981;6:354-364.
9. Hukuda S, Mochizuki T, Ogata M, et al. The pattern of spinal and extraspinal hyperostosis in patients with ossification of the posterior longitudinal ligament and ligamentum flavum causing myelopathy. *Skeletal Radiol.* 1983;10:79-85.
10. Kamioka Y, Yamamoto H, Tani T, et al. Postoperative instability of cervical Ossification of the Posterior Longitudinal Ligament and cervical radiculomyelopathy. *Spine.* 1989;14:1177-1183.
10A. Key CA. On paraplegia depending on disease of the ligaments of the spine. *Guy's Hospt Rep.* (Series 1) 1938;3:17-31.
11. Klara PM, McDonnell DE. Ossification of the posterior longitudinal ligament in caucasians: diagnosis and surgical intervention. *Neurosurgery.* 1986 19:212-216.
12. Kojima T, Waga S, Kubo Y, et al. Anterior cervical vertebrectomy and interbody fusion for multi-level spondylosis and ossification of the posterior longitudinal ligament. *Neurosurgery.* 1989;24: 864-872.
13. Kubota T, Kazuhumi S, Kawano H, et al. Ultrastructure of early calcification in cervical ossification of the posterior longitudinal ligament. *J Neurosurg.* 1984;61:131-135.
14. Lee T, Chacha PB, Khoo J. Ossification of the posterior longitudinal ligament of the cervical spine in non-Japanese Asians. *Surg Neurol.* 1991; 35:40-44.
15. McAfee PC, Regan JJ, Bohlman HH. Cervical cord compression from ossification of the posterior longitudinal ligament in non-orientals. *J Bone Joint Surg Br.* 1987;69B:569-575.
16. Miyazaki K, Kirita Y. Extensive simultaneous multisegment laminectomy for myelopathy due to the ossification of the posterior longitudinal ligament in the cervical region. *Spine.* 1986;11:531-542.
17. Nakano N, Nakano T, Nakano K. Comparison of the results of laminectomy and open-door laminoplasty for cervical spondylotic myeloradiculopathy and ossification of the posterior longitudinal ligament. *Spine.* 1988;13:792-794.
18. Nose T, Egashira T, Enomoto T, et al. Ossification of the posterior longitudinal ligament: a clinicoradiological study of 74 cases. *J Neurol Neurosurg Psychiatry.* 1987;50:321-326.
19. Ohtani K, Nakai S, Fujimura Y, et al. Anterior surgical decompression for thoracic myelopathy as a result of ossification of the posterior longitudinal ligament. *Clin Orthop.* 1982;166:82-88.
20. Ohtsuka K, Terayama K, Yanagihara M, et al. A radiological population study on ossification of the posterior longitudinal ligament in the spine. *Arch Orthop Trauma Surg.* 1987;106:89-93.
21. Ono M, Russell WJ, Kudo S, et al. Ossification of the thoracic posterior longitudinal ligament in a fixed population. *Radiology.* 1982;143:469-474.
22. Pennes DR, Martel W, Ellis CN. Retinoid-induced ossification of the posterior longitudinal ligament. *Skeletal Radio.* 1985;14:191-193.
23. Portha C, Coche G, Moussa K, et al. Ossification of the posterior longitudinal ligament after cervical irradiation. *Neuroradiology.* 1982;24: 111-113.
24. Pouchot J, Watts CS, Esdaile JM, et al. Sudden quadriplegia complicating ossification of the posterior longitudinal ligament and diffuse idiopathic skeletal hyperostosis. *Arthritis Rheum.* 1987;30: 1069-1072.
25. Sato M, Turu M, Yada K. The anterior-posterior diameter of the cervical spinal canal in the ossification of the posterior longitudinal ligament. In Japanese. *No Shinkei Geka.* 1977;5:511-517.
26. Shinomiya K, Furuya K, Sato R, et al. Electrophysiologic diagnosis of cervical ossification of the posterior longitudinal ligament myelopathy using evoked spinal cord potentials. *Spine.* 1988;13 1225-1233.
27. Terayama K. Genetic studies on ossification of the posterior longitudinal ligament of the spine. *Spine.* 1989;14:1184-1191.
27A. Terayama K, Kurokawa T, Seki H. Nationwide Survey Report of OPLL. In: *Disease Designations*

by Ministry of Health & Welfare. *Report of the Proceedings of Studies of the Research Committee on PLL Ossification.* (1975) Tokyo. Ministry of Health and Welfare. 1976;8-33.
28. Tominaga S. The effects of intervertebral fusion in patients with myelopathy due to ossification of the posterior longitudinal ligament of the cervical spine. *Int Orthop.* 1980;4:183-191.
29. Tomita K. Total decompression of the spinal cord for combined ossification of the posterior longitudinal ligament and yellow ligament in the thoracic spine. *Arch Orthop Trauma Surg.* 1990; 109: 57-62.
30. Tomita K, Kawahara N, Baba H, et al. Circumspinal decompression for thoracic myelopathy due to combined ossification of the posterior longitudinal ligament and ligamentum flavum. *Spine.* 1990;15: 1114-1120.
31. Tomita K, Nomura S, Umeda S, et al. Cervical laminoplasty to enlarge the spinal canal in multi-level ossification of the posterior longitudinal ligament with myelopathy. *Arch Orthop Trauma Surg.* 1988;107:148-153.
31A. Tsukimoto H. Pathological case reports of hyperostosis in the cervical spinal canal which caused myelopathy. *J. Jpa Orthop Assoc.* (Tokyo) 1960;34:107. Abstract.
32. Tsuyama N. Ossification of the posterior longitudinal ligament of the spine. *Clin Orthop.* 1984;184: 71-84.
33. Yamamura IA. Clinico-pathological study of the ossifying process in cervical posterior longitudinal ligament. In Japanese. *Saigaiigaku.* 1975;18:651-662.
34. Yamashita Y, Takahashi M, Matsuho Y, et al. Spinal cord compression due to ossification of ligaments: MR imaging. *Radiology.* 1990;175:843-848.
35. Yonenobu K, Ebara S, Fujiwara K, et al. Thoracic myelopathy secondary to ossification of the spinal ligament. *J Neurosurg.* 1987;66:511-518.
36. Yu YL, Leong JCY, Fang D, et al. Cervical myelopathy due to Ossification of the Posterior Longitudinal Ligament: a clinical radiological and evoked potentials study in six Chinese patients. *Brain.* 1988;111:769-783.

CHAPTER 13

Natural History and Nonoperative Management

Harold J. Weinberg, MD, PhD

Degenerative disease of the cervical spine produces two distinct clinical syndromes. Cervical radiculopathy is the consequence of nerve root entrapment by a combination of spondylosis and/or disk disease. Cervical myelopathy occurs secondary to spinal cord compression by the same pathologic processes.

The natural history of these two entities has never been fully clarified, but those studies that are available indicate some general prognostic trends and permit the formulation of a rational approach to conservative management. Many nonoperative modalities can be used in both radiculopathy and myelopathy. Their success rate in radicular disease is excellent, but when spinal cord compression occurs surgery is generally the preferred management.

Natural History

Study of the natural history of a disease implies an analysis of the short- and long-term clinical features, with no intervening treatment of any kind. This has not been done to any significant degree for cervical radiculopathy because the pain and weakness caused by the condition cannot be ignored by physicians when various successful means of therapy exist.

In a study of 51 patients with radiculopathy by Lees and Turner,[7] only 5 patients were believed to have received either no treatment at all or simply bed rest, and 3 of these improved. Ten patients who were followed for more than 10 years had either a complete recovery or were left with only mild symptoms. Of the 41 patients studied for less than 10 years, 19 made a complete recovery within a short period of time and 12 were left with slight intermittent symptoms. Eleven of 51 patients were left with moderate or severe symptoms (22%). In this study done in 1963, a number of nonsurgical modalities were used and it is reasonable to assume that with the addition of some newer modalities the conservative success rate can be even higher.

Although there has been speculation on a differential effect of nerve root compression depending on the level of involvement, this has not been carefully studied. Thus, the concept that C6-7 innervated muscles can tolerate compression better than C5 or C8-supplied muscles has been considered but never proven.[11] Patients who present with cervical radiculopathy and are followed for prolonged periods do not tend to develop cervical myelopathy. This suggests either a different pathophysiology or distribution of lesions, and requires the natural history of cervical spondylotic myelopathy to be studied separately.

One of the earliest attempts to describe the natural history of this disease was the study of Clarke and Robinson[5] in 1956. In their series of 120 patients, 26 were untreated. The mean time to diagnosis was 3 years and the maximum survival without any treatment was 18 years. The disease was shown to have an ultimately poor prognosis in their patients, but evolved over many years. In 75% of cases, the disease was episodic. In 5%, the disease began with abrupt neurologic deficit followed by gradual deterioration. In the remaining 20%, there was slow progression starting from the onset.

Multilevel spondylotic disease is reported to be associated with a much greater likelihood of clinical deterioration as compared to patients with single-level myelopathy. Bradshaw[2] found in his study of 78 patients with spondylotic myelopathy that only those with single-level lesions responded well to conservative treatment. Unfortunately, more than 50% of these patients deteriorated again after a year.

Others have remarked upon the delay in diagnosis. Roughly 50% of the patients in the large study published by Brain and his colleagues[3] were not diagnosed until symptoms had been present for longer than 1 year. This is probably a consequence of the natural history of the disease: many patients stabilize or actually improve within the first year, and therefore fail to seek medical attention that could document the myelopathy. Although 11 of 14 conservatively-treated patients improved and none deteriorated, the selection between the surgical and nonsurgical groups was not controlled, so that little can be learned of natural history in this analysis. Overall, the study concluded that old age, severity of the spinal cord compression on radiographic studies, the number of levels of involvement, and the duration of symptoms all had a negative impact on prognosis. Future studies could not confirm all of these conclusions.

Lees and Turner[7] studied 44 patients with myelopathy and evidence of cervical spondylosis on radiographic imaging studies. All patients had Babinski signs. Of these patients, 34 were followed for more than 5 years and 22 for longer than 10 years. Almost all the patients developed symptoms after the age of 40. The authors followed each patient's natural history and then plotted the duration of symptoms versus time. The major temporal pattern was of an attack followed by stability or improvement. Most patients would have subsequent attacks over the years and then remain static for some time. Usually a residual loss of function occurred after each attack. Only a few patients had progressive decline. The authors concluded that spondylotic myelopathy is a condition characterized by prolonged periods free of the development of new symptoms, punctuated by random exacerbations lasting about a year.

The patients were further studied as to their degree of disability. Four patients were considered mildly disabled, with only upper extremity involvement. Fifteen were believed to have moderate disability of the arms and legs, and over the years these patients tended to remain clinically stable. Twenty-five patients had severe disability, and some of these improved to a moderate level of disability. Only 2 patients died as a consequence of spinal cord dysfunction.

Unfortunately, this again tells us little of natural history because 33 of the total number of patients received treatment of some kind, either a collar or surgery. The 11 untreated patients were in the mild to moderate category and did extremely well with intervals of up to 30 years without deterioration. The remainder of the patients were more severely affected and were treated with varying degrees of success. Of the 28 conservatively (nonsurgically) treated patients, 4 deteriorated, 7 stabilized and 17 improved.

Nurick[8] studied 91 patients, 37 of whom were treated conservatively. In this group, 27 had mild symptoms at the onset and 18 of 27 remained that way. This result was not statistically different from his group treated surgically. Looking at those patients who were mild in nature and failed conservative therapy, patient age greater than 60 years was the most important factor. This study confirmed the finding of Lees and Turner[7] that in most cases of myelopathy there was an initial decline followed by a stable period. Thus, the degree of disability may be established early and not change for a prolonged period of time. Most cases are mild and remain that way. The final conclusion of this study was that the condition was generally benign and nonprogressive except in patients of age 60 years or more in whom it can be more rapidly progressive.

More dynamic analyses appeared more recently. Barnes and Saunders[1] studied 45 patients with myelopathy, with a mean follow up of 8.2 years. They found that those who deteriorated tended to be women with increased cervical mobility, and suggested that mobility should be measured as a way of assessing and selecting patients who will need surgery. They found that radicular symptoms in the arms, sensory symptoms in the legs, sphincter dysfunction, age, and relation to trauma had no impact on the prognosis as sole parameters. However, all patients who did deteriorate had a combination of radicular symptoms in the arms and sensory symptoms in the legs, and were more likely to be female.

This study showed a significant difference in terms of total range of neck and head movement in those patients who worsened with time. Sixty-two degrees of range seemed to be the critical value. Recurrent neck movement moves the spinal cord up and down and stretches it by 10% during flexion. Stretching across ridges may have significant impact upon cord function, and thus the focus of treatment should be on restriction of movement either by immobilization or surgery. Since the natural history of this illness is most often an early deterioration followed by a long period of stability, it would be very useful for the clinician to have criteria to determine which patients would benefit from an early surgical intervention, particularly within the first year. The studies suggesting measurement of neck mobility as a criteria for early surgery deserve more interest from clinicians.

No study has definitely demonstrated that the degree of canal compromise on imaging studies correlates with prognosis. The number of levels affected may be more important. Age over 60 years was indicative of poor prognosis in some but not all studies. Certainly the severity of clinical deficit would be a factor influencing a choice of operative treatment, since conservative management seems not to reverse this condition to any significant degree when the patient has significant dysfunction. Similarly, a patient whose myelopathic symptoms progress despite conservative treatment should be considered for operation.

The occurrence of neck or head trauma prior to the development of symptoms of spondylotic myelopathy has been mentioned often but never adequately studied. In one study[3] of 45 patients, 16 had some relationship between neurologic symptoms and trauma. Of these, only 8 developed symptoms immediately after trauma. In 6, the trauma occurred months or years prior to the onset of symptoms. In the remaining 2, some symptoms developed prior to the trauma, which then caused a deterioration in these symptoms. This study only focused on chronic spondylosis, so the impact of acute disk herniation on myelopathy was not analyzed.

Overall, it is most probable that any injury superimposed on pre-existing asymptomatic spondylosis may cause spinal cord damage. One aspect of this problem relates to the increased population of young patients found to have asymptomatic spondylotic disease on magnetic resonance imaging (MRI) studies ordered to clarify a cause for cervical radiculopathy. This group has not been studied independently, but it would seem reasonable to undertake conservative measures and only consider surgical intervention if signs or symptoms of cord compression develop.

In one older study[9] of spondylosis, it was found that in random patients older than 50 years of age, 50% had radiographic evidence of spondylosis. This figure was 75% in patients over the age of 65. Sixty percent of patients over age 50 had some neurologic abnormality attributable to cervical spine disease. The average age at onset of symptoms was 49 years in this study, with a range of age 14 to 70 years. Application of conservative therapy to the young asymptomatic patient may significantly reduce the number of patients who develop symptomatic disease as they age.

The goal of conservative treatment of cervical root disease is to rapidly relieve symptoms and allow the patient to function normally. Usually a combination of modalities must be used to accomplish these goals. The effectiveness of any approach depends upon the intensity of the pain, the degree of limb weakness, and severity of the neurologic signs and imaging findings. Treatment must focus on removing the contact between the structural lesion and the nerve root.

Natural history data indicate that this is usually a self-limited illness and treatment should be directed toward those symptoms that can be affected with minimal risk. Even after significant weakness, recovery can occur without surgery. Electromyography (EMG) may have a role here. Two to 3 weeks after symptoms develop, if an EMG shows no evidence of denervation a neuropractic lesion is possible and the prognosis is excellent. A finding of denervation on EMG, while indicating a more severe nerve entrapment, has not been shown to result in a significantly worse recovery although the rate of recovery may be prolonged.

A multicenter trial of different types of therapy by the British Association of Physical Medicine was published in 1966.[4] Traction, collar, advice on posture, placebo physical therapy and placebo medication were studied. There was a 75% or greater rate of improvement in all patients except for those taking placebo medications. Increasing age and increased frequency of attacks correlated with the worst response to therapy. Unfortunately, this study did not distinguish between patients with cervical spondylosis and other causes of neck and arm pains, but this success rate coincides with that seen in other more focused studies. For example, Bradshaw[2] found that 11 of 13 patients with radicular pain experienced relief by wearing a firm plastic collar.

The conservative treatment of myelopathy is another matter entirely. Conservative treatment with immobilization would improve or stabilize symptoms in less than 50% of patients at best.[13] Even this improvement can be transient, and any signs of progressive myelopathy or of a neurologic dysfunction interfering with daily activities should be an indication for a surgical opinion.

Modes of Therapy
Collar

Immobilization is a fundamental principle of the treatment of a musculoskeletal problem; in cervical spine disease immobilization is generally accomplished by the use of a collar. The rationale of immobilization is to decrease intervertebral motion that can further press on nerve roots or the spinal cord. In addition, limitation of movement may reduce soft tissue and joint space swelling present in the involved areas that may contribute to pain and mucle spasm. Two basic types of collars are used: a soft collar, generally made from foam, provides a moderate degree of limitation of flexion, extension, and rotation, and a plastic collar which is considerably more immobilizing.

Radiographic studies of the cervical spine in several positions provide guidance as to the proper position for the collar. The repeated act of flexion and extension can damage the spinal cord as it moves up and down across spondylotic ridges. The size of the foramen increases in flexion and decreases in extension by approximately one-third. In extension, the ligamentum flavum becomes folded and buckled and this reduces the anteroposterior diameter of the spinal canal and can worsen myelopathy. The nerve roots become stretched with flexion and can develop increased angulation.

The ideal position of the neck in cervical spine degenerative disease is with the neck in slight flexion, avoiding the extreme flexion which stretches the cord and roots. The collar should fit under the occiput and rest on the trapezius. Some plastic collars are more extensive and include attachments to the chin and/or chest wall. Plastic collars provide better immobilization of the spine but have the disadvantage of being hotter and requiring more custom fitting than soft collars. There is no controlled study to indicate that more severe cervical disease should be treated with a firmer collar.

Use of a collar is clearly much more effective in treating radiculopathy than in treating myelopathy. In Roberts' study[10] of 24 patients with spondylotic disease causing myelopathy documented by myelography, patients were given 2 to 3 weeks of bed rest in the hospital followed by immobilization with a plastic collar. Of these patients, 29% improved, 38% were unchanged, and 33% worsened. Those who deteriorated tended to have a longer duration of symptoms and were classified as moderately severely involved. Based on this study it was felt that if no clinical improvement occurred by 5 months, surgery should be undertaken.

Bradshaw[2] found that those patients who improved with a collar had single-level myelopathy rather than multilevel disease. These patients were also treated with exercises and muscle relaxants, so the effect of collars alone could not be assessed. Clarke and Robinson[5] studied 16 patients with myelopathy treated with a collar and found a 50% success rate. They recommended a 3-month trial of collar before surgery and if there was no deterioration, another 3-month trial if necessary. Surgery was suggested at any point that clinical deterioration occurred.

The chronic use of a collar has negative aspects. After wearing a collar for a few months, the neck muscles can atrophy and weaken and there can be contraction of stretched muscles, leading to cervical instability. For this reason, once the initial muscle spasm resolves and pain is decreased, which usually takes 1 to 2 weeks, the use of the collar should be tapered. The collar should be used mostly for driving or in situations where neck movement might be excessive. The collar should also be worn at night to preclude the awkward neck positions that may occur during sleep.

Review of the literature suggests that the use of a plastic, truly immobilizing collar for more prolonged periods of time during the initial attack is a fundamental aspect of immobilization. If treatment is begun with a soft collar, it would be reasonable not to consider surgery unless a firm collar has been used as well. This approach should be applied particularly for radicular disease. In patients with mild disease, simply keeping the head in a position of maximal comfort for 15 to 20 minutes at a time may give relief from radicular symptoms. Bed rest provides some immobilization, but proper head position must be taught. The patient should not sleep prone, but stay supine with the head slightly flexed. A cervical pillow of some type may be useful in this regard.

Cervical Traction

Cervical traction is a treatment used for cervical radiculopathy. Traction cannot be performed unless the neck muscles are very loose. Other modalities such as analgesics, heat, or massage, may have to be used first to decrease pain and reduce severe spasms. At a minimum, traction is another means of immobilization, but it may also separate vertebrae, opening foramina and flattening disks by stretching the posterior longitudinal ligament. It may also reduce friction and inflammation at the facet joints. Because of the risk of producing additional compression on the cervical spinal cord in certain positions, it should not be employed unless it is clear that myelopathy or significant spinal canal narrowing is not present. It should generally not be used unless bed rest and a collar have failed, as these modalities are sufficient to control radicular symptoms.

Some patients may be made worse by traction even when done properly. It has been suggested, although it has not been proven, that such deterioration is indicative of an underlying disk herniation. Traction is usually applied via a sling mechanism. The pull should be across the occiput with a chin strap providing a counter balance. Some force is felt through the chin, resulting in frequent dysfunction of the temporomandibular joint.

There are different theories regarding the best direction of traction. Some suggest that any position that is comfortable to the patient should be used. Others suggest either extension or flexion. As noted before, extension can narrow the canal and foramina, so the ideal position would be one of slight flexion. Traction using skull calipers has been used on occasion but is infrequently employed for obvious reasons.

Traction may be applied continuously or intermittently. Continuous traction generally requires hospitalization or adequate home support. This is generally done with a pulley-weight system over a door, using a halter around the occiput and chin. In the hospital, intermittent traction can be given with the patient supine or sitting. Traction is generally begun with a 10-pound weight. Since it takes 30 to 60 pounds to move the cervical vertebrae, this lower weight may only be a means of maintaining bed rest. If the 10-pound weight is tolerated, the weight can be raised to 20 pounds for 15 minutes at a time, 2 to 3 times a day; this may allow additional relaxation of neck muscles, and may straighten the cervical lordosis. In acute radiculopathy, relief of pain can be almost immediate. Since this is at a weight level where actual vertebral involvement does not occur, the loosening of muscle spasm must in some way contribute to the relief. Unfortunately, this pain relief only lasts as long as the traction is applied.

It is unclear whether traction actually helps. The British Association of Physical Medicine in 1966[4] studied the effect of 20 minutes of traction (weight not specified) in a "most comfortable" position, and documented several hours of relief without producing any long-term benefits. This suggests that continuous traction could work as a nonpharmacologic therapy. Another study[12] found that traction of 15 pounds for 10 minutes had no advantage over a collar.

So what is the role of traction? While spasm and pain can be reduced with local and pharmacologic measures, mild traction can immobilize the neck and lead to less spasm, and thus relieve pain transiently. The amount of weight needed to actually separate vertebrae to reduce compression (approximately 45 lbs) is too large for routine home use and would necessitate hospitalization.

Heat/Cold

Application of heat to the neck has some role in reducing pain by decreasing muscle spasm. This can be accomplished by radiant heat or diathermy; the relief of pain in this way can help to allow better exercise tolerance and improved traction. Hot packs and infrared lamps produce local skin analgesia, but can't penetrate to the subcutaneous level. These modalities affect superficial nerve endings and may work by activating the endorphin systems. Another theory as to heat's mode of action is that there may be an increase in blood flow to the involved area, leading to decreased muscle ischemia and pain from spasm.

Application of heat at home may be accomplished via either dry heat pads or a moist heating apparatus. Alternatively, a hot shower applied through a cloth or towel can be recommended. The application should be intermittent to avoid burning the skin. Some believe that a rapid change in temperature is more important than the actual temperature achieved. Interestingly, in some cases of severe muscle spasm ice packs may be more helpful to the patient.

Ultrasound

Ultrasound techniques have no real role in the treatment of acute pain from neck dysfunction, or in preparing neck muscles for traction, because they do not produce local analgesia as does superficial heat treatment. They cause deep heating delivered as sound waves; while this may relax deeper muscles prior to stretching them, this is not one of the usual modes of treatment for cervical disease. There is no significant use for ultrasound in root disease, and some believe it may worsen the situation.

Massage

Massage may foster muscle relaxation, with a decrease in local pain and spasm. It is unclear how massage works, but there may be a relationship to central pain-mediating pathways. By reducing spasm and pain it may allow for traction more effectively. Unfortunately, the beneficial effects are transient.

Manipulation

Many patients have derived benefit from neck manipulation. In theory, manipulation could be equivalent to a form of traction, but there is no pathologic evidence to suggest that significant spine movement occurs with externally applied forces except in cases of severe trauma. The technique should never be used in cases of myelopathy or when there is focal radicular deficit. The complications of neck manipulation can be disastrous. Vascular injury of the vertebral artery may occur when the neck is extended and turned to the side, narrowing the contralateral vertebral artery. Cerebrovascular events are rare, given the large number of manipulations performed. Even though it is a rare complication, given the self-limited and generally benign nature of radiculopathy it is difficult to justify taking any risk at all.

Transcutaneous Electrical Nerve Stimulation

Transcutaneous electrical nerve stimulation (TENS) is used in many pain disorders. It may work by activing endorphins. TENS is effective in some, but not all, patients with neck pain, and is a benign procedure although not inexpensive.

Injection

Local anesthetic or steroid injections into the paraspinal muscles can reduce muscle spasm and increase mobility. Injections are given at the most tender and painful sites. This is best done over the posterior spinal and neck muscles. Some workers feel that the best criteria for success is a transient increase in pain during the injection. Since the injection can provide benefit for longer than the duration of expected local anesthesia, the activation of the endorphin system or interference with pain reflex arcs may come in to play.

Facet joint blocks have been tried in patients with degenerative disease causing chronic pain exacerbated by neck movement. One approach is to inject bupivacaine .25% with a depot steroid preparation, using fluroscopic control. In root disease with secondary root edema from spondylosis or disk, epidural injections of lidocaine and steroids have been reported to help some patients, but must be done by a highly-trained individual.

Medical Therapy

Given the natural history of root disease, pain relief is the prime goal of most conservative plans. Although many nonsurgical modalities have been discussed, use of pharmacologic agents is frequently sufficient to alleviate the symptoms, usually in combination with a collar. The three basic types used are analgesics, anti-inflammatory agents, and muscle relaxants. There should be no reluctance to rapidly alleviate pain with oral analgesics such as acetaminophen with codeine. Muscle relaxants can be helpful since muscle spasm and its consequent pain is often a considerable component of cervical spine dysfunction. The most commonly used medications include carisoprodol, methocarbamol and diazepam. Cyclobenzaprine is particularly effective and well tolerated. Therapy is begun with a dose of 5 mg every 8 hours and increased to 10 mg every 8 hours if no significant sedation occurs. A 10-day trial is recommended.

In view of the underlying pathology in

cervical spine degenerative disease, the use of anti-inflammatory agents seems rational. Nonsteroidal agents can be given for 10 days to 2 weeks. No evidence indicates that any one of these medications is more effective than others in relieving cervical radicular symptoms, so one is best advised to rely upon experience with individual drugs and their side-effect profile. If patients have an upper extremity motor deficit or if their pain does not respond rapidly to the above regimen, prednisone 60 mg a day is given for several days followed by a tapering course over 10 to 14 days.

The medical regimen just described is designed for the treatment of patients with radiculopathy, and no clear-cut benefit can be expected in myelopathy. The use of steroids and a collar may provide some transient relief of myelopathic symptoms, but is unlikely to affect the natural history in severe disease.

The final issue to address is the treatment of the patient with cervical spondylosis who has been effectively managed through the acute attack. The patient with cervical spine disease should be taught how to hold the neck to avoid positions that may compromise neural structures. Sudden neck movements should be avoided. Ideally, the patient should keep the neck in slight flexion with the chin tucked in. Long-term improvement of posture is important. For example, drooping of the shoulders often leads to a compensatory neck hyperextension. Consideration should be given to a shoulder brace to train the patient to keep the shoulders up and back.

The patient should sleep on a hard bed. When getting up, strain on the neck should be avoided by rolling off to the side first. The patient should not sleep prone because it keeps the neck rotated and strained. When reading or writing, material should be kept in a place where the neck is not excessively flexed or extended. Reading in bed should not be done with the neck markedly flexed. A car seat should be kept as close to the wheel as possible to avoid hyperextension. Men should avoid shaving with the neck extended.

Exercises are often recommended in the setting of recent radiculopathy. Exercise should be avoided at the onset of acute pain. Once pain subsides, one can focus on shoulder mobilization and muscle strengthening exercises of the neck and arm. By elevating the shoulder girdle, shoulder exercises may reduce traction on the nerve roots. These exercises consist of various stretching maneuvers involving the shoulder. Exercises focusing on neck muscles may improve support of the cervical spine, decreasing mechanical stress. Since excessive mobilization of the spine is not useful, and may be harmful, exercises should be done isometrically. In cases of radiculopathy with significant limb weakness, exercises are useful to restore normal function.

References

1. Barnes MP, Saunders M. The effect of cervical mobility on the natural history of cervical spondylotic myelopathy. *J Neurol Neurosurg Psychiatry.* 1984;47:17-20.
2. Bradshaw P. Some aspects of cervical spondylosis. *Q J Med New Series.* 1957;26:177-208.
3. Brain WR, Northfield D, Wilkinson M. The neurological manifestations of cervical spondylosis. *Brain.* 1952;75:187-225.
4. British Association of Physical Medicine. Pain in the neck and arm: a multicentre trial of the effects of physiotherapy. *Br Med J.* 1966;1:253-258.
5. Clarke E, and Robinson PK. Cervical myelopathy: a complication of cervical spondylosis. *Brain.* 1956;79:483-510.
6. Green D, Joynt RJ. Vascular accidents to the brain stem associated with neck manipulation. *JAMA.* 1959;170:522-524.
7. Lees F, Turner JWA. Natural history and prognosis of cervical spondylosis. *Br Med J.* 1963;2:1607-1610.
8. Nurick S. The natural history and results of surgical treatment of the spinal cord disorder associated with cervical spondylosis. *Brain.* 1972;95:101-108.
9. Pallis C, Jones AM, Spillane JD. Cervical spondylosis: incidence and implications. *Brain.* 1954;77:274-289.
10. Roberts AH. Myelopathy due to cervical spondylosis treated by collar immobilization. *Neurology.* 1966;16:951-954.
11. Schlesinger EB. Intervertebral disks. In: Rowland LP, ed. *Merritt's Textbook of Neurology.* 8th ed. Philadelphia, Pa: Lea and Febiger; 1989:407.
12. Steinberg VL, Mason RM. Cervical spondylosis: pilot therapeutic trial. *Ann Phys Med.* 1959;5:37-47.
13. Symon L, Lavender P. The surgical treatment of cervical spondylotic myelopathy. *Neurology.* 1967;17:117-127.

Index

Bold italic numbers indicate figures, illustrations, and tables.

A

AAI, see Atlantoaxial impaction
AAS, see Atlantoaxial subluxation
Acetaminophen with codeine, 165
Acromegaly, 41
AIDS myelopathy
  cervical spinal cord involvement, 38
Allen, K.
  "window", 105
ALS, see Amyotrophic lateral sclerosis
Allografts, 78, 84, 121-123, *122*. See also Bone grafting fibular, 156
American Rheumatism Association scale, 131, *132*
Amyloidosis, 41
Amyotrophic lateral sclerosis (ALS), 44, 45. See also Motor neuron disease and Anterior horn cell disease.
  spondylotic myelopathy and, 7
Anesthesia
  SSEP responses and, 63, 64
Ankylosing spondylitis (AS), 141-148
  clinical manifestations, 142
  definition and epidemiology, 141
  diagnostic criteria, 142, *143*
  etiologic factors, 141, 142
  natural history, 145
  radiographic features, 143-145
  spinal complications of, 145
  surgical correction of flexion deformity, 146, *147*, 148, *148*
Ankylosis, 143, 144. See also Ankylosing spondylitis.
Annulus, 121
Anterior cervical plating, 79
Anterior decompression
  ossification of the posterior longitudinal ligament and, 155, 156
Anterior horn cell disease, 37, 44, 45. See also Motor neuron disease
Anterior interosseous nerve, 41
Anterior operation for cervical spondylotic myelopathy (anterior cervical decompression and fusion), 73-88
  compared with posterior approach, 92
    spine stability, 94
  graft complications, 83-85
  injuries to soft tissue and vascular structures, 82, 83
  injuries to spinal cord or nerve roots, 80-82
    etiology of neurologic deficit, 81
    incidence, 80
    management, 81, 82
  outcome, 86-88
    anterior cervical diskectomy and interbody fusion, 86
    anterior decompression without bone grafting, 86, 87
    anterior decompression utilizing corpectomy, 87, 88
    demographic and epidemiologic factors, 88
  technique, 73-79
    adjunctive instrumentation, 79
    bone grafting, 78, 79
    bone removal, 75-78, *75-77*
    closure and postoperative management, 79
    corpectomy, 79
    intubation and operative positioning, 74
    operative incision, 74
    perioperative preparation, 73, 74
    soft-tissue dissection, 74, 75
Anterolisthesis of vertebral motion segments
  forward translation of the head and, 3
Anti-inflammatory agents, 166
Arthritis, rheumatoid, see Rheumatoid arthritis
Arthrodesis, 126, 134-137
Articular disease, 131
AS, see Ankylosing spondylitis
Atlantoaxial impaction (AAI), 128, *128*, 129, *130*, 131, 133-136
Atlantoaxial stability, 126
Atlantoaxial subluxation (AAS), 126, *126-128*, 128, 131-134, 136, 137, 145
Atlas of Standard Radiographs, 142
Autogenous fibula, fusion with, 156
Autograft fusion, 121, 123, see also Bone grafting
Awake fiberoptic intubation, 107
Axial symptoms
  of benign cervical disk disease and spondylosis, 1, 2
Axilla, 110

B

Babinski reflex, 40, 45
Babinski signs, 160

Basilar impression, 132
Basilar invagination, *129*
Benzodiazepines, 116
Bipolar cautery, 110
Bolus injections of barbiturates
    SSEP potentials and, 64
Bone
    pathophysiology of, 11-13
    remodeling, 12
Bone grafts
    after bony decompression, 78
    anterior approach and, 118-123
    complications, 83-85
        collapse, 84, 85, *85*
        displacement, 84
        nonunion or pseudoarthrosis, 85
Bone marrow
    changes seen on MR imaging, 12
Brachial plexus nerve
    entrapment neuropathies, *42*
    injuries, 37, 43, 44, *44*
Brachioradialis reflex
    in myelopathy, 7
British Association of Physical Medicine traction study, 164
Brooks fusion, 135, *135*
Bupivacaine, 165

C

Carisoprodol, 165
Carotid artery injury, 82
Carpal tunnel syndrome
    myelopathy and, 7
    rheumatoid arthritis and, 41
Cartilage, 10
Cartilaginous tissue, proliferation of, 154
Caspar, W., instrumentation, 84
    distraction pins, 78, 120
    measuring calipers, 78
    retractors, 75, 120
Cauda equina syndrome, 145
Cerebrospinal fluid fistula, 82
Cerebrospinal fluid leak, 112
Cervical orthosis, 84
Cervical disk, soft, see Soft cervical disk
Cervical spine disease,
    signs, 37
Cervical spondylosis, see also Radiculopathy
    evaluation, *38*
Cervical spondylotic myelopathy (CSM), see also Anterior operation for cervical spondylotic myelopathy, Myelopathy, Posterior operation for cervical spondylotic myelopathy
    terminology, 91
Cervical spondylotic radiculomyelopathy, 91
Cervical spondylotic radiculopathy, 105-112, see also Posterior operation for cervical spondylotic radiculopathy, Radiculopathy
Cervical stenosis with myelopathy
    motor neuron disease compared, 45
Cervical sympathetic chain injury, 83
Cervicobrachalgia
    syndrome triad with radiculopathy and myelopathy, 6
Cervicomedullary junction, 133
Chamberlain's line, *128, 129*
Chlamydia, 141
Chondrogenesis
    caused by substances present in muscle, 13
Chondroitin sulfate
    in cartilage, 10
Cloward
    instruments, 75, 123
    technique, 75, 86-88, 118, 121
Collagen
    in cartilage, 10
    in disk, 11
Collar
    use in cervical spine disease, 162, 163, 165, 166
Computed tomography (CT)
    ankylosing spondylitis and, 143, 144
    anterior operation and, 75
    dentate ligament section and, 97
    diagnostic use, 17-25, 46, 47
    herniated disk and, *25*
    normal anatomy on, 17-20, *18, 19*
    postmyelographic, see Computed tomography following myelography
    spondylotic disease and, 20
    technique, 17
    with intravenous contrast, 21, 22, *22*
Computed tomography following myelography (CTM), 22-25
    delayed, 24
    disk herniation and, 25, 115, *115*
    foraminal narrowing and, *3*
    normal anatomy and, 23, *23*
    ossification of the posterior longitudinal ligament and, 153
    rheumatoid arthritis and, 133, *133*
    spondylotic changes and, 23, 24
    technique, 22, 23
Coronal bowstring effect, 96, 97, *97*
Corpectomy, 79, 84, 87
Corticosteroids, see also Steroid injections
    in neurologic deficit following operation, 81
    oral, 116

Index

preoperative use, 73
severity of cervical spine involvement by rheumatoid arthritis and, 131
topical, 116
Cotrel-Dubousset rod, 136
Cranial settling, see Atlantoaxial impaction
Crohn's disease, 142
CSM, see Cervical spondylotic myelopathy
CT, see Computed tomography
CTM, see Computed tomography following myelography
Cubital tunnel entrapment neuropathy
myelopathy and, 7
Curettes
anterior operation and, 77, 81, 120
posterior operation and, 109
Cutaneous receptors, 49
CVA, see Ischemic cerebrovascular disease
Cyclobenzaprine, 165
Cyclophosphamide, 45
"Cystic necrosis", 24, 32, see also Myelomalacia

D

Decompressive procedures, for atlantoaxial instability, 136
Degenerative disease of the cervical spine, see also Radiculopathy, Myelopathy
modes of therapy, 162-166
natural history, 159-162
Demyelinating disease, 39, see also Motor neuron disease, Myelopathy
Dentate ligament section (DLS), 96-98
Diabetes mellitus
median neuropathy and, 41
ossification of the posterior longitudinal ligament and, 151
Diazepam, 165
Diffuse idiopathic skeletal hyperostosis (DISH), 145, 151
Direct needle stimulation of annulus fibrosis or facet joints reproducing axial pain, 1
DISH, see Diffuse idiopathic skeletal hyperostosis
Disk degeneration, see also Soft cervical disk
cause of disability, 1
single-level, 1
Disk herniation
causing neck pain, 1
lateral cervical, 2
posterolateral, 114
seen on computed tomography, 20, 21, *21*
seen on computed tomography following myelography, 25, *25*
Disks, intervertebral

pathophysiology in cervical spondylosis, 11
seen on computed tomography, 20
Diskectomy, cervical, 116, 118, 119, 121, *122*, 123
"Diskogenic" neck pain, 113
Diskography
reproducing axial pain, 1
Distal compartment entrapment, see "Double crush syndrome"
DLS, see Dentate ligament section
Dorsal root ganglia, 13
"Double crush syndrome"
cervical radiculopathy and, 44
myelopathy and, 7
Drilling
in anterior operation, 75
in bone grafting, 78
in bone removal for foraminotomy, *108*, 109, 110, 117
in wide laminectomy, 155
minimizing spinal cord trauma, 81
Dura, ossification of, 154
Dural root sleeve, 107, *108,* 109
Dural sheath, 110
Dural tears, 82
Dysesthesias
in myelopathy, 7
Dysphagia
from osteophyte compression, 1

E

Elastic fibers
disk and, 11
Electromyography (EMG), 45, 46
cervical spine disease, 162
upper extremity weakness, *46*
EMG, see Electromyography
Endotracheal intubation, 83, 106
Enterobactericceae, 141
Enthesopathy, 144
Enzyme systems
in cartilage, 10
in annulus, 11
Epidural veins, 110
Esophageal injury, 83
Ethanol abuse, chronic
neuropathy and, 41
Exercises
treatment for radiculopathy, 166

F

Facet arthropathy and overgrowth and foraminal narrowing, 3
Facet hypertrophy
in cervical spondylosis, 9

Facet joints
  block injections, 165
  foraminotomy and, 109
  on computed tomography, *19*, 20
Facetectomy, 106, 110
Fasiculations
  in spondylotic myelopathy, 6, 7
Fibular grafts, 78
Fischgold and Metzger's line, *128*
Flexion deformity
  surgical correction, 146-148, *148*
Focal canal stenosis, 110
Foraminal spur (hard disk)
  radicular signs and symptoms, 2, 3
  narrowing, 3
Foraminotomy, 95, 105-112
  bone removal, 107-110
  incision, 107
  patient position, 107
Forceps, micropituitary, 118
Forestier's disease, 145
Fractures in late-stage ankylosing spondylitis, 145
Frykholm, R., 105, 110
Fusion, see Bone grafting

G

Gadolinium-DTPA, 32, *32*
Gait abnormalities
  and myelopathy, 7
Gallie H-graft, 135
Ganglion seen on computed tomography, 19
Glucose intolerance, 151
Gluticorticoids, 12
Grafts, see Bone grafting
Granulation tissue, 134
Gray zone, 94, *94*, 95
Guillain-Barre syndrome
  neuropathy and, 41
Guyon's canal, 42

H

Halifax interlaminar clamps, 135
Halo orthosis, 134
Headache
  from C2 entrapment, 2
  with chronic disabling neck pain, 2
Headlight, 120
Heat/cold
  treatment for muscle spasm, 164
Hemilaminectomy, 110
Herniated disk, see Disk herniation
HLA antigen studies, 151
HLA-B-27, 141
Hoffman's sign
  in myelopathy, 7
  ossification of the posterior longitudinal ligament and, 154
Horner's sign, 46
Horner's syndrome, 44, 83, 123
HTLV-I-II-III
  spinal cord involvement, 39
Hyperextension of neck, 107
Hyperreflexia in myelopathy, 7
Hypotension
  SSEP potentials and, 63
Hypothermia, intraoperative
  SSEP potentials and, 63

I

Ileocolonoscopy, 142
Iliac crest
  in bone grafts, 78, 99, 118, 119, 122
Imaging (diagnostic) of degenerative disease, 17-34
  studies compared, 32-34
    for cervical disk herniation, 115
Investigation Committee Report on OPLL, 151
Impactor, 79
Indomethacin, 145
International Ten Twenty System, 56-58, *58*
Interoperative lateral film, 107
Interosseous muscle wasting, 37, *43*
Interspinous spinal evoked potentials, 55
Intubation,
  with anterior operation, 74
Ischemic cerebrovascular disease (CVA), 38

J

Joint disease
  diagnosis of, 37
Joint inflammation
  and cartilage, 10

K

Keratin sulfate
  and cartilage, 10
  and disk, 11
Kerrison punches, 117
Kerrison rongeurs, 76, 78, 98
Key
  first report of ossification of the posterior longitudinal ligament, 151
"Keyhole" foraminotomy, *3*, 105, 117, 118
Klebsiella, 141
Kyphosis, see also Kyphotic deformity
  "effective" cervical, 93-96, *94*, *95*
  foraminotomy and, 118
  thoracic, 141
Kyphotic deformity, see also Kyphosis
  ankylosing spondylitis and, 146, *147*
  grafting to reduce incidence, 87

Index

"kinking", 126
postoperative, 101, 123

L

Laminar hypertrophy
  in cervical spondylosis, 9
Laminectomy
  choice of approach
    dentate ligament section plus, 96-98
    fusion plus, 98
    with posterior root decompression, 110
    with ventral osteophyte excision, 98
  compared to anterior decompression, 73, 92, 93
  inappropriate length, 101
  inappropriate width, 100
  ossification of the posterior longitudinal ligament and, 154
  technique, 98, *99*
Laminoplasty, open-door, 155, *155*
Lateral radiograph, 120, *120*
Lateral spurring
  seen on computed tomography following myelography, 23
L'Hermitte's sign, 39, 74
Ligaments
  changes in cervical spondylosis, 13
Ligamentum flavum
  hypertrophy, 13
  in extension, 162
  infolding during hyperextension, 5, 80
  ossification, 13
  removal of, 110
  seen on computed tomography, 19, 20
  seen on computed tomography following myelography, 23
Lordosis, "effective" cervical, 93-96, *94*
Loupes, 109, 120
Lower extremity complaints
  in myelopathy, 7
Lower motor neuron dysfunction
  compared with upper motor neuron, *38*
Lumbar stenosis
  and myelopathy, 7
Lupus erythematosus myelopathy
  spinal cord involvement, 39
Luque rectangles, 136
Luque rods, 146

M

McGregor's Line, 128, *128, 129*
McRae's Line, *128*, 129
Magerl, technique of, 135
Magnetic motor evoked potentials (MMEPs), 54
Magnetic resonance imaging (MRI)
  asymptomatic spondylotic disease shown on, 161
  bone marrow changes shown on, 12
  cervical radiculopathy and, 161
  compared with other imaging techniques, 25
  cord and root involvement in spondylosis shown on, 9
  dentate ligament section and, 97
  diagnosis of demyelinating disease, 39
  disk degeneration shown on, 1
  herniated disk on, 2, *31*, 32, *32*, 33, 115
  normal anatomy on, 26, *27*, 28
  ossification of the posterior longitudinal ligament and, 153
  spondylotic changes shown on, 9, 28-32, *29, 30*
  technique, 26
  T1-weighted, 26, *27, 29, 30, 130, 153*
  T2-weighted, 26, *27*, 32, *32, 114, 115, 153*
Manipulation
  somatosensory evoked potentials and, 64
  use in cervical disease, 165
Massage
  use in cervical disease, 165
Mayfield three-pin head piece, 62, 107
Mechanoreceptors, 49
Median nerve, 41, 42, *42*
  potentials, 56, *56*
Mediastinal widening, 83
Mediastinitis, 83
Meningiomas of foramen magnum
  producing myelopathy, 39
  spondylosis and, 7
Mennell's sign, 142
MEPs, see Motor evoked potentials
Methocarbamol, 165
Methylmethacrylate, 135
Methylprednisolone, 81
Meyerdink retractors, 107
Micro-curettes, 120
Micro-nerve hooks, 120
Microscissors, 99
"Mimics" of degenerative disease of the cervical spine, 37-47
Mitsui interlaminar clamps, 135
MMEPs, see Magnetic motor evoked potentials
Mononeuropathy, *38*, 41-44
Monoradiculopathy, cervical, 114, 121, 123
Motor complaints
  in myelopathy, 7
Motor evoked potentials (MEPs), 54
Motor neuron diseases, see also Upper motor neuron dysfunction,
  Lower motor neuron dysfunction
    evaluation of, *38*
    spondylotic myelopathy and, 7
MR, see Magnetic resonance imaging
MRI, see Magnetic resonance imaging
Multiple sclerosis

signs and symptoms, 39
spondylotic myelopathy and, 7
Muscle afferents, primary, 1
Muscle relaxants
   use in cervical spine disease, 165
Muscular dystrophy
   myotonic, 45
Myelogram
   lateral cervical, *5*
Myelomalacia, 24, 30
Myelopathy, cervical spondylotic
   central cervical disk herniation and, 113, 114
   clinical manifestations, 1-7
   diagnostic imaging compared, 32, 33
   natural history, 5-6, 159-162
   ossification of the posterior longitudinal ligament and, 154
   postoperative, 122
   rheumatoid arthritis and, 133
   signs and symptoms, 4-7
Myeloradiculopathy, *114*
   ossification of the posterior longitudinal ligament and, 155

N

Nerve roots
   C5, 123
   seen on computed tomography, 19
Neural foramen
   after decompression, 108
   seen on computed tomography, 19
Neuralgic amyotrophy, 44
Neuroactive peptides
   in dorsal root ganglia, 13
Neurofibromas
   producing myelopathy, 39
Neuromuscular blockade
   somatosensory evoked potentials acquisition and, 64
Neuropathy
   diagnosis, 41
New York criteria for ankylosing spondylitis, 142, *143*
Nitrous oxide
   somatosensory evoked potentials amplitudes and, 64
Nociceptors, 49
Nonsteroidal anti-inflammatory agents (NSAIDS), 116
NSAIDS, see Nonsteroidal anti-inflammatory agents

O

Odontoid, 132, *133*
OPLL, see Ossification of the posterior longitudinal ligament
Ossification of the posterior longitudinal ligament (OPLL), 151-157
   classification, 152, *152*, 153

clinical presentation, 154, 155
imaging studies, 152, 153, *152, 153*
incidence and epidemiology, 151, 152
pathology and pathophysiology, 153, 154
postoperative progression, 156, 157
somatosensory evoked potentials and, 60, 64
treatment, 155-157
Osteoblasts, 11-12
Osteoclasts, 11-12
Osteogenesis, 13
Osteophytes
   anterior operation and, 75-77, 86
   destruction of cartilage and, 10
   operation with neck in extension and, 73
   posterior operation and, 109, 110
   seen on computed tomography following myelography, *24*
   seen on magnetic resonance imaging, 30, *30*
   spondylotic, 114
Osteophytic ridges ("hard disks")
   on computed tomography, 20, @20
   posterior operation and, 106
Osteophytosis
   in cervical spondylosis, 9
Osteoporosis
   caused by glucocorticoids, 12
   rheumatoid cervical spine disease and, 132
Osteosclerosis, 132
Osteotome, 110
Osteotomy, 146, *147*, 148, *148*

P

Pain
   atypical, facial, 3
   radicular, postoperatively, 112
Pancoast tumor, 44
Pannus, *127, 130,* 134
Paraplegia
   ossification of the posterior longitudinal ligament and, 154
Paresthesias
   brachial plexus injuries and, 44
   in myelopathy, 7
Parsonage-Turner syndrome, 44
Peripheral neuropathies
   etiology, 40, *40*, 41
   evaluation, 38
PGE_2, 12
Phalan's sign, 41
Philadelphia collar, 79, 107
Pisohamate tunnel, 42
"Platybasia", see Basilar impression
PLL, see Posterior longitudinal ligament
Posterior decompression

Index

ossification of the posterior longitudinal ligament and, 156
Posterior longitudinal ligament (PLL), 76-78, 120, 153, 154. See also Ossification of the posterior longitudinal ligament
Posterior occipitocervical fusion, 136
Posterior operation for cervical spondylotic myelopathy, 91-101.
See also Laminectomy
cervical fusion, 99, *100*
dorsal operative approach, 96-98
failure, 99-101
mechanisms of spinal cord distortion, 96
patient selection criteria, 92-96
rationale, 91, 92
Posterior operation for cervical spondylotic radiculopathy, 105-112. See also Foraminotomy
advantages and disadvantages, 105, 106
anesthesia, 106, 107
case selection, 106
complications, 111, 112
outcome, 110, *111*
surgical approach, 107-110, *108, 109*
Posterior tibial recordings, 56, *56*
Posterolateral compression, 20
Postmyelographic CT, see Computed tomography following myelography
Posture
treatment for cervical spondylosis, 166
Prednisone, 166
Primary lateral sclerosis
Prolapse, subligamentous, 118
and spondylotic myelopathy, 7
Prostaglandins, see also PGE2
and osteoclasts, 12
Proteoglycans
and cartilage, 10
and disk, 11
Pseudoarthrosis, 84, 85, 122, 145
Pseudobasilar invagination, see Atlantoaxial impaction
Pseudobasilar settling, see Atlantoaxial impaction
Psoriasis, 145

R

RA, see Rheumatoid arthritis
Radial nerve, *42,* 43
Radiculitis, 123
Radiculopathy,
clinical manifestations, 1-7
compared with myelopathy, 91
diagnostic imaging techniques compared, 33, 34
evaluation, *38*
magnetic resonance imaging and, *34*
myelopathy and, 159
ossification of the posterior longitudinal

ligament and, 154
postoperative worsening, 122, 123
unilateral, 113, 114, see also Monoradiculopathy
signs and symptoms, 2-4
Radiographs, 107
of atlantoaxial region in rheumatoid arthritis, *128, 137*
Radionuclide studies, 145
Ranawat method, 128, *128, 129*
Recurrent laryngeal nerve injury, 82, 83, 119, 122
Redlund-Johnell method, 128, *128*
Reiter's syndrome, 145
Retractors, 75, 79, 107, 120
Retrocorporeal venous plexus
seen on intravenous contrast computed tomography, 21
Rheumatoid arthritis (RA)
of carpal tunnel, 41
of cervical spine, 125-137
atlantoaxial region, 126-129, *126-130*
clinical features and natural history, 129-131
management, 133-137
pathology, 125, 126
radiology, 131-133, *132, 133*
Rheumatoid granulation tissue, see Pannus
Rheumatoid subcutaneous nodules, 131
Robinson and Smith technique, 118, 119, 121.
See also Smith-Robinson operation
Roentgenograms
fusion assessment, 78
Rome Symposium on Population Studies in Relation to Chronic Rheumatic Diseases, 142, *143*
Rongeurs
anterior operation and, 76, 77, 81
cervical laminectomy and, 98
pituitary, 120
posterior operation and, 117
wide laminectomy and, 155

S

Sagittal bowstring effect, 96
Salmonella, 141
Schilling's test, 40
Segmental deficits
and myelopathy, 6
Sensory complaints
causes, 37
in myelopathy, 7
in radiculopathy, 3
SEPs, see Spinal evoked potentials
Shear force
and myelopathy, 5
Shigella, 141
Skull calipers
use in traction, 164
Smith-Robinson operation, 75, 87, 88, 120, see

also Robinson and Smith technique
Soft cervical disk disease, see also Soft disk herniation
   clinical presentation, 114, 115
   imaging, 115
   management, 115, 116
   natural history, 113, 114
   nonoperative treatment, 116
   surgical treatment
      anterior approach, 118-123
      posterior approach, 117, 118
Soft disk herniation, 110
Somatosensory evoked cortical potentials, 54-58
Somatosensory evoked potentials
   (SSEPs), 49, *49*, 54, 55
   acquisition parameters, *55*
   early components, *57*
   factors affecting acquisition, 63-64
   in cervical surgery, 66-70
      monitoring and outcome, 67, 68, 74
      intraoperative, 60-62, *61*, 66, 69, *69*, 70, *70*
         anesthesia technique, 61, 62
         electrophysiology, 68, 69
         monitering protocol, 60, 61
   median nerve responses, 56, *56*
   monitoring techniques, 53-58
   neuroanatomy, 49, 50
   physiology, 50, 52
   posterior tibial responses, 56, *56*
   predictors of post-traumatic outcome, 60
   preoperative, 58-60
      prophylaxis, 66
   responses to changes, 64-66
      false negatives, 65, 66, 70
      false positives, 64, 65, 70
   resuscitative measures, 66
   schematic nerve, *52*
   spinal cord injury in animal models and, 53
Spastic paraparesis
   and spondylotic myelopathy, 7
Spinal canal
   narrowing, seen in myelopathy, 5, *5*
   seen on computed tomography, 17, 18
Spinal cord
   compression, 96
   ossification of the posterior longitudinal ligament
      and, 154
   pathways, 50. *50, 51*
   seen on computed tomography following
      myelography, 23
Spinal dura, *108,* 110
   ossification of, 154
Spinal evoked potentials (SEPs), 54. See also
   Somatosensory evoked cortical potentials,
      Somatosensory evoked potentials
   interspinous, 55

Spinal instability
   complication of posterior facetectomy, 111
Spinal osteotomy, see Osteotomy, spinal
Spondylosis of cervical spine
   as cause of disability, 1
   chronic, 161
   definition, 9
   distinguished from soft disk herniation, 110
   etiology, 9
   in upper cervical roots, 3
   neurogenic factors, 13
   pathophysiology of bony and ligamentous changes, 9-13
      normal versus pathologic changes, 9, 10
Spurling's sign, 115
SSEPs, see Somatosensory evoked potentials
Steroid injections
   use in cervical spine disease, 165
Subarachnoid space
   seen on computed tomography following
      myelography, 23
Subaxial region of the spine
   abnormalities of, 128, 129, *130*
Sublaminar wires, 134
Subluxation, 133
Substance P, 13
Syndesmophyte formation, 144, *144*
Syndrome of Morvan, 39
Synovitis, 144. See also Rheumatoid arthritis.
Syringomyelia
   upper extremity symptoms, 39
Syrinx formation
   computed tomography following myelography and, 23
   magnetic resonance imaging and, 30

T

Temporomandibular joint dysfunction, 3
TENS, see Transcutaneous electrical nerve stimulation
Tetraplegia
   ossification of the posterior longitudinal ligament
      and, 154
Thermoreceptors, 49
Thoracic duct, 119
Tinel's sign, 41
Tomaculous neuropathy
   symptoms, 41
Traction
   cervical, 163, 164
   skeletal, 134
   using skull calipers, 164
Transcutaneous electrical nerve stimulation (TENS)
   use in neck pain, 165
Trigger-point injections, 116
Tumors
   upper-extremity weakness and, 39

Index

U

Ughtoff's sign, 39
Ulcerative colitis, 142
Ulnar nerve, 42, *42, 43*
Ultrasound, 116
    use in cervical disease, 164
UMN, see Upper motor neuron dysfunction
Upper extremity weakness
    evaluation, 38
Upper motor neuron (UMN) dysfunction, 37-40
    cerebral and spinal cord, 37, 38
    cervical cord diseases, 39, 40
    compared with lower motor neuron dysfunction, *38*
Upward migration of the odontoid, see Atlantoaxial impaction
"Useless hand syndrome of Burdach", 39

V

Valsalve maneuver, 115
Vascular disease
    diagnosis of, 37
Vasculitis, systemic, 41
Vasoactive intestinal peptide (VIP), 13
Vertebrae
    C2
        ankylosing spondylitis and, 144
        posterior arch, 107
    C5 root dysfunction, 3, 4
    C6, C7, C8, and T1 radiculopathy, 4
Vertebral arteries
    injury, 82, 112
    seen on computed tomography, 19, 20
Vertebrobasilar vascular insufficiency, 1
Vertical subluxation of the axis, see Atlantoaxial impaction
VIP, see Vasoactive intestinal peptide
Vitamin B^{12} deficiency, 40
Vocal cord paralysis, 123

W

Wake-up test, 53, 54
Whipple's disease, 142

The index for *Degenerative Disease of the Cervical Spine* was prepared by Susan Cuthbert, M.A.

Previously Published Books in the *Neurosurgical Topics* Series

Management of Posttraumatic Spinal Instability
   Edited by Paul R. Cooper, MD

Malignant Cerebral Glioma
   Edited by Michael L.J. Apuzzo, MD

Intracranial Vascular Malformations
   Edited by Daniel L. Barrow, MD

Neurosurgical Treatment of Disorders of the Thoracic Spine
   Edited by Edward C. Tarlov, MD

Contemporary Diagnosis and Management of Pituitary Adenomas
   Edited by Paul R. Cooper, MD

Complications of Spinal Surgery
   Edited by Edward C. Tarlov, MD

Neurosurgical Aspects of Epilepsy
   Edited by Michael L.J. Apuzzo, MD

Complications and Sequelae of Head Injury
   Edited by Daniel L. Barrow, MD

Practical Approaches to Peripheral Nerve Surgery
   Edited by Edward C. Benzel, MD

Cerebrovascular Occlusive Disease and Brain Ischemia
   Edited by Issam A. Awad, MD

Neurosurgery for the Third Millennium
   Edited by Michael L.J. Apuzzo, MD

For order information call (708) 692-9500.